4/8/93

Work, Stress, Disease
and Life Expectancy

WILEY SERIES ON STUDIES IN OCCUPATIONAL STRESS

Series Editors

Professor Cary L. Cooper
Manchester School of Management,
University of Manchester
Institute of Science and Technology

Professor Stan V. Kasl
Department of Epidemiology
School of Medicine
Yale University

Further titles in preparation

Work, Stress, Disease and Life Expectancy

Ben (C) Fletcher

Hatfield Polytechnic, UK

JOHN WILEY & SONS

Chichester · New York · Brisbane · Toronto · Singapore

Copyright © 1991 by John Wiley & Sons Ltd,
Baffins Lane, Chichester,
West Sussex PO19 1UD, England

Other Wiley Editorial Offices

John Wiley & Sons, Inc., 605 Third Avenue,
New York, NY 10158-0012, USA

Jacaranda Wiley Ltd, G.P.O. Box 859, Brisbane,
Queensland 4001, Australia

John Wiley & Sons (Canada) Ltd, 22 Worcester Road,
Rexdale, Ontario M9W 1L1, Canada

John Wiley & Sons (SEA) Pte Ltd, 37 Jalan Pemimpin #05–04,
Block B, Union Industrial Building, Singapore 2057

Library of Congress Cataloging-in-Publication Data:

Fletcher, Ben (C)
    Work, stress, disease, and life expectancy / Ben (C) Fletcher.
        p.   cm.—(Wiley series on studies in occupational stress)
    Includes bibliographical references.
    Includes index.
    ISBN 0-471-91970-5
    1. Medicine, Psychosomatic.   2. Stress (Psychology)   3. Job
stress.   I. Title.   II. Series.
    [DNLM: 1. Diseases—etiology.   2. Life Change Events.   3. Life
Expectancy.   4. Occupational Diseases—psychology.   5. Stress,
Psychological—complications.   WA 400 F612w]
RC49.F58   1991
616.9′8—dc20
DNLM/DLC
for Library of Congress   91–166
                                                                   CIP

Lritish Library Cataloguing in Publication Data:

A catalogue record for this book
is available from the British Library.

ISBN 0-471-91970-5

Printed and bound in Great Britain by Courier International Ltd, Tiptree, Essex

Contents

Contents

Editorial Foreword to the Series

This book, *Work, Stress, Disease and Life Expectancy*, is the eighteenth* book in the series of *Studies in Occupational Stress*. The main objective of this series of books is to bring together the leading international psychologists and occupational health researchers to report on their work on various aspects of occupational stress and health. The series will include a number of books on original research and theory in each of the areas described in the initial volume, such as Blue Collar Stressors, The Interface Between the Work Environment and the Family, Individual Differences in Stress Reactions, The Person–Environment Fit Model, Behavioural Modification and Stress Reduction, Stress and the Socio-technical Environment, The Stressful Effects of Retirement and Unemployment and many other topics of interest in understanding stress in the workplace.

We hope these books will appeal to a broad spectrum of readers—to academic researchers and postgraduate students in applied and occupational psychology and sociology, occupational medicine, management, personnel, and law—and to practitioners working in industry, the occupational medical field, mental health specialists, social workers, personnel officers, lawyers and others interested in the health of the individual worker.

CARY L. COOPER
University of Manchester Institute of
Science and Technology
STANISLAV V. KASL
Yale University

* Five earlier titles are now out of print.

Preface

Few doubt that psychological factors play an important role in mental health and physical disease: lay-people place stress and tension above traditional risk factors such as smoking, blood pressure and cholesterol levels as causes of heart attacks (Shekelle & Liu, 1978). Recent years have also seen an explosion of medical research which takes account of the psychological dimension, and there are many thousands of learned articles on stress and illness.

Few people also doubt that occupational stress has significant effects on psychological well-being. The literature on work stress is growing apace, although it has only recently started to take serious account of the physical disease consequences.

This book is an attempt to bridge the gap between the psycho-medical literature and the research on occupational stress. It does not attempt to integrate all the relevant literature, or to critically evaluate all the studies included: such an exercise would require a book many times the size of this one.

The first chapter outlines and discusses a number of central models of stress, either because they have been very influential or because they are particularly relevant to the workplace and have been applied to the prediction of illness. This chapter also describes a new model, the Catastrophe or Configural Model, which attempts to incorporate the advantages of previous models and make new testable predictions.

Chapter 2 outlines and evaluates the research on the role of life events in illness. Life events research has contributed a great deal to the area, and the methodologies spawned from it are probably more widespread and influential than seems at first sight. It is for this reason that the chapter considers life events research from a methodological perspective. The literature has much to teach us about how to tackle (and not tackle) the relationship between stress and health. The chapter also provides a backcloth against which to evaluate some of the life events research detailed in subsequent chapters.

The next three chapters consider the research attempting to show that psychological factors compromise the immune system, and are implicated in the onset of cancer and coronary heart disease: the two killers responsible for most deaths.

Chapter 3 discusses the possible role of psychological factors in immune system functioning. Although the chapter does include reference to studies relevant to the workplace, the major thrust of it is to convince the reader that psychological stressors can have major health consequences as revealed by direct immunocompetence measures. Without the demonstration of such a link, much of the research investigating stress and disease would be left in a scientifically unacceptable vacuum. This is an exciting area of research for this reason alone. It is also in a state of relative infancy.

Chapters 4 and 5 pay particular attention to the role played by personality factors in cancer and heart disease. The concept of type A coronary-prone behaviour has received considerable attention in relation to work issues, despite its somewhat shaky scientific validity. The relationship between other psychological stressors and disease is also considered in some detail.

Chapter 6 attempts to bring the research discussed in the previous chapters into a wider context by illustrating some of the hidden consequences of work. It shows how work stress spills over into the home environment and what effects this may have on the well-being and life expectancy of marital partners. It discusses my own research on the transmission of occupational stressors between marital partners, and tries to show that specific disease risks may be communicated through psychological mechanisms. It reinforces the view that the distinction between work and home may not be very clear-cut in terms of health effects.

Chapter 7 is a rather descriptive chapter which provides information on the epidemiology of illness with specific reference to work: how many people in a workforce are likely to be suffering at any point in time, and at what level in the organisation they will be. A version of this chapter has been published before (Fletcher, 1988a), although this has been expanded and updated.

There are many controversies within the pages of this book. Many are given less space than they deserve. Many issues are also embedded within other issues and could not be made explicit; the book makes quite dense reading as it is. I have tried to be impartial and for this reason have discussed some studies and issues in great detail. There are a number of general points I would like the reader to bear in mind when reading the book:

1. Stress is poorly defined (although this book attempts to help here). It is essential, however, that stress is not considered to imply that causes or effects are 'consciously apprehended' by the individual, or that stress is equated with 'negative affect'. People should not be considered to know either when they are 'under stress' or what is stressing them. They *may* know, but verbal reports in the area of stress should be treated with the same caution (if not more) as they are given in cognitive psychology (e.g. Ericsson & Simon, 1980; Fletcher, 1983a). People can construct sensible, but not necessarily useful, *a priori* explanations, but stress effects are likely to be more complex than these. To say that people do not 'consciously apprehend' stressors, however, does not imply that they do not 'cognitively apprehend' them in the sense that their cognitive systems register and are modified by them. It also does not imply that questionnaire and interview data are worthless. On the contrary, it implies only that models of stress must be subtle enough to construe responses in a theoretically justified way.

2. By their very nature, psychological factors are general in their effect. A stressor is also a contaminant in the sense that it can bias how other things are perceived. The search for ever more specific causes of diseases does not easily admit of wide-ranging bedfellows whose actions may be revealed in many different psychological as well as physical guises. This is one reason why the burden of proof to implicate psychological factors in disease is great. However, the search for 'causes' of disease is misplaced to some degree. Many factors are likely to be involved in the onset of an illness, just as there is no single cause for hypertension; only a mosaic of contributing factors. It is also too easy to confuse concomitants of illnesses as having some causal role, they may merely be aspects of the disease syndrome. Descriptions of cause at one level may be inappropriate at another, just as treatments are. What is needed is a wider perspective on the illness process which includes a due contribution for psychological factors. Some physical diseases may be the general dysfunctional outcome of a wide battery of assaults on the person, including psychological ones. 'Causes' may also be embedded in other causes: what 'causes' a person to smoke is as much part of the lung cancer and heart disease puzzle as how smoke has its effects on the organism. Psychological 'causes' may merely be temporally more distant.

3. It is for these and other reasons that psychological research in this area is difficult. It is a harder scientific jigsaw puzzle to demonstrate that psychological factors are involved in the genesis of disease than to isolate biological or physical environmental risk factors. Psychological factors may be protective as well as injurious. Nonetheless, current research is tackling these problems and the weight of evidence (rather than any particular demonstration) seems to favour a causal role for psychological factors. My suspicion is that they will be shown to be increasingly important.

I hope this book is of value to the reader. It should provide useful reading for those in the area of health psychology, stress research, occupational health, medicine and those in the caring professions who have paramedical training. I have also used it successfully as a course text with final-year undergraduates in both psychology and biology, as well as on postgraduate taught courses in occupational psychology.

My thanks to Fiona Jones for all her help in the preparation of this book.

BEN (C) FLETCHER
St Albans, UK

Chapter 1
Models of Stress and Disease

Psychology is an inexact science. Stress is difficult to operationalise. These are matters of fact. They do not, however, make the enterprise of examining the role of stress in disease any less worthwhile or less useful. Certainly psychological investigation is not the only area where imprecision occurs. Consider, for example, why about one in 500 Americans is fitted with a cardiac pacemaker (Parsonnet, 1982). Such pacemakers are invaluable aids for those with such conditions as acquired complete heart block and bradyarrhythmia. The operation necessary to fit them is relatively major, although routine. Recent evidence, however, suggests that only 44% of pacemaker implants are definitely indicated by medical evidence, and that unwarranted implantation is widespread (Greenspan *et al.*, 1988). Psychological researchers do not need to excuse imprecision in their own science, although they, like medics in their own field, must provide explanations of it. This book attempts to do that in relation to stress and health.

This chapter outlines a number of influential general models of stress and disease and then details several important models of occupational stress which have been developed to examine the link between work and health. The final section outlines a new model which capitalises on the strengths of those described and makes new testable predictions.

As a preliminary to outlining any specific models it will be useful to make some elementary distinctions since the word 'stress' can cause confusion. In this book the term 'stressor' refers to the precursors or independent variables which may be the causes of dysfunction or ill-health. The term 'strain' is used to denote the dependent variables which are the consequences of being in an environment which contains sufficient stressors. Strain may be physiological or psychological, short-term (temporary elevation of physiological levels or minor illness) or long-term (disease or death). Although 'being under stress' may be considered the same as showing strain, the latter term does not imply that the process is in any way attentionally heeded: indeed strains may be physiological, behavioural or medical as well as psychological. One truism in the stress literature is that individuals differ in the way they perceive and react to potential stressors. It has been common practice, therefore, to consider 'moderating' or 'mediating' variables. These are often aspects of the individual's personality or environment which change the likelihood that any stressor or constellation of stressors gets translated into strain. Different models of stress hypothesise different relationships between stressors, moderators, mediators, and strains.

GENERAL MODELS

A number of experts, under the auspices of the Institute of Medicine/National Academy of Sciences in the United States, collaborated in an assessment of the role of stress in human health (Elliot & Eisedorfer, 1982). In their report they highlighted the need for closer collaboration and understanding between behavioural scientists and biomedical researchers. Both are essentially concerned with a common pathway—the brain, or the influence of higher nervous processes—yet there has been something of a rift in research efforts·

> In the biological sciences, investigators have tended to use stressors primarily as experimental tools.... Investigators in the psychological and social sciences have demonstrated strong associations between certain psychosocial events and physical and mental illness...[and] used 'stress' as a causal explanation...without trying to elucidate the physiological and psychological mechanisms through which such stressors may act (p. 18).

This book attempts to provide an understanding of the role of psychological factors in the genesis of disease (rather than how they affect the course of the disease or in what ways and how well people cope with it). A necessary prerequisite in these investigations is to be able to model the processes that lead to the clinical manifestations of the disease or its medical precursors. This chapter outlines some of the models important for our understanding of how psychological factors might affect the onset of pathological changes in the diseased person. There are many 'models' of stress. Only a few central ones will be considered here, and they have been chosen because they have had a major impact on subsequent conceptualisation of the process of disease, or because they make a particularly important contribution to some aspect of the process. These are not biological or medical models of specific diseases. Some of these will appear in later sections. Instead they are general models which may be applied to the genesis of a number of disease classifications. One reason for this bias is the belief that most diseases may have a psychological etiology as well as a specific physical one. Whilst it seems likely that the same psychological stressors will have different disease outcomes it is not axiomatic that they necessarily do. Indeed, it seems probable that increasingly sophisticated psychomedical research will reveal greater and greater specificity of disease outcome for the effects of psychological factors.

There is a need for models even if they do lead to conceptual misunderstandings and a plurality of definitions. We are faced with the problem that people become ill. The illness (or its precursors) is the outcome of interest to us. What has caused the illness? The answer is not usually a simple one. More often than not only weak guesses can be made. One reason for our lack of progress in this area is the reliance on simple notions of 'cause'. What is needed is a way to model the multifaceted *influences* of various factors on the disease without taking the view that some 'cause' the disease and others play a minor role: knowledge is simply not advanced enough to be certain (or even simply to have good grounds for suspicion) that factors which have not been researched in much depth (i.e. psychological ones) do not play a major role in the onset or development of a disease. There are two major reasons for taking this stance.

First, our medical understanding of the major causes of death (cancer and heart disease) is poor *when considered against the criterion of true cure (as opposed to relief of symptoms)*. Keys *et al.* (1972), for example, a major proponent of the importance of dietary factors in heart disease, suggest that less than 50% of the coronary heart disease incidence in men can be explained by a combination of all the traditional risk factors. Of course, even the explicable portion of the incidence may be influenced by psychological factors. The need for models is not an academic or abstract need because our ability to cure people (and possibly to relieve symptoms more successfully) is dependent upon understanding the entire mosaic of related influences. Even if the effects of psychological factors on the disease process are subtle, or cannot easily be measured because we do not know what or how to measure them, it is fallacious to conclude that the factors are less important or less influential.

Second, we must make sure that we are asking the right questions. A simple causal model probably leads to the wrong ones. Page (1977), who published an influential 'mosaic' theory of essential hypertension, felt that the chief value of the theory was "that it gives an answer to the wrongly phrased question: What is the cause of essential hypertension? The causes are many because of the inter-relationships of the many dynamic regulatory mechanisms" (p. 587). Treatment of the mechanisms, not of the blood pressure, is required. The shortsightedness of taking a restricted outlook on disease etiology is well put by Obrist (1981), the well-known cardiovascular psychophysiologist, in his discussion of the use of cardiovascular indices of behavioural states:

> Why should evolution place so much responsibility on the cardiovascular system when we have evolved such a complex central nervous system to carry out these matters of behaving? I am beginning to believe that, to whatever extents cardiovascular adjustments are uniquely sensitive to behavioural events (independent of metabolic processes), they are but ripples on the wave and can be inundated by the wave (p. 200).

We need to know about the moon to understand the motions of the sea, and to understand disease we need to know about people (as well as their bodies). Unless we learn more about the set of etiologically significant factors, and how the processes relate to one another, we cannot hope to develop cures and successfully preventative procedures. This is another reason we need to model the processes.

Models of the multifaceted influences of disease are important for less obvious reasons. For example, they serve to definitionally outline woolly concepts such as psychological 'stress' and related terms (e.g. stressor, strain). The term 'stress' is often used to denote the influence of psychological (or at least non-physical) factors on the organism, but is used in a number of different ways. For some researchers the term is too vague to be useful. Obrist (1981), for example, writes:

> Throughout this monograph, I have intentionally refrained from using the concept of stress.... The term is ambiguous. It has negative connotation with regard to its possible consequences.... Its measurement can be circular.... Finally...there are some individuals who demonstrate little or no cardiovascular response to our experimental procedures while still others demonstrate appreciable responsiveness (p. 2).

Other researchers take the view that there is order in the chaos.

Stressors and Strains

Mason (1975) has outlined four different roles for psychological stress:

1. Stimulus-based definitions in which stress is defined by the measurement of the effects of an environmentally manipulable variable (see Figure 1.1 and Table 7.1 for a list of such stressors relevant to the work situation). Much of the research on occupational stressors is based on cross-sectional and correlational studies for which a stimulus-based outlook is an axiomatic assumption.
2. Response-based definitions where stress is defined by demonstrable effects on the organism. Stress is exhibited strain. Strain can be shown in many different ways (physiologically, psychologically, behaviourally, medically, for example). Selye's General Adaptation Syndrome (e.g. 1983) is an example of a physiological response-based model.
3. Stimulus–response interactions, in which stress is an abstract or non-functionally defined term which *may* have strain or response consequences. The emphasis is on potential effects in just the same way that a pathogen may result in clinical manifestations.
4. Psychologically mediated definitions which make reference to the whole spectrum of interacting factors including social and coping effects and *how* events and factors are *perceived*. For example, Lazarus and his co-workers view stress as "the person's appraisal of the *relationship* between the input and its demands and the person's agendas (e.g. beliefs, commitments, goals) and capabilities to meet, mitigate, or alter these demands in the interests of well-being" (Lazarus *et al.*, 1985, p. 770).

Other ways of defining stress have been in terms of an upset of equilibrium, a physiological reaction, a psychological reaction, or a medical manifestation (Elliot & Eisendorfer, 1982), although these can be considered examples of simple response-based models with restricted application.

The different models are not mutually exclusive, but should be treated as being complementary. The final 'configural model' described in this chapter attempts to integrate aspects of them all. Different types of models have different uses in different circumstances, as will become apparent.

One use of models is to bring order and prediction to a range of findings which are complex and variable. There is probably a greater need for models in psychomedical investigations than in straight medical or biological research. One difficulty with psychological research in disease is that the findings are generally less consistent than (say) endocrine responses to physical stressors (Mason, 1975). This does not imply that psychological stressors are less important; it is probably a reflection of the fact that their influences are more complex.

Models have to be evaluated against evidence, as well as having a functional or definitional role. Any general model of disease which considers psychological or psychosocial factors needs to account for a range of accumulated evidence concerning:

- the observed interrelationships between stressors and strains;
- the prevalence and incidence patterns of strains;
- the individual differences in the pattern of responses;
- the effects of acute and chronic stressors, or the changes that occur over time;
- the positive and negative effects of stressors;
- the associated effects of an organism being under a given level of strain;
- how an individual's perception affects the relationships between stressors and strains;
- the interrelationships between the various strain measures should be predictable and sizeable unless there are *a priori* reasons to predict otherwise;
- commonality between the human and animal studies.

KAGAN & LEVI'S MODEL

In 1974 Aubrey Kagan and Lennart Levi published a review of the role of what they called 'psychosocial stimuli' in disease, in *Social Science and Medicine*. Essentially they propose that external psychosocial stressors (which are stimuli that originate in social arrangements and relationships and act through higher nervous system processes) and the individual's psychobiological programme (influenced by genetics and early environmental influences) additively determine the psychological and physiological stress reaction. These reactions may lead to mental and physical precursors of disease which, if they persist, lead to the clinical manifestations of the disease and eventual death. This sequence of events is affected or mediated by interacting variables (mental or physical, intrinsic or extrinsic factors which promote or prevent the process that might lead to disease). The system is a cybernetic one with continuous feedback between each of the elements.

The model has several advantages. The continuous feedback provided by the interacting variables allows for changes in the organism's responses over time: the acute effects of stressors may be different from their chronic effects as the system adapts to the changes. In addition, they allow for learning through the same mechanisms. The model explicitly predicts that individual differences in response to a stressor will be present for one of three reasons: genetic differences, differences in personality due to the influence of early environmental factors, and differences in the stress reaction due to variations in how the stressor is perceived and evaluated (intrinsic mental factors can 'alter' effects of stressors). One particular advantage of the framework is that it posits the influence of psychological factors at several different layers. Of major importance here is that it differentiates extrinsic psychosocial stressors from psychological mediation of stressors: those which are outside the control of the organism and those which are a direct consequence of the organism's intrinsic attentional evaluation. Thus strain is not simply a function of either how the organism perceives the environment or how the external environment is organised. The model can explain the positive and negative effects of a stressor by presuming that the exogenous stimuli can be overlaid by the individual's endogenous perception of it. This is an important property of the model, since it can be used to interpret how an individual's coping mechanisms can modify the effects of a stressor. For example, animals which are subjected to electric shocks will show stress-induced pathology. If the shock is predictable, however, the pathology will be less severe (Weiss, 1970). Animals will even choose a shock that is three times more intense, and lasts up to nine times longer, if it is signalled than if it is unpredictable (Harsh & Badia, 1975).

Kagan & Levi (1974) present a considerable amount of evidence within the framework of their model. They suggest that a number of psychosocial stimuli seem to have pathogenic effects in some individuals including an *excess or deprivation* of:

- parental care;
- social and economic circumstances, including group and interpersonal contacts, status and affluence;
- freedom of action.

They also consider that being ill is itself a stressor.

The pathogenic effects of these psychosocial stimuli are expressed through mental, physiological and social processes. Kagan & Levi present evidence to show that the combination of stressors and the individual's stress response determines the likelihood of disease and its precursors. They pay particular attention to the neuroendocrine response of the individual (the hypothalamic adrenal–medullary and sympathetic pituitary adrenal–cortical axes) and conclude that "causation of disease by psychosocial stimuli is unproven but at a high level of suspicion" (p. 236) for thyrotoxicosis (Graves' disease), cardiac pathologies including hyperproteinaemic responses, arrhythmias, and myocardial oxygen consumption changes, essential hypertension, gastrointestinal tract disorders including motility disorders and peptic ulcers, and suicide in the young. Since 1974 a much greater weight of evidence has been accumulated in relation to these and many other pathologies.

Kagan & Levi's conceptualisation has been important in structuring a considerable amount of succeeding work (e.g. Henry & Stephens, 1977; Steptoe & Mathews, 1984). Its major weakness, however, lies in its lack of predictive power. Whilst it raises many useful issues which have subsequently been pursued, it fails to outline how the important mechanisms have their action: it does not offer any clues as to how the precursors of disease change functional morphology; it does not explicitly classify different types of psychosocial stressors, or psychological mediators, in terms of their effects on the individual; it does not specify any limit to the extent of psychological influences in physical dysfunctions; nor is it specific about the role of psychological processes. It is a conceptual framework rather than a predictive model (Warr, 1980). As such psychological variables have the function of mopping up whatever physiological or physical factors cannot explain. They can be attributed with as much or as little influence as is necessary and their role is therefore a secondary one.

SELYE'S GENERAL ADAPTATION SYNDROME

For Selye (e.g. 1936, 1946, 1976, 1983) 'stress' (strain) is an adaptive *response* which can be caused by exogenous (environmental) or endogenous (intra-individual) stressors. It is a physiological concept which requires that anything which affects the individual's neuroendocrine system is *necessarily* defined as a stressor. Selye (1976) considered that the physiological effects on an organism should be considered "the objective indices of stress and the basis for the development of the entire stress concept".

Selye's model, the General Adaptation Syndrome (GAS), proposes that when an individual is exposed to a stressor of a physical or psychological nature they may show up to three successive types of response, depending upon the intensity and chronicity of the stimulus and the coping mechanisms the individual can employ:

1. *Alarm reaction.* This is the initial response to any stressor to which the organism is not adapted, and has two phases:
   - the shock phase or immediate response, which would be indicated by various bodily symptoms such as tachycardia and increased respiration caused by various hormonal changes;
   - the countershock phase or rebound reaction, in which the level of neuroendocrinal activity is increased to cope with the extra bodily requirements to maintain the alarm reaction. Acute strain reactions and diseases would reveal themselves during the alarm reaction, and the individual may die.
2. *Stage of resistance.* If the individual remains alive they will show resistance or adaptation to the stressor with bodily reactions which are in contradistinction to those of the alarm reaction. For example, there is an increase in corticoid-

containing lipid storage material, anabolic activity and haemodilution. Changes in morphology with chronic stressors will have pathogenic consequences and with continued exposure to stressors (which do not need to be the same ones that caused the original reaction—indeed they may have previously been neutral in their effects, but become conditioned after being paired with the stressor) the organism will show loss of adaptive capacity and demonstrate the final phase.

3. *Stage of exhaustion.* The body's ability to adapt to stressors is finite (although there will be individual differences due to genetic differences and previous environmental learning). If the stressors are not removed (or their effects diminished) the organism will become exhausted as the vital bodily reserves of hormones drop to a pathological level, a return of symptoms, and death will ensue after damage at organ sites.

Although any type of stressor has a similar effect on bodily functions, Selye proposes that there are four classifications based on the two axes of degree and type of stress:

eustress—good stressors,
distress—bad stressors,
hyperstress—too much,
hypostress—too little.

Mason (1968) has proposed that it is the *novel, strange or unfamiliar* aspects of the environment that are common to the different stressors. It is something of a difficulty for Selye's physiological approach that the perception or awareness of threat may be necessary for the animal to demonstrate a stress response (Fleming, Baum & Singer, 1984; Mason, 1975): the suggestion of psychological primacy sits uneasily for Selye.

Selye's major claim is that strain is the common denominator of the adaptive reactions and that there is absolute *nonspecificity* of response:

> It is difficult to see how such essentially different things as cold, heat, drugs, hormones, sorrow and joy can provoke an identical biochemical reaction in the organism. Yet this is the case; it can now be demonstrated by highly objective quantitative biochemical determinations that certain reactions of the body are totally nonspecific and common to all types of exposure (Selye, 1973).

Stress research, therefore, is concerned with nonspecific actions, whilst classical medicine has generally been concerned with specific effects. Medicine ignores the "syndrome of just being sick" or the "stereotyped syndrome that characterises diseases as such" (Selye, 1983, p. 2).

The claim of absolute nonspecificity is a strong one which has been criticised as lacking empirical support to date. Mason (1975), for example, has not been able to show that any single hormone responds to all stimuli in an absolutely nonspecific manner, and Selye (1983) considers that "we still know virtually nothing about the nature of the first mediator" (p. 9) of the strain response, although "Whatever the nature of the first mediator...its existence is assured by its effects" (p. 6). These difficulties in identifying a physical causal precursor of the GAS do not in my view produce any difficulties for the model. The thrust of this book lies in the suggestion that psychological factors can take the place of these 'first mediators'. There is no necessity that these psychological factors require emotional or attentional mediation in the way suggested by Mason (1975, p. 25). If it is possible that psychological factors have primacy as the causal core of bodily responses, it is not surprising or necessary that these psychological reactions should have *single and unique* physiological and neurochemical correlates.

Selye's model is important in the analysis of disease for a number of reasons. First, given that any factors which affect hormone levels can be considered as stressors, if it can be shown that psychological variables have such effects they are given the same status as physical stressors. The door is open for psychological factors to play a significant role in the disease process. In his early writing the role of these factors was not considered important: "in 1936, I gave little thought to the psychological or sociological implications, for I saw stress as a purely physiological or medical phenomenon" (Selye, 1983, p. 1). This perspective has changed as evidence has accumulated to the point where it is likely that psychological stressors "play(s) some role in the development of every disease; its effects—for better or worse—are added to the specific changes characteristic of the disease in question" (Selye, 1983, p. 12). Mason (1975), in his historical view of the stress field, wrote "It is now known that *emotional stimuli rank very high among the most potent and prevalent natural stimuli capable of increasing pituitary–adrenal cortical activity*" (p. 23) and that physical stressors (e.g. heat, exercise) elicit "*an appreciable degree of emotional disturbance*" (p. 24).

Second, the GAS specifies how the course of the disease may develop if the stressor is chronic, as well as outlining the mechanism of the acute initial reaction.

Third, as has already been suggested, psychological variables do not need to be attentionally mediated in order to have strain consequences. That is, an individual does not have to perceive the stressor as being unpleasant, or beyond their capacities to cope with it, in order for it to have an effect: if it produces a neuroendocrine response it is a stressor. This approach does have the obvious weakness that it produces a circularity of definition for its central term 'stress'. This does not, however, affect its status in implicating psychological factors in disease.

A criticism of Selye's work has often been made that it makes no specific predictions concerning which physiological responses will occur to what stressors. In this sense the model is not specific enough (see Fisher, 1984, for further discussion of the stimulus–response specificity issue). There is, perhaps, a more critical difficulty. Selye (1983) recognises that diseases "cannot be ascribed to any one pathogen but to 'pathogenic constellations'; they belong to what we have called the *pluricausal diseases*" (p. 13). His conceptualisation, however, allows only physiologically based responses to act as indices of the pathogenic constellations.

The model is a response-based model and has to presume that *anything* which serves to produce a reaction is a stressor (and, therefore, a cause of any ensuing disease). As McGrath (1970) and Cox (1978) have pointed out, physiological indicators of strain are useful only when one knows that a change in the recorded level is actually caused by a stressor and not some other stimulus, or random fluctuation, which, *a priori*, the investigator would not label a stressor. Moreover, if diseases and illness have multifactorial causes these causes are likely to have multifactorial effects, including psychological ones.

MODELS OF OCCUPATIONAL STRESS AND DISEASE

The models discussed so far provide a simple framework for considering in a relatively neutral and non-theoretical manner, the relationship between stressors and psychological and physical diseases. Figure 1.1 presents a typical example of occupational stress based on numerous similar conceptualisations (e.g. Cooper & Marshall, 1976; Cooper, 1986; French *et al.*, 1982; Schuler, 1982). Such models make no real attempt to predict the prevalence and incidence of disease, or chart the subtle interactions between their many variables, or to facilitate the conceptual understanding of what occupational stress is. They are useful, however, as thumbnail sketches to envelop and list the critical factors which any predictive model should deal with, and to provide a chart of the current state of knowledge (and belief). Epidemiological models of chronic disease (e.g. Medalie, 1985), which may be considered even less predictive, take account of a considerably greater number of factors (e.g. social networks, family system, age, sex, geographical, cultural and political factors).

A number of interactive models of occupational stress have been produced in recent years which can be empirically tested and also have pragmatic implications for redesigning jobs to reduce health risks. Such models are particularly useful because they provide a general framework within which to consider the possible effects of a whole range of *possible* stressors, even if the particular stressor–strain relationship has not been specifically tested. If the broad dimensions of the model are shown to be empirically justifiable, the specific stressors that might be subsumed under their umbrella are given some degree of credence.

TAKING ACCOUNT OF SUPPORT AND DECISION LATITUDE

It is clear that work demand is not equivalent to work strain, although it is itself a major occupational stressor. For example, underutilisation of abilities, and other work factors which imply lack of demand, are among the more powerful predictors of strain. It has also been shown that higher levels of strain are associated with lower-level unskilled jobs (e.g. Chapter 7; Fletcher, 1988a). One resolution to this apparent

11

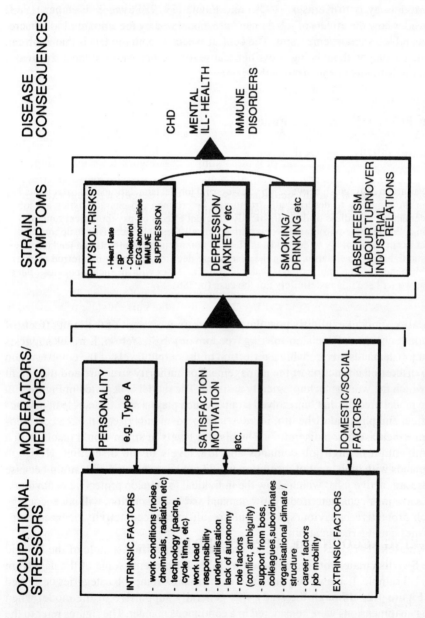

Figure 1.1   A stressor–strain model (reproduced by permission from Fletcher, 1988a)

paradox is to postulate that another work dimension moderates the relationship between work demand and strain. This necessitates examining variables together.

Models by both Karasek (1979) and Payne (1979; Payne & Fletcher, 1983) consider how the effects of job demand are moderated by the amount of job discretion and job support/constraint. The central aspect of both models is that a job can be demanding without being stressful because some other aspect of the job provides resources to meet or neutralise the demands.

The Effect of Decision Latitude

Karasek (1979) suggests that:

> Failure to distinguish between job stressors and job decision latitude is also reflected in the tendency to describe all structurally determined job characteristics as 'job demands' regardless of their drastically different effects on psychological functioning. While the environmental determinacy of all these characteristics supports the uniform terminology of demands, the lack of homogeneity of effects can lead to substantial misinterpretation, as in the case where decision authority is referred to as a 'demand'.... The implication is that job strain increases with all such 'demands', but as we will see this is definitely not the case (p. 286).

Karasek's model explicitly postulates that strain is a result of the joint effects of work demands and decision-making freedom or job discretion. Karasek suggests that job demands are probably a reflection of the output levels of the company, and job discretion a function of the management or authority structure and the extent to which the work is technologically assisted. The model is depicted in Figure 1.2. The model predicts that 'unresolved strain', which plays a significant role in psychological and physical ill-health, increases as job demands rise without a commensurate increase in job discretion. The highest levels of strain would result from a combination of high job demands and low levels of job discretion. High job demands with high level of discretion would not be associated with strain because these are 'active jobs' which allow the individual to develop protective behaviours. 'Passive jobs', characterised by low demand and low discretion, will not encourage such protective behaviours and would result in reduced activity, learned helplessness, and a rise in strain.

Karasek (1979) tested the model on a random stratified sample of the US and the Swedish male working population. Table 1.1 presents some of the data from the US sample. It shows only the data for the four extreme job categories described in Figure 1.2, although the study was generally supportive of the model when the two dimensions were considered in a continuous manner. The figures refer to the percentage of men demonstrating the particular strain considered for each of the four categories of job. The study is based entirely on self-report survey data.

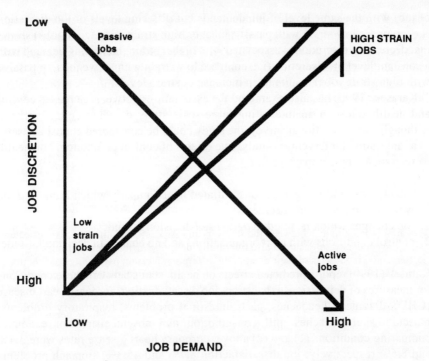

Figure 1.2   Karasek's job strain model (adapted from Karasek, 1979)

Table 1.1.   Strain levels for four job categories for US males (figures taken from Karasek, 1979)

	Job category			
Strain measure	Low strain job	High strain job	Passive job	Active job
Depression	11.1	51.3	27.9	26.9
Exhaustion	7.4	32.5	9.6	25.0
Job dissatisfaction	18.5	55.3	40.9	13.8
Life dissatisfaction	7.1	29.3	19.7	1.5
Tranquilliser/sleeping pill consumption	2.3	13.9	4.5	8.7
Sick days off	14.0	46.2	38.8	17.8

The figures refer to the percentage of men in each of the job categories who exhibited significantly elevated levels on the strain measure

As can be seen from Table 1.1, the predictions with respect to the 'unresolved strain' diagonal of the model are strongly supportive of the proposed interaction between job demands and job discretion. The protective effect of the activity level is also in the predicted direction for four of the six strain measures. A comparison of jobs with the same level of job demands but differing levels of job discretion (i.e. compare low strain with passive jobs, or high strain with active jobs) shows that decreasing discretion is associated with higher strain; increasing demand with a constant level of discretion (i.e. compare low strain with active jobs, or passive with high strain jobs) results in an increase in strain levels.

Karasek (1990) has also examined the associations between increased control and health status in an interesting large-scale study of white-collar workers. Although a cross-sectional survey, the study could be considered almost as useful as a longitudinal intervention study. The effects of control or autonomy on health were assessed by comparing:

1. job changes and reorganisations initiated by a company which *increased* the workers' job decision latitude;
2. job changes which resulted in *decreased* decision latitude;
3. control conditions with no reorganisations and no change in decision latitude.

Karasek (1990) reports predicted effects on health status between these conditions for measures of depression, exhaustion, job dissatisfaction, coronary heart disease (CHD), dizziness, headaches, gastrointestinal problems, respiratory problems, muscular–skeletal aches, pill consumption and absenteeism. For example, comparing conditions (1) and (2) above, coronary heart disease rates were 3.4% and 8.6% respectively; job dissatisfaction 8.7% and 45.3%; stomach problems 16.9% and 24.4%; depression 13.7% and 27.8%. Moreover, those who had reported decreases in job control were more likely to have had at least four absences from work in the preceding year (10.7% vs. 5.0%).

The model has recently been applied to an examination of job satisfaction, burnout, depression and psychosomatic symptoms amongst hospital and nursing-home employees. Landsbergis (1988) shows that the level of these strains was significantly greater in those jobs where workers perceived they had a high workload and little decision latitude, even after controlling for the effects of hours worked, shift, age, sex, education and number of children. There were also no differences in strain levels between 'active' and 'passive' jobs, nor was activity level of the job related to both discretion and demands, as predicted. The study did fail, however, to find any relationships between the job characteristics and CHD risk or smoking behaviour.

A laboratory-based examination of the model by Perrewe & Ganster (1989) also provided limited support. One hundred and twenty-five subjects did a mail-sorting task under different levels of workload and control. Perceived demand had no impact on the physiological indicators (pulse rate and skin temperature), although demand was related to anxiety and job satisfaction. Low discretion was associated with higher anxiety (but not satisfaction or physiology) under higher demand conditions (but no effect of discretion was present at low demand).

Such findings have important implications for practice as well as models of stress, because they imply that redesigning work to increase job discretion should have benefits for workers even if the overall level of job demands remains unchanged. Such benefits have been observed when either an individual's or a group's level of decision authority has been increased (e.g. Wall, Clegg & Jackson, 1978; Wall & Clegg, 1981; Kemp *et al.*, 1983). The importance of worker autonomy and responsibility is an implicit aspect of some major theories of motivation (e.g. Herzberg), as well as underpinning the Job Characteristics Model of Hackman & Oldham (1976), which has been very influential in the job redesign literature.

Karasek's model has also been applied to the prediction of endocrine, metabolic and cardiovascular activity. Karasek, Russell & Theorell (1982) review the physiological evidence and discuss the relationship between catabolic (strain) and anabolic (regeneration) processes relevant to cardiovascular functioning. They suggest that when demand is high, but discretion low, adrenal–cortical and adrenal–medullary activity will be high with elevations in cortisol and adrenalin. Catecholamine activity is increased in situations of high demand. Cortisol secretion, on the other hand, seems to be elevated in situations where discretion or control is low. High levels of serum catecholamines have been linked with increased coagulability of the blood (Ardlie, Glew & Schwartz, 1966), myocardial degeneration (Bassett, Strand & Carincross, 1978), and atherosclerosis (Carruthers, 1969; Haft, 1974). With high demand but low discretion there would be concomitant increases in heart rate, blood pressure and decrease in the ratio of high density lipoproteins (HDL) to low density lipoproteins (LDL). High demand, however, can be characterised in the right work situations as healthy high activity if job discretion is also high. In this situation adrenalin would show rapid return to baseline levels following exposure to stressors, with consequent lowering of heart rate and blood pressure and increase in HDL/LDL ratio.

It is unclear how well the model predicts (as opposed to hypothesises) actual coronary heart disease risk factors. In a large-scale study of casual blood pressure, for example, Fletcher & Jones (1990, 1991) report that the work factors in the model did predict a range of psychological strain measures. Diastolic and systolic blood pressure, however, consistently resulted in negative (i.e. non-predicted but significant) relationships, when the traditional blood pressure risk factors were controlled.

Karasek's model has been applied to the prediction of the prevalence and incidence rates of coronary heart disease in both the USA and Sweden (Karasek *et al.*, 1982). A subsample from the US Health Examination Survey (HES) of 2159 white males from 180 different occupations were rated according to the degree of job demand and job decision latitude. The assessment of myocardial infarction was based on the assessment of a clinical panel of doctors who were provided with ECG, chest X-ray, medical history and blood chemistry results. In the first of the Swedish studies the assessment of job demands and decision latitude was based on self-report questionnaire responses. The 1461 individuals who showed no evidence of self-reported cardiovascular symptoms (chest pain, dyspnoea, high blood pressure, heart weakness) were followed up six years later. Standardised odds risk ratios were determined for both job demands and decision latitude in multiple regressions which included some normal CHD risk factors. Low decision latitude was associated with a 2.0 and 1.4 excess risk respectively, and a demanding job with 1.5 and 1.3 excess risk. Two further studies using CHD–case control methods supported the view that the *interaction* between these work factors has important consequences for the prediction of CHD. In one study all cases (334) of myocardial infarction in 40–64-year-old men in Stockholm over a two-year period were matched with at least two infarction-free controls. The 'job characteristics' of 118 different jobs were assessed by interviews with another sample of 3876 men (Alfredsson, Karasek & Theorell, 1982). An analysis of the job characteristics that distinguished the low from the high CHD jobs showed that low control combined with high demand (or a rushed work tempo) was a significant discriminant in which the "excess risk predicted exceeded the mere *summation* of high demand or low control" (Alfredsson *et al.,* 1982, p. 166). It should also be noted that these work factors were consistently found to be predictors of CHD despite very marked differences in methodologies and end-disease points. In fact the average CHD risk of low job discretion was around 1.72, which is roughly equivalent to the effects of high serum cholesterol levels.

It is unclear why there are apparent inconsistencies when the model is applied to CHD and the risk factors. It seems likely that this is, in part, due to the different action of acute and chronic stressors, how the measurements of the job factors are taken (i.e. by scaled questionnaires given to individuals or by independent ratings of the jobs by others), and the interaction between the various risk factors themselves and how they relate to the stressors.

Interestingly, Karasek (1978) has applied the job demand–discretion to the prediction of eight factors of leisure activities obtained by the Varimax rotation of items used in a national stratified sample of Swedish adults. The model predicts that workers' leisure time activity levels will vary according to the 'activity diagonal' shown in Figure 1.2. If the level of job 'activity' has a direct effect on pursuits outside the work environment, the model predicts that jobs with low discretion and low demand ('passive jobs') would be associated with much lower participation in political and leisure activities than jobs high in demand and discretion ('active jobs'). In general the survey found that the more active the job the more active the leisure pursuits. The amount of Variety in Leisure, Total Active Leisure and Total Political Activity all confirmed this hypothesis. A comparison of *non-participation* rates of people whose jobs were high demand/high discretion with those with low demand/low discretion produced the following:

Variety in Leisure: 9.4% vs. 40%
Total Leisure Activity: 24.6% vs. 49.6%
Total Political Activity: 33.9% vs. 61.6%.

There were, however, important exceptions to this pattern. For example, reading adventure magazines and window-shopping were more likely in low activity jobs

(71.2% vs. 53.8%). In addition, although 'Elite Political Activity' revealed a strong active job–active leisure link (22.8% vs. 75%), 'Mass Political Activity' did not (45% vs. 48.1%). In fact, the jobs with high demand but low discretion (what Karasek calls the 'heavy' or 'high strain' jobs) had the lowest non-participation rates (30%).

Clearly Karasek's (1978) data have severe limitations for making causal assertions. They do, however, suggest that work factors affect non-work activity. Chapter 6 considers the spill-over from work to home in greater detail.

The Demands–Supports–Constraints Model

Payne (1979) has developed a model of stress similar to that of Karasek, but more appropriate as a model of occupational stress because it is useful for predicting strain levels within an occupationally homogeneous group as well as between different occupational groups (Payne & Fletcher, 1983). The model also forms the basis of a measure of occupational stressors and strains, known as the *Cultural Audit* (Fletcher, 1989). The model proposes that strain is the result of the lack of balance between three work factors:

1. *Job demands*—this is the degree to which the work environment contains stimuli which peremptorily require attention and response. It is much more encompassing than Karasek's (1979) concept of demand, which largely measures the role overload aspects of jobs. The stimuli might be technical, intellectual, social or financial. Job demands represent the things that have to be done and the environment in which the individual is placed. Table 1.2 presents some common job demands.
2. *Job supports*—this is the degree to which the work environment contains available resources which are relevant to the demands of the individual or the group. These supports may be technical, intellectual, social, financial, etc. For example, being part of a happy cohesive workforce may make the job demands easier to cope with. Psychological support has been shown to moderate the relationship between stressors and strains (House *et al.*, 1979; Payne & Jones, 1987).
3. *Job constraints*—jobs are made much harder by the lack of relevant resources, which are usually finite in supply. Such constraints can act to prevent the individual maximising the benefits of the supports, as well as affecting how individuals can cope with the demands. Thus constraints are those aspects of the working environment which prevent the worker or group from coping with the demands. Table 1.2 shows some common supports–constraints (for operational reasons, supports and constraints are treated as a single bipolar dimension).

According to the demands–supports–constraints model of stress, strain results from a lack of balance between the three variables. Thus, high job demands are not stressful (i.e. they do not lead to strain) if the job also provides good levels of support and low constraints. In fact, high demands can be positively good in the right circumstances because they provide stimulation and utilise the worker's abilities—underutilisation of abilities and boredom are amongst the most potent stressors and also usually occur in work environments where supports are low and constraints high. One obvious practical implication of the model is that highly demanding jobs can be made less stressful without reducing the level of the demands: instead the level of supports can be increased or the constraints reduced. The model has implications for redesigning work to reduce the amount of strain in an organisation whilst at the same time boosting efficiency.

Table 1.2.   Work stressors as demands or supports–constraints (adapted from Fletcher, 1990)

Work demands	Work supports–constraints
Job pressure	Being clear about role
Having too much to do	Job discretion, autonomy or control
Having too little to do	Quality of relationships with:
Being responsible for people	Boss
Responsibility for things (equipment)	Colleagues
Demands from others	Subordinates
Conflicting demands/roles	Union membership
Over–under-promotion	Role ambiguity
Keeping up with others/organisations	Variety level/skill utilisation
Organisational climate	Social perception of job
Office politics	Participation in decisions
Organisational structure	Payment/reward system
Organisational/job changes	Quality of equipment
Major decisions	Physical working conditions
Expectancies of others/organisation	How work is planned/managed

This model has been tested on a whole array of occupational groups (e.g. managers, teachers, nurses, taxi drivers, students, lorry drivers, health visitors, social workers, ministers of religion) and has been shown to have predictive value (e.g. Fletcher & Morris, 1988; Fletcher & MacPherson, 1989; Jones, Fletcher & Ibbetson, 1991; Payne & Fletcher, 1983). It is important to note, however, that the central concept of support does not simply refer to social or interpersonal aspects, although these are known to reduce the effects of stress. It also includes such job factors as being clear about the task in hand and having a measure of autonomy and discretion over how the work is ordered and executed. Fletcher & Jones (1990, 1991) showed that support factors did increase predictability over and above Karasek's demand and job decision latitude dimensions for a range of dependent variables including depression, free-floating anxiety, life and job satisfaction.

THE VITAMIN MODEL OF OCCUPATIONAL STRESS

This model, proposed by Warr (1987), has been developed to provide a framework within the context of mental, rather than physical, ill-health. It suggests that the biological analogy of the vitamin requirements of the body is useful for under-standing why occupational stressors produce strain. It can be considered a version of the simple environmental stressor–strain models such as Kagan & Levi's (1974) model. Although it can take account of some individual differences, it is essentially a 'situation-centred' rather than a 'person-centred' model (Gergen & Gergen, 1982).

The vitamin model proposes that a person's health is affected by environmental psychological factors in a way analogous to the effects of vitamins. Vitamins are necessary for proper body functioning and vitamin deficiency produces bodily dys-functions. Beyond a certain level of intake, however, vitamins do not have any addi-tional beneficial effect: their positive effect plateaus at a constant level (e.g. as for high doses of vitamins C and E) and may even have negative toxic consequences (as for very high doses of vitamins A and D). The relationship between intake and health is decidedly non-linear, as depicted in Figure 1.3. Warr (1987) identifies nine work stressors which he proposes affect mental health in a similar way. The nine psychological 'vitamins' are shown in Table 1.3, and Warr reviews the research on mental health and work which generally supports his framework. Table 1.3 also shows the presumed effect of high 'dosage' of the stressor in terms of whether there is an Additional Decrement (as for vitamins A and D) or a Constant Effect (as for C and E).

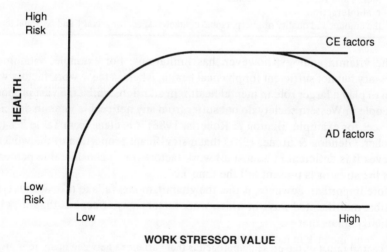

Figure 1.3   Warr's (1987) vitamin model analogy between work stressors and health (reproduced by permission)

The model may provide a useful framework with which to consider different jobs in terms of their mental health consequences. If so, it is also likely to have ramifi-cations for physical well-being. At minimum it provides a useful guide for job description, comparison and an outline of good practice. It also provides a welcomed framework within which to consider where improvements in jobs should be aimed.

Work, Stress, Disease and Life Expectancy

Table 1.3.   Environmental work stressors identified by Warr (1987) in the context of the vitamin model of stress (reproduced by permission)

CE (constant effect) stressors
1. Financial remuneration
    income in terms of needs and comparisons with others
2. Physical work environment
    safe work, ergonomically sound, reasonable environmental and physical conditions
3. Social position
    work role providing sufficient esteem and meaningfulness

AD (additional decrement) stressors
4. Job discretion and control
    control over job content, timing and pace of work
5. Skill factors
    degree to which job allows current skills and opportunity to acquire new skills
6. Variety in job
    intrinsic job variety or diversity, degree of repetition, and cycle time
7. External job demands/goals
    level and pattern of job demands (time and load), conflicts between demands, degree
    of task identity or visibility
8. Job clarity
    degree to which feedback is given or available, ambiguity in relation to work require-
    ments and future developments
9. Social interaction
    the amount and quality of interpersonal contact, respect for privacy and personal territory

The vitamin analogy, however, has limitations. For example, vitamins are necessary but not sufficient for physical health, whereas these work factors would seem to play a larger role in mental health. In addition, whilst the vast proportion of people in Western society do not suffer from any noticeable vitamin deficiency (but see, for example, Benton & Roberts, 1988) it is clear from Table 7.1 (from Fletcher, Glendon & Stone, 1987) that a significant proportion of the workforce believes it is deficient in almost all work factors (i.e. a considerable percentage feels the stressor is present 'all the time').

More important, however, is that the vitamin model fails to take account of the possible multifaceted ways in which work factors may affect health. Warr (1987) explicitly states that

A central thrust of the present approach is that variations between many jobs are of no psychological consequence. Variations in those occupational environments which fall in the middle range...are thought to be irrelevant to mental health. Rather than studying these environments, it is more important to concentrate attention on jobs which fall at the extremes of the nine environmental dimensions, especially those with very low values (p. 21).

I suggest that this approach may be fundamentally flawed. The model is not itself empirically tested. Instead support for it comes from a (very sound) literature review showing that the nine environmental factors do act *in isolation* as predicted by the vitamin model. For the model, as developed, there should be no interrelationship or interaction between the different factors. Moreover, the whole constellation of a job as measured and described by the nine features should not have any impact *over and above* their individual contributions. It is possible (and, and as we shall see later, likely) that the *profile* of a job in terms of the important job stressors probably has *more* impact on well-being than all the separate factors considered separately and additively.

INTERACTIVE MODELS OF OCCUPATIONAL STRESS

Models of occupational stress differ from physiological models of stress inasmuch as they are not neutral or assumptive about what is meant by the term 'stress': the models attempt to provide a predictive as well as descriptive account of strain levels which may be observed in the workplace. These psychological models should not be considered as being incompatible with the environment-based models outlined so far, because their purpose is somewhat different. They attempt to take account of important *individual differences* which the previous models do not do so explicitly. They have developed because more recent research has shown that physiological and medical indices of bodily dysfunction need to take account of psychological variables if they are to be maximally predictive. Whilst physical factors (e.g. temperature, pathogens, exercise) may account for the majority of the variance in exhibited body functioning, a significant residual is contributed by psychological variables (e.g. Payne & Rick, 1986b). These psychological factors may have different effects on different people for a number of reasons including:

1. Individuals may perceive the same stressors in different ways because their circumstances differ. For example, one person may have a more supportive family or boss than another and may, therefore, react differently to work stressors. This category of conditional suggests that the researcher needs to take account of a more complex set of environmental or contextual matters in order to predict strain levels adequately: differences between individuals can be ironed out by painting a richer picture of the environment in which they are placed.
2. Individuals may perceive the same stressors in different ways because they differ in how they see the world.
3. Individuals may be more or less reactive to given environmental conditions because they have differentially biased functional systems (e.g. genetic factors, physiology, different relevant histories).

Differences Between People

There are many different work environments, and we have seen that some of the work factors intrinsic and extrinsic to the work environment can affect mental and physical health. There are, however, many differences between people and any comprehensive model of occupational stress must take account of how different people respond differently in the same situation. We shall see in later chapters how some of these differences have been linked to well-being. The purpose of this section is to outline a general framework within which to consider how some of these individual differences affect strain levels within an organisation.

Perhaps the most comprehensive interactive model of this type is the *person–environment (P-E) fit model*. This has been developed and tested most extensively by researchers from the Institute of Social Research at the University of Michigan (e.g. Caplan *et al.*, 1975; French *et al.*, 1982; Van Harrison, 1978). The basic framework for the model is shown in Figure 1.4.

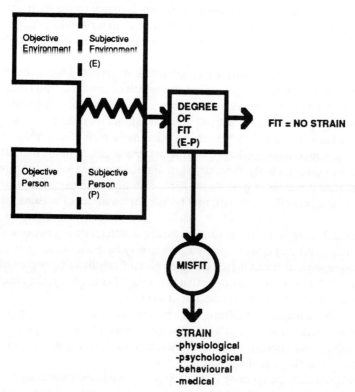

Figure 1.4   The person–environment fit model of stress

The essential distinction to note is that between *objective* and *subjective* environments. The objective elements refer to the outside world independent of the person's perceptions of them. They are the 'situation-centred' aspect (Warr, 1987), or reality as it is. The subjective elements refer to the person's perception of themselves and the environment. Their perceptions may or may not be accurate assessments of the world and themselves. French, Rogers & Cobb (1974) use the term 'contact with reality' to denote the degree to which the objective and the subjective assessment of the world are matched, and the term 'accuracy of self-assessment' to denote the relationship between the objective and subjective person.

Clearly, if the objective person and the objective environment do not 'fit' in a particular work context there is propensity for strain (for example, if an unskilled person is required to do a skilled job). The resulting strain level, however, is not a function of the interrelationship between these objective factors, as it might be considered to be in a totally situation-centred or environment-driven conceptualisation of stress: a person may have developed strategies to cope adequately with any misfit between the objective elements. What is of primary concern for predicting the level of strain is the degree of *misfit* between the person's perception of the environment and their perception of themselves. (It should be noted that there is no requirement in the model that these evaluations have to be explicitly considered by the person.)

In the early versions of the model, Van Harrison (1978) considered two dimensions which were central:

1. Motive-supply. This refers to the capacity to which a job supplies fulfilment of the individual's motives.
2. Ability-demand. This refers to the relationship between the demands of the job and the individual's abilities to meet the demands.

One of the strengths of the model is that it can explain why such factors as underutilisation of abilities, or lack of autonomy, are very important stressors, and why unskilled workers have higher strain levels than professionals. The model posits that it is the degree of misfit *per se* between the person and the environment elements of each dimension that is causally related to strain levels. Thus, an inadequately demanding job, as well as an overdemanding job, should produce strain. In addition, a job which supplies more than an individual's requirements for motives, as well as one which supplies less, will produce strain in certain circumstances. The model is also designed to predict more minor variations in health in essentially healthy populations, as opposed to more catastrophic acute breakdowns.

Data from Caplan *et al.*'s (1975) large study of 2030 workers from 23 different occupations included stressor measures which have allowed an in-depth analysis of the P-E fit model in the prediction of psychological and physiological strains (Van Harrison, 1978; French *et al.*, 1982). The essential test of the model is whether the discrepancy between person (P) and environment (E) measures of each dimension is a better predictor of strain than either the P or E measures considered separately. Van Harrison (1978) presents such data for one central aspect of work: job complexity which was derived from multiple items which measured such aspects as the presence of a fixed work routine, the number of tasks which had to be handled at any one time, and the variety of people that had to be dealt with. The workers had to rate the complexity of their job and their preferred level of complexity.

The P-E misfit was derived from the difference between these subjective assessments of the job. For the six strains considered (job dissatisfaction, boredom, somatic complaints, anxiety, depression and irritation) the predicted U-shaped curves were obtained. In addition, the P-E misfit measure significantly correlated with all of the strain measures, whilst less than half of the P or E correlations were significant. In multiple correlations, the addition of the misfit measure to the P and E measures significantly increased the amount of variance accounted for on each of the strain indices. Van Harrison (1978) suggests that careful consideration should be given to matching the person to the job at the time of hiring, that the fit should be periodically checked, and that future expectancies will probably play a significant role in P-E misfit-induced strain.

The model has been subjected to the most detailed analysis by French *et al.* (1982). P-E fit was measured on eight dimensions:

1. *Income*: the discrepancy between actual earnings and the amount the person felt they should have been paid.
2. *Overtime*: the amount of overtime worked in comparison to the amount the person would have liked to have worked.
3. *Length of service* in the job compared to the length of time the worker felt they would need to be in that job to become fully trained.
4. *Education* level of the person compared to the level of formal education they felt was necessary to do the job well.
5. *Job complexity*, including P-E misfit in terms of contact with different types/groups of people, task variation, number of parallel jobs/roles.
6. *Workload*, which included P-E fit in terms of how fast and hard the work required the person to work, the number of projects/tasks, overall workload and time to do the job.
7. *Responsibility for people*, which assessed the fit in terms of responsibility for the future of others, their morale, and their welfare.
8. *Role ambiguity*, which referred to clarity of job objectives, the person's clarity and ability to predict the expectations of others, and clarity of job responsibilities.

The measures of strain included seven *psychological* aspects (job dissatisfaction, workload dissatisfaction, boredom, somatic complaints, depression, anxiety and irritation), ten health-related strains (based on smoking behaviour, caffeine consumption, obesity and dispensary visits), physical illness (cardiovascular disease, peptic ulcers, gastrointestinal problems and respiratory infections), and eight physiological measures (systolic blood pressure, diastolic blood pressure, heart rate, cholesterol, T3 and T41 thyroid hormones, uric acid and cortisol levels).

The correlational results showed support for the P-E fit model on each of the eight dimensions. For example, misfit on each of the dimensions correlated with *workload dissatisfaction*, seven of the dimensions correlated with *job dissatisfaction* (not income), six with *boredom* (not overtime or income), five with *depression* (not responsibility for persons, overtime, or length of service). *Somatic complaints* were correlated with lack of P-E fit on job complexity and workload. The physiological strains were also predicted by the model in some cases. For example, *T3* correlated with the job dimensions job complexity and workload; *serum uric acid* levels with income and length of service; and *systolic blood pressure* with role ambiguity and workload.

The P-E fit model does, of course, predict curvilinear relationships between each work dimension and strain measure (i.e. too much and too little produces strain). Stepwise multiple regressions were used to determine the amount of strain variance accounted for by such curvilinear relationships *over and above* the variance linearly predicted by the component P and E measures. Results showed that the P-E relationship accounted for more of the strain variance on over half the occasions when a strain indicator was predicted by the linear measure. P-E fit for *job complexity* was the most successful work dimension in predicting strain, accounting for an extra 14% of the variance for workload dissatisfaction. It should be noted, too, that although the additional variance accounted for was rather modest (ranging from 1.5% to 14%) the measures used, and the narrow scoring range, may have been somewhat limiting. It is also important to note that the P-E fit model has generally been applied to quite broad job dimensions, across a wide variety of jobs (e.g. the 23 occupations in the NIOSH study), with relatively crude strain measures. Even though the broad framework does not account for a large proportion of the predictable strain, more detailed refinements of the model and measures are possible. For example, misfit on some dimensions may be more important than others, the aggregate of misfit on a broad dimension may not itself predict strain well because only some of the component dimensions contribute, only some job dimensions may produce specific strains and not others, and fit–misfit on a job dimension may be occupation-specific in its effect. Whilst none of these possibilities has been adequately tested, previous stress research would suggest they may be applicable to the P-E fit model. The model's framework could cope with such contingencies.

THE CONFIGURAL OR CATASTROPHE MODEL

So far we have seen that models of stress can provide useful frameworks for organising different aspects of the literature. To summarise the preceding sections any all-embracing model of occupational stress must be able to predict:

1. *Individual differences* in the perception of work stressors, and how the stressors affect different people. It must take account of how different people perceive themselves and their job.
2. *Strain is not simply a function of job (and other) demands* (although an excess of demand and other factors can result in strain.
3. Jobs which do not supply a *sufficiently enriched environment* produce strain.
4. Strain results from the *interplay between various dimensions*.

5. The impact of stressors should not be considered general: *specific stressors can have specific strain effects.*
6. *Work and domestic factors are not independent.*
7. The effects of potential stressors may *vary over time* even though the level of the stressors may not.
8. *The stressed person perceives the world differently from the unstressed person.* Moreover, when suffering from strain the same individual may perceive previously unstressful factors as real stressors.

The models of occupational stress considered so far predict aspects 1–5 above to a greater or lesser extent. For example, the vitamin model proposes that strain results from the absence or excess of any of the nine stressors or 'vitamins', and demand is only one such stressor. The level of resulting strain depends to some extent on the levels of all nine stressors, although a deficit or excess of any one vitamin stressor may have specific health consequences (Warr, 1987, is not explicit about how far the vitamin analogy can be taken). The model does not, however, adequately deal with the differences between individuals except by asserting that 'enduring personal characteristics' interact with the vitamin stressors: the model proposes that differences in (e.g.) baseline mental (and, by implication, physical) health have an impact on the effects of the stressors. The vitamin analogy seems to break down because it does not specify particular stressor–strain mechanisms in the same way that vitamin excess or deficiency mechanisms can be isolated.

The aspect of stress which most models do not cope with adequately is that potential stressors are not constant in effect, even for the same individual. For example, points 7 and 8 above suggest that some stressors may not play as large a *causal* role in strain as others, since their apparent effect varies with the context of other stressors. Fletcher & Payne (1980b) have distinguished between *primary* and *secondary stressors*. The former could be considered the 'true' causes of stress, or at least to play a major role in determining the level of strain. Secondary stressors, on the other hand, are environmental factors which become associated (and hence correlated) with strain but only because the individual's threshold for them has become lowered by the strain arising from the primary stressors. In other words, the secondary stressors are contingent on the pre-existence of strain caused by other factors. To all intents and purposes, cross-sectional studies will not reveal any differences between primary and secondary stressors unless the individual's level of strain is taken account of. Indeed, secondary stressors may seem to play a more important causal role because they will be associated with the last-presenting examples.

There is some support for the notion that the stressed person perceives the world differently, as predicted by this distinction. Payne (1979), Fletcher & Payne (1980b) and Fletcher & Jones (1990) present evidence that the statistical relationship between variables is dependent upon the levels of strain. For example, Payne (1979) divided his sample of managers into a high strain and a low strain group, depending upon their score on the General Health Questionnaire. The high strain group showed correlations between self-esteem and number of years with employer, job pressure, satisfaction with boss, with colleagues, how time-consuming they found work and that the important things were the most difficult. None of these were significant for the low strain group. The high strain group also showed correlations between work satisfaction and a number of demands, supports and constraints which were not present for the low strain group. It should be noted, too, that the two samples did not differ much in terms of strain since the managers were labelled 'high strain' if they were in the top quartile of GHQ scores. Fletcher & Jones (1990) extended the distinction between primary and secondary stressors by showing that the relationships between variables were different for those with elevated blood pressure, compared to those with normal levels. Since high blood pressure is considered largely asymptomatic this would support the idea that the primary/secondary stressors effects are not mediated solely by psychological variables.

Pearlin (1989) also distinguishes between primary and secondary stressors in those situations where

one event leads to another event or triggers chronic strains; strains, for their part, beget other strains or events. Thus clusters of stressors may develop, each cluster being made up of a variety of events and strains. Furthermore, the clustered stressors may be formed by problems that originated in different institutionalised roles...occupational strains may create marital strains, and so on (p. 247).

Pearlin goes on to say that the distinction

will help to distinguish between people who may be similar with regard to their exposure to one stressor but who differ appreciably with regard to the array of stressors to which they are exposed. Such discrimination can go far in explaining why people who seem to be alike with regard to the problems they face differ sharply with regard to the intensity and range of stress outcomes that they manifest (pp. 248–9).

Figure 1.5 presents one conceptualisation of such *catastrophe* or *configural* effects, which also takes account of the home–work interface.

This is called a configural or catastrophe model because the basic predictions it makes are related to the idea that a condition of strain can result from a small (even less than noticeable) change in the central variables (the demands–support–constraints, or the perceived fit). The net result of the small change is to alter the relationships (but not the isolated values, except in the one variable) between the stressor variables in the model so that their sum is nudged over some threshold value. Any environmental factor which causes an increment in strain over threshold may not, in isolation, itself be a powerful predictor of strain. The effect of the change, however, is to reconfigure or flip the system into the state of being definitely under strain (i.e. the strain is no longer subclinical) and if this situation persists chronic health problems are more likely (as in the Kagan & Levi, 1974, conceptualisation discussed earlier). When the internal state is reconfigured the person perceives the

Phase 1:Pre-catastrophe
(example with only five dimensions for two roles)

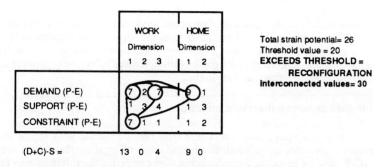

	WORK Dimension			HOME Dimension		
	1	2	3	1	2	
DEMAND (P-E)	7	2	7	9	1	Total strain potential= 11
SUPPORT (P-E)	8	3	4	9	3	Threshold value = 20
CONSTRAINT (P-E)	7	1	1	1	2	Node threshold value = 10
						BOTH BELOW THRESHOLD
(D+C)-S =	6	0	4	1	0	

Phase 2: Support on dimensions work 1 and home 1 reduced by a total of 15.

	WORK Dimension			HOME Dimension		
	1	2	3	1	2	
DEMAND (P-E)	7	2	7	9	1	Total strain potential= 26
SUPPORT (P-E)	1	3	4	1	3	Threshold value = 20
CONSTRAINT (P-E)	7	1	1	1	2	EXCEEDS THRESHOLD = RECONFIGURATION
						Interconnected values= 30
(D+C)-S =	13	0	4	9	0	

Figure 1.5   The configural model of stress

environment as being overall more stressful because the isolated variables in the model become interconnected as a result of the catastrophe (in the example in Figure 1.5 the total value of the connected nodes is 30, whereas the highest value of any nodes in the pre-catastrophe state is only 9, and the total 'strain potential score' is 25). This reconfiguration will make factors stressful which were not so previously. Aspects that can precipitate a catastrophe would include any, some, or all of the following:

- an increase in any demand (home or work) (the D values),
- an increase in any constraint (the C values),
- a decrease in any support (the S values),
- a change in the person's perception of themselves (the P values),
- a change in the person's perception of the environment (the E values),
- failure to cope with sub-threshold strain for an extended period.

The model makes a number of testable assumptions:

1. Strain is the result of the perceived overall demands and constraints exceeding the person's perceived capabilities and supports.
2. There are a number of strain-relevant *dimensions* within a number of separable *environments* (e.g. work, home). These dimensions could be considered aspects of each environment which are necessary for well-being (e.g. they could be considered analogous to Warr's vitamins).
3. Each demand, support and constraint relevant to each dimension is determined by the person's evaluation of their environment and themselves in relation to that demand, support or constraint. The outcome of this evaluation can be assigned value and represents a single *node* within Figure 1.5 (shown as numbers).
4. The *strain potential* for each dimension is the resulting value from the interplay between the P-E misfit values (shown as a node in Figure 1.5) of the demands plus constraints, minus supports relevant to that dimension.
5. Overall strain potential is the sum of the values from all dimensions.
6. The strain potential value of any one dimension can itself be high enough to produce a manifestation of actual strain (e.g. anxiety, elevated blood pressure, catecholamine secretion). This does not happen in the majority of people. It is normally the sum of 'sub-threshold' strain potential values that determine the level of strain.
7. Any node which itself is above some critical value (10 in the example) is afforded particular attention by the individual. It is definitely attentionally heeded and can, therefore, be verbally described. (Although it may be that the node itself does not produce strain because its effect is being moderated by another node of that dimension.) It should be noted that 'attentionally heeded' does not imply cause or even attribution of cause by the individual.
8. The relationship between overall strain potential and observed strain is linear up to some threshold value (20 in the example).
9. When the strain potential value reaches the threshold, the system is reconfigured as a result of the 'catastrophe'. The consequence of this is that all relevant nodes which have a high enough individual potential (5 in the example) become actively interrelated or interconnected (shown by the connected lines in the example), thus destroying dimensional independence (and dimensional 'safety' for those with low individual strain potential).
10. Strain can be manifested in various ways including psychological, behavioural, physiological, social and medical.

A number of predictions are made by this model over and above the sum of the constituent models from which it is derived:

1. The result of a minor change in one of the variables (which reconfigures the system into catastrophe) can be very different from the occurrence of some major

stressor (e.g. a spouse dying). This is because the major event may not result in any change in the perceived relationship between the elements because in and of itself the major events command the primary focus of the individual. The minor change may not itself command any attention.

2. This last point also makes it more understandable why many stressors may not be consciously heeded in terms of their significance or their effect on well-being.

3. Because the model proposes that individual demands, supports and constraints are related to strain in some additive manner prior to catastrophe, and also because the mathematical relationship between the variables and strain changes with reconfiguration, the strength of their statistical associations with strain variables would not be very great. This is because, at a number of levels, the role any variable plays in strain is moderated by several variables/factors. For example, demandingness for one aspect of work is affected by the P-E fit equation, and the effect of the resultant 'demand residue' is then moderated by the levels of support and constraint relevant to that variable. Therefore, one would only expect to account for a reasonable proportion of the predictable variance in the strain scores when each element of the model is taken account of, as well as their interrelationships.

4 The catastrophe can result in cross-boundary (e.g. home and work) contamination, as well as linkage between variables within one boundary (e.g. as in phase 2 of Figure 1.5). Prior to catastrophe the areas may well have been largely independent.

5. If the pre-catastrophe situation returns, the strain will not necessarily disappear because the network of connections would have been established, resulting itself in a changed perception of the situation (which would make it more complex to change the values in isolation).

6. It may be that nodes can remain connected, even when the system returns to a sub-threshold level. This would have the effect of allowing for a learning history. Thus, an organism has a catastrophe history which may play a role in future situations (e.g. one could consider that, once activated, the network pathways are primed for a certain length of time thereafter).

7. If the organism has gone over threshold, the addition of a high demand-relevant support, or the removal of the specific demand, will not necessarily be effective in reducing strain (because of the interconnections that have been made). If, on the other hand, the organism is at a sub-threshold level, the removal (or support) will be helpful.

8. One might expect personality differences in how individuals react to similar environments for a number of reasons including:
   - differential perceptions of the environment and of themselves (i.e. P-E fit);
   - differences in the perceptions and effects of demands, supports and constraints;
   - the setting of different threshold values;
   - the reactiveness of the system to respond to stressors and return to base levels.

The preceding discussion of previous models provides support for some of these predictions. Others will be considered in the remaining chapters. The next chapter evaluates the evidence that the sum total of life events (some of which are of minor importance when considered alone) may affect disease susceptibility. Chapter 3 presents evidence that psychological factors can markedly affect mechanisms which are the guardians against many diseases: the immune system. It is necessary to demonstrate that subtle psychological factors affect the 'nuts and bolts' workings of the immune system, rather than relying on demonstrations that there are chronic disease consequences from stress. The other chapters then explore aspects of the model in relation to the major diseases.

Chapter 2
Life Events and Disease

It has been said that to be alive is to be under to stress. Events that do occur in most of our lives, however, do differ in apparent stressfulness. An aim of this chapter is to outline the methodology that is often used in the so-called 'life events literature', to highlight some of the practical and theoretical difficulties inherent in investigating the relationship between stress and disease. The chapter is specifically concerned with the life events literature. However, the methodological considerations are applicable to all subsequent chapters in this book.

For the purposes of this chapter it is necessary to define what is meant by the concept of a life event. Paykel & Rao's (1984) working definition will suffice: "by a life event we mean a discrete change in the subject's social or personal environment. The event should represent a change, rather than a persisting state, and it should be an external verifiable change, rather than an internal psychological one" (p. 73). More on this later.

In this field the term *'stressful life event'* is often used instead of the more neutral *'life event'* (e. g. Dohrenwend & Dohrenwend, 1984; Kasl, 1983). The former term has the connotation that the person to whom the life event occurs not only perceives the event but also subjectively views it as being emotionally or somehow stressful. (Consider the title of one review paper by Andrews & Tennant (1978), for example: "Being upset and becoming ill: An appraisal of the relation between life events and physical illness".) Whilst it is probably true that major events are so perceived it will be noted that according to the catastrophe model outlined at the end of Chapter 1 this is not necessary for an event to precipitate strain. Indeed the significance of the life events literature is precisely that even minor events have their own (unnoticed) independent influence on the disease process.

The question concerning the causal significance of life events in disease is often considered from a slightly different perspective (Kasl, 1983):

1. Are stressful life events characteristics of the environment, or are they characteristics of different types of people?
2. Do the methodological and measurement problems in this area preclude any demonstration of a causal role for life events in disease?
3. Are life events merely associated with illness in a non-causal way because of the mediation of some other factor (e.g. the illness itself)?

Each of these questions suggests different ways of approaching the central problem of evaluating the etiological significance of life events in disease.

The purpose of this chapter is to consider general and methodological questions, without specifically being addressed to particular diseases. The issues relevant to specific diseases have been discussed elsewhere (e.g. Wells, 1985, discusses this in relation to coronary heart disease; Paykel & Rao, 1984, in relation to cancer).

Amongst the first researchers to do large sample work on life events and illness were Hinkle and his co-workers in the 1950s in the Bell Telephone Corporation (e.g. Hinkle & Plummer, 1952; Hinkle & Wolff, 1957; Hinkle *et al.* 1958). They observed that individuals with illnesses involving more organ systems tended to report more life events, and that the number of reported illnesses was linked with the number of reported life episodes. Individuals in 'unsatisfactory' life circumstances tended to report clusters of apparently unrelated syndromes which were not related to pathogen exposure, nutritional factors or leisure behaviour. They also reported that a small proportion of people were responsible for the majority of illness shown in their sample population. Whilst these studies were extremely important in establishing probabilistic links between life events and disease they are retrospective, they do not quantify or differentiate between life events in anything but the crudest form and their measurement of many of the important variables was necessarily imprecise.

HOLMES AND RAHE'S SEMINAL WORK

In 1967 Holmes & Rahe published a seminal paper which produced a ratio scaled schedule of 43 broad-spectrum recent life events. These life events referred to changes that may occur in a person's domestic or work situation, including changes in personal or interpersonal relationships and habits—essentially changes for which some psychological adjustment is necessary on the part of the person.

The importance of this work was that it established for the first time a self-report questionnaire assessment of the magnitude of the *potential psychosomatic impact* of a number of events, some of which everyone is likely to experience from time to time. Furthermore it could be applied efficiently to large samples of ordinary people to establish a quantified estimate of the recent life changes they had experienced. This *Social Readjustment Rating Scale* (SRRS), based on a *Schedule of Recent Experiences* (SRE), provided a quantifiable estimate of two categories of events: those which reflect a person's lifestyle and those which are indicative of occurrences of particular events.

The items Holmes & Rahe used are shown in Table 2.1, together with the magnitude estimates derived from their original 394 subjects. Subjects had been asked to rate the 43 items (derived from clinical experience of over 5000 patients since 1949) "as to their relative degree of necessary readjustment" (p. 213). It should be borne in mind that the scale is necessarily based on common life experiences for application to general population samples. There will, of course, be individual differences both in what people experience and how much the experiences impact. A small proportion of individuals are responsible for most of the illness rates and the great majority of the illnesses are minor in nature. There are many rare events which are not (explicitly) on the list which may have major impact (e.g. being a bystander at a gory accident, being in a plane hijack), and the categories of events on the list each cover a wide range of occurrences of potentially different magnitudes (e.g. enforced and voluntary retirement). It should also be noted that there is no assumption that individuals experiencing these events should perceive them as having any impact on them: the occurrence of the life event is all that is required.

Table 2.1 shows the mean number of occurrences of each event reported by 199 hospital patients based on their reports of the preceding 10 years (from Holmes & Masuda, 1974). Even for these hospitalised patients, occurrence rates are not high (indeed the mean magnitude of items reported was 29.1 Life Change Units). If such life changes are related to subsequent illness, the presumption follows that, *on the average*, such illnesses are caused by quite minor readjustments in everyday living as well as more major events. The events rated as being of high magnitude are not common (for example, Holmes & Holmes, 1970, report a −0.71 correlation between magnitude and frequency. The Pearson correlation between LCU score and occurrence rates shown in Table 2.1 is −0.313, $p<0.05$), and annual rates/magnitude = −0.478).

Holmes & Rahe pioneered a number of retrospective and prospective studies to attempt to establish a causal role for life events in physical illness. For example, 88 young hospital physicians (22–33 years old) were asked to report on their major health and life changes for the past 10 years (note that some would have been reporting events occurring at the age of 12). It was found that those who scored between 150 and 199 LCUs (*mild*) reported that 37% of 'life crises' (defined as clusters of LCUs exceeding 150 in any one year) were associated with health changes, with the number rising to 51% for *moderate* LCU scores (200–299) and 79% for *major* LCU scores (in excess of 299). When followed up after nine months, the life events of the preceding 18 months showed that 49% of the high LCU physicians reported having suffered a disease whilst only 25% of the moderate LCU group and 9% of the mild LCU group reported such illnesses (from Holmes & Masuda, 1974).

In a study of 2424 naval personnel Rahe (1968) found that high LCU scorers (those whose LCU score fell into the top 30% derived from pre-cruise assessments) had nearly 90% more *first* illnesses in first month of a six-month cruise period than the 30% with the low LCU scores. Over the six-month period the high risk group recorded 2279 illnesses (i.e. 3.1 each) compared to the 1583 (2.2 each) of the low risk group.

The Schedule of Recent Experiences has been shown by Holmes & Rahe to predict both minor illnesses such as colds, backache, cuts, bruises, stomach aches (e.g. Holmes & Holmes, 1970), major onsets such as myocardial infarction (e.g. Rahe & Paasikivi, 1971; Theorell & Rahe, 1971) and even the injuries suffered by American football players in college (Holmes & Holmes, 1970). This implies that psychological mediation may play a significant role in the whole gamut of illness

Table 2.1. Social Readjustment Rating Scale items with their associated Life Change Unit scores (from Holmes & Rahe, 1967, Table 3); frequency of occurrence of life changes in a 10-year period (derived from Holmes & Masuda, 1974, Table 7); and the mean annual frequency of life events of 2321 people from Masuda & Holmes, 1978 (Table 3)

Life event	LCU score	Occurrences per subject (hospital patients, over 10-year period)	Annual frequency (healthy individuals)
Death of spouse	100	0.06	0.03
Divorce	73	0.17	0.03
Marital separation	65	0.55	0.14
Jail term	63	0.31	0.26
Death of close family member	63	1.15	0.17
Personal illness or injury	53	3.98	0.48
Marriage	50	0.36	0.07
Fired from work	47	0.09	0.09
Marital reconciliation	45	—	—
Retirement	45	0.22	0.05
Change in health of family member	44	1.26	0.40
Pregnancy	40	—	—
Sex difficulties	39	0.80	0.26
Gain of new family member	39	1.19	0.18
Business readjustment	39	0.54	0.12
Change in financial state	38	1.57	0.41
Death of a close friend	37	1.22	0.21
Change to different kind of work	36	1.38	0.30
Change in number of arguments with spouse	35	0.63	0.22
Mortgage over $10 000	31	0.42	0.06
Foreclosure of mortgage or loan	30	0.90	0.04
Change in responsibilities at work	29	1.33	0.25
Son or daughter leaving home	29	0.47	0.10
Trouble with in-laws	29	0.39	0.15
Outstanding personal achievement	28	1.01	0.42
Wife begins or stops work	26	0.66	0.16
Begin or end school	26	0.57	0.18
Change in living conditions	25	0.99	0.31
Revision in personal habits	24	1.00	0.34
Trouble with boss	23	0.51	0.17
Change in work hours or conditions	20	1.58	0.49
Change in residence	20	3.67	0.79
Change in schools	20	0.34	0.16
Change in recreation	19	1.53	0.34
Change in church activities	19	0.74	0.19
Change in social activities	18	1.40	0.35
Mortgage or loan of less than $10 000	17	1.65	0.38
Change in sleeping habits	16	1.34	0.42
Change in number of family get-togethers	15	0.80	0.26
Change in eating habits	15	1.32	0.40
Vacation	13	4.49	0.71
Christmas	12	—	—
Minor violations of the law	11	1.23	0.41

and in how individuals behave subsequent to events that occur. Their research has spawned a massive literature by other researchers investigating almost every disease and psychological disturbance. One particularly good example using the Life Events approach is provided by Kemeny *et al.* (1989). This was a prospective study of the role of psychological factors in herpes simplex, which measured immune system functioning (T-lymphocyte levels of CD4+ [helper–inducer cells] and CD8+ [suppressor–cytotoxic cells]), as well as disease recurrence rates. It considered major life events as well as daily hassles, the effects of anticipated stress (i.e. that which the subject felt would occur), the residual stress effects (i.e. when the preceding events had been accounted for), as well as the stress of having herpes itself. The study confirmed the link between the immune system measures and the recurrence of the herpes simplex virus by showing that CD8+ levels were indeed lower one to two weeks prior to recurrence. Although the measures of life events were not related to recurrence rates, and major life events score only showed a modest correlation of -0.36 with CD4+ levels ($p>0.05$), daily hassles did correlate significantly with CD8+ levels, as did residual and anticipated stress scores. Although showing only suggestive evidence of the role of stress and life events in the disease process, the study does highlight many of the links in the causal chain which need to be made before life events studies can make a real contribution in this arena.

In a discussion of the relationship between life events and episodes of physical illness Mechanic (1974) wrote:

> It is clear that stressful life events play some role in the occurrence of illness in populations. But any statement beyond this vague generalisation is likely to stir controversy. The important issues in understanding how life events interact with social psychological, biological, and intrapsychic variables require specification of *what events* influence *what* illnesses under *what* conditions through *what* processes (p. 87).

The problem, as far as Mechanic perceives it, is not in the generation of theories but in the construction of measurable, practical and communicable tools to test the theories. The Schedule of Recent Experiences and the Social Readjustment Rating Scale heralded a major advance because they offer an answer to these problems. Whether such tools and similar ones (e.g. the Daily Hassles Scale of Kanner *et al.*, 1981) can provide evidence of a life events–illness link has been the subject of considerable debate. Some of the issues involved will now be considered.

METHODOLOGICAL ISSUES IN LIFE EVENTS RESEARCH

> The recent popularity of life events research has little to do with its theoretical or conceptual underpinnings in view of the fact that substantial discussion of the complexities of a social-stress hypothesis regarding illness and health predates the appearance of this particular body of work.... What may account for the attraction of life events research is the methodology identified with it (Liem & Liem, 1984, p. 234).

It is for this reason that Holmes & Rahe's work has been so influential. Their original list of life events has acted as the basis of many other instruments which have been developed subsequently (see Rahe, 1984) They *measured* life events and illness. It is also on methodological grounds that their work has come in for considerable criticism: does their technique reliably and validly measure what it purported to? What is essentially under scrutiny is whether life events are truly *environmental factors* and whether they can be considered as risk factors in illness on the same footing as other traditional risk factors (e.g. smoking, cholesterol).

In discussing this issue it is important to distinguish two classes of difficulty. The first concerns those which are inherent in the specific measuring instrument (and hence the derivable theory) that was used by Holmes & Rahe. The second are those difficulties applicable to Holmes & Rahe's work (and its derivatives), but only in so far as they are criticisms of a whole approach to a particular problem of which their work is an example. One criticism of the latter kind is their use of paper-and-pencil questionnaires which some researchers do not consider appropriate in this area (e.g. Paykel, 1983). An example of the former is their use of magnitude estimation to derive the life event weightings, which has been criticised (Dohrenwend *et al.*, 1978; Shrout, 1984).

What Counts as 'Significant'?

Rabkin & Struening (1976) point out that large sample studies are characteristic of life events research, and that the resulting statistical correlations are rather small ("may account at best for nine per cent of the variance in illness", p. 115). In Rahe's work, for example (1974, Rahe & Arthur, 1978), the correlations between life events and illness criteria were around 0.12. It should be noted, however, that this does not imply that the association is of no practical significance, as some have suggested (Andrews & Tennant, 1978; Rabkin & Struening, 1976). Given that one is measuring only a small proportion of psychologically relevant factors, accounting for a consistently predictable (albeit small) proportion of the variance is quite respectable.

The clinical importance of the life events should be weighed against other risk factors. One major consideration is that 'life events' as defined by this body of work are both acute and infrequent, which sets them apart from many traditional risk factors such as smoking and cholesterol levels. In addition, as Craig & Brown (1984) have pointed out, less than 1% of the variance is explained by the link between lung cancer and smoking: many people who develop lung cancer smoke, but there are many more smokers who do not have cancer (see Chapter 4 for a discussion of how psychological factors interact with physical risk factors in the onset of cancer). Similarly, the tubercle bacillus is a necessary agent in the onset of tuberculosis, but it is not sufficient by any means (see Chapter 3). Rahe (1984) suggests that there has been a tendency to overgeneralise the role of traditional risk factors in illness and to underemphasise the fact that those with risk factors such as elevated cholesterol stay healthy for extended periods of time. Perhaps there has also been a tendency to underplay the role of life events. This has not been helped by the acknowledged difficulty of accurately measuring life events and their temporal relationship to illness onset. Whilst the measurement problem is of primary importance, it is wrong to assume that measurement inaccuracies will invariably *inflate* apparent associations. Indeed, as we shall see below, failure to take account of many mediating variables increases measurement error, increases the variance, and probably diminishes the likelihood of obtaining strong associations. Error is double-edged. Psychological phenomena may be more difficult to measure than biological indices. This does not make them less important.

It is difficult to evaluate the relative contribution of psychological risk factors such as life events against more traditional physiological and behavioural risks. The primary reason for this is our lack of understanding of the relationship between mind and body. It does not follow that we are justified in assuming that psychological stress cannot be isolated from physical stress and, therefore, that physical stress is of primary importance. Indeed, the argument could be justifiably reversed. It is more a matter of being constrained by a biomedical orientation in medicine than by the logical construction of an evidential base. Only bias and prejudice can decide some issues.

The statistical difficulty outlined above makes interpretation difficult, and has led to the development of alternative estimations of risk such as 'attributable risk' (how much of a given illness can be attributed to given risk factors), 'relative risk' (the increase in likelihood of suffering an illness given exposure to the risk factor) and 'brought forward time' (the degree to which a risk factor promotes premature illness) (see Craig & Brown, 1984; Paykel, 1978). Whilst each of these methods of assessing risk side-steps the philosophical dilemma, they do provide useful alternatives for describing risk.

What Constitutes a Stressful Life Event?

Life events just happen (although we may be partly responsible for some). Whether or not they are stressful (i.e. produce illness and disease) is an empirical question. That life events have to be adjusted to is more a matter of the way the world is organised than a matter of choice. Holmes & Rahe viewed the required *change* (psychological, physiological, behavioural) as the potential stressor. It did not matter much how the person was affected psychologically, or what people felt about a particular event that occurred (therefore one did not need to use elaborate data collection techniques such as interviews, etc.). All that was important was that the event (or enough events) happened to *them*. Holmes & Rahe (1967) noted that "only some of the events are negative or 'stressful' in the conventional sense, i.e. are socially undesirable. Many are socially desirable and consonant with the American values of achievement, success, materialism, practicality, efficiency, future orientation, conformism and self-reliance" (p. 217). For them it was how many of the changes people experienced which needed to be measured accurately. If people experienced sufficient life change they would have a high risk of becoming ill. This was what Holmes & Rahe (1967) empirically tested and found evidence for.

A number of researchers have criticised the stance that *life change* is the causal nexus in the life events–illness chain. Instead they propose that only change which is undesirable in some way has any causal status. This too is an empirically testable claim, even if a little circular (only changes which are stressful produce stress). It could, in principle, be tested (albeit inadequately) with measures derived in the same way as the SRE. Thus, one must be careful to distinguish theoretical disagreements from concern about whether the instruments used do indeed show what they purport to. The former requires methodological changes in procedure to gather different kinds of arbitrating evidence, whilst the latter suggests that the collected evidence is inadequate to test the hypothesised view.

The idea that life change *per se* is stressful has been questioned in a number of ways.

The SRE measured both desirable and undesirable events without differentiation. For Holmes & Rahe the impact of the events was presumed critical in inducing change and propensity to illness. For them each item in the SRRS was an event which required "a significant change in the ongoing life pattern of the individual. The emphasis is on change from the existing steady state and not on psychological meaning, emotion, or social desirability" (Holmes & Masuda, 1974, p. 46). A study by Dohrenwend (1973) did indeed produce evidence to support the view that change measures were better predictors of psychiatric impairment than those based on undesirability (although a reanalysis by Andrews & Tennant, 1978, suggests the difference was not statistically significant). It does appear that desirable changes are unrelated to some kinds of illness (Gersten *et al.*, 1977; Miller, Ingham & Davidson, 1976; Paykel, 1974). Andrews & Tennant (1978) developed a 67-item life event list from the SRE and Paykel, Prusoff & Uhlenhuth's (1971) scale. From this they derived measures of life change and life event distress. When these scales were administered to a random sample of Sydney households (*n*=863) they found that the distress scale was associated with the later onset of neurotic impairment (as measured by Goldberg's, 1972, General Health Questionnaire) and that the change score added nothing to the prediction of impairment despite the independence of the two scales.

These results have led some researchers to propose that it is necessary to develop scales which separate positive from negative events (e.g. Sarason & Sarason, 1984, 1985), or which differentiate 'desirable', 'neutral' and 'undesirable' (Hough, Fairbank & Garcia, 1976), or which scale life events along some subject-based evaluative criterion such as the degree of 'upsettingness' (Paykel *et al.*, 1971). Whilst this may appear an attractive option, any subject-based evaluation leaves open the likelihood of confounding 'cause' and 'effect' measures (see below): the evaluation of what is undesirable or upsetting may be confounded with the psychological outcome measures themselves.

The effects of measurement confounding suggest there is insufficient evidence to justify abandoning the notion that change *per se* may have strain consequences; undesirable change may indeed be a better predictor of psychologically related illness, as the above studies suggest. This does not, however, imply that the same is true of physical diseases. Psychologically relevant events may have direct organic consequences which are not mediated by emotion, affect or felt meaning. Sarason & Sarason (1985), for example, have suggested that "It is possible that the totality of life changes affects the body's physiological homeostasis, whereas only negative life changes are associated with personal dissatisfaction and a lowered sense of well-being" (p. 224). Much of the evidence presented elsewhere in this book would support such a notion. There is some evidence that 'upsettingness' rather than 'adjustment' is important in some 'physical' diseases such as myocardial infarction or back pain (e.g. Lundberg, Theorell & Lind, 1975; Lundberg & Theorell 1976) but considerably more research is required here. A relevant point is that even if undesirable life events are correlated with serious physical illness such as myocardial infarction (e.g. Pancheri *et al.*, 1980) this does not entail that it is the undesirability that mediates the life events effect. One needs to parcel out the relative contributions of desirability and change in order to establish their independent effects. Moreover, it is necessary to ensure that the events which were rated as undesirable were perceived so before their occurrence, to be sure that the felt undesirability of the event is not a consequence of the effects of the change the event has induced in the person. One particular problem, however, is to have objective indices of 'undesirability' or 'distress'. Not only will different individuals have different views of the desirability of life events, but independent judges do not show concordance with subjects' ratings (Rahe, 1978).

One instrument which attempts to measure both positive and negative life changes, and allows the subject to rate both the desirability and impact of life events, is Sarason's Life Experiences Survey (Sarason, Johnson & Siegel, 1978; see also Sarason & Sarason, 1984, 1985). This is a 47-item self-report measure, 34 of which are similar to the SRE, although the items are themselves more detailed. The subjects can also refer to life events that are not on the list. Studies which have employed this instrument have tended to show that negatively evaluated events are correlated with illness to a more robust extent than positive events, although physical illness which does not have a recognised psychosomatic component has received scant attention.

Life Event Categories

Paykel has argued that different types of event have qualitatively different effects in terms of illness. If so, it may not be sensible to cling to the view that only the magnitude of the required adjustment is of importance in illness. More details of the types of experienced events are required, as well as their classification into 'event categories'. These different event categories may show illness-specific relationships.

For example, Paykel *et al.* (1969) studied the occurrence within the previous six months of four types of event categories in depressives and matched controls. Only the occurrence of 'exits' (the departure of a person from the immediate social sphere of the subject) and 'undesirable' events discriminated the two groups. 'Entrances' (the addition of a person in the immediate social sphere of the subject) and 'desirable' events showed no such pattern. Paykel, Prusoff & Myers (1975) examined 53 patients who had attempted suicide, and compared them to depressive and general population controls. Using Paykel's 61-item Life Events measure, interviews revealed that suicide attempters had experienced more undesirable events than either set of controls, with no differences in desirable event experiences. They experienced more entrances and exits than the general population controls, and more entrances than depressives. The suicide group experienced more events than the general population controls in each activity except 'work', as well as more 'health' and 'legal' events than depressives.

This type of research does imply that the type of event category may be related to the particular disorder under scrutiny, and that such categories may have useful and specific predicted capacity beyond measuring simply the amount of life change.

What Constitutes a Life Event?

The SRE assumes that there is no difficulty in identifying what constitutes a life event: the questionnaire explicitly lists them. It does not, however, qualitatively distinguish between different types of event except in terms of LCU loading. It may be that different events have different types of effect dependent, for example, on their chronicity. Cohen (1981), for example, lists four different types of stressor: acute time-limited events, stress event sequences, chronic stressors, and chronic but intermittent stressors. We know that such different categories of stressors may produce quite different types of strain responses in animals (see Chapters 3 and 4). Holmes & Rahe's work is primarily confined to a consideration of event sequences, and largely ignores the other types of stress events.

Second, the SRE does assume that life events are clearly and unambiguously identifiable by the subject. This assumption is questionable. One reason for this concerns the use of retrospective reporting, which will be discussed below. A separate problem is that of deciding whether a given event has occurred. Only a quarter of the SRE events are unambiguous occurrences. The others require subjects to make quite subtle judgments: "For instance, in assessing an argument with someone close, one needs to define the relationship, and the magnitude and persistence of a dispute which will cross the threshold to be an event worth recording, rather than a trivial occurrence" (Paykel, 1983, p. 342). Such open judgments are likely to be affected to a marked degree by individual differences and intra-individual mood changes, etc.

Third, a major assumption of the SRE as a measuring instrument is that the list of life events is relatively universal in its applicability (although there are amended lists for special groups). That is, it can be used with confidence on most people. This can be questioned. Individual differences and group differences (e.g. ill vs. healthy) cast doubt on this universality principle.

Life Events as Symptoms

A further assumption of the life events research is that the occurrence of the events is independent of any illness or disease condition. It is the accumulation of external life event changes which is supposed to lead to the predisposition for illness, and not an illness which predisposes the individual to experience the life events. Hugdens (1974) has criticised life events work because the events referred to are often *symptoms* or consequences of being ill, rather than causes of illness. In other words we create some of the events. He suggests that those events which are possible consequences of the illness should be excluded, otherwise causal attributions cannot be made at all reliably. In his view this would mean excluding 29 of the 43 in Holmes & Rahe's list, 32 of 61 in Paykel *et al.*'s (1971) long list and 18 of 33 from the shorter version. This would decimate these instruments.

Dohrenwend & Shrout (1985) have discussed this issue of confounding at length in relation to the Hassles Scale of Kanner *et al.* (1981), which is a scale meant to measure everyday 'hassles' or minor events ("irritating, frustrating, distressing demands and troubled relationships that plague us day in day out" [Lazarus & DeLongis, 1983, p. 247]). It is suggested that the hassles are themselves very similar to psychological symptoms. Therefore, the reason that the hassles score correlates so well with psychological symptoms is because "Nothing correlates with symptoms like other symptoms" (p. 780). Dohrenwend & Shrout (1985) go on to show that the Hassles Scale, which is purported to have eight dimensions, has only one second-order factor which itself accounted for the strong associations found previously (see also Lazarus *et al.*, 1985).

This type of confounding has been observed in other areas of health psychology where the psychological stressors and the health outcome measures are both self-report. Watson & Pennebaker (1989), for example, show that some self-report health measures reflect a pervasive disposition towards negative affectivity which is also highly correlated with the evaluation of stressors, including the Hassles Scale (frequency and intensity scores). Since this negative affectivity was not itself related to actual or long-term health status, the associations between stressors and strains are probably being markedly overestimated in studies which do not take account of the affectivity dimension. What this paper also implies is that either the events or the outcomes need objective measurement. This is at least more likely if only life events, and not their desirability, are considered.

This criticism makes it more important to use techniques of information-gathering which allow accurate dating of the events and the onset of illness, as well as objective measures of health status. Paykel & Rao (1984) have suggested that we might deal with this problem in one of three ways. First, we might confine the investigation to those life events which unambiguously antedate the illness. Second, the events resulting from illness could be independently separated from others by detailed scrutiny of the contextual circumstances by experts (Brown *et al.*, 1973). We will discuss this procedure below. Third, it is possible to use consensus judgments for event lists to distinguish causal from consequential events (Tennant & Andrews, 1977).

'Sick role' Contamination

Closely related to the last point is the issue raised by a number of commentators who have suggested that life event scores may be associated with care-seeking behaviour, or taking on a 'sick role', rather than the onset of actual illness (e.g. Craig & Brown, 1984; Dohrenwend & Dohrenwend, 1984; Mechanic, 1974; Rabkin & Struening, 1976). This difficulty is partly a consequence of having unclear or imprecise criteria for illness. As Minter & Kimball (1978) have suggested, many people have the symptoms of illness but do not visit a doctor. Thus, if the criteria for illness are derived from medical records, or from self-motivated attendance, any observed association of 'illness' with life event scores will simply be a reflection of the specific sick role being adopted, and not the presence of an organic disorder. Life events may change a person's threshold for complaint. Satin (1972), for example, found that almost 90% of admissions to an emergency unit reported a recent life stress, and suggests that the physical disorder simply provides the ticket for admission. Ward, Bloom & Friedel (1979) also showed that tricyclic anti-depressants can alleviate physical pain.

The marked association between physical symptoms of illness and affective states (Lipowsky, 1975) makes it difficult to resolve the sick role problem in life event research. Craig & Brown (1984) suggest that some resolution is provided by classifying somatic symptoms into three different groups:

1. morphological or physiological changes in specific organs or organ groups;
2. those clearly related to psychological disturbance, such as muscle tension in anxiety;
3. 'physical' symptoms without underlying physiological or structural changes (e.g. irritable colon syndrome).

Clearly, such classification would go some way to reducing the problem, although the categories are fuzzy and may partly be confounded by how advanced disease conditions are.

Life Event Clusters

Brown & Harris (1978) have argued that life events are not additive or independent. Indeed, Brown (1981) has found, using his own Bedford College instrument, that "when an assumption of additivity is built into the measurement of life events and difficulties the estimate of their causal importance is reduced by at least one half" (p. 464). There are several aspects of this relevant to life events research. The first point is that a major event (e.g. marriage) is often followed by a number of other significant changes, although these changes may also occur independently of the event (e.g. moving house, change in financial state, mortgage, change in number of arguments, change in social activities, pregnancy, etc.). Thus the same event has different consequences depending upon the context in which it occurs. The techniques developed by Brown and his colleagues are designed to account for contextual effects and will be outlined below. They are, however, fundamentally different in emphasis to the self-report questionnaire work of Holmes & Rahe. If events are not additive it makes little sense adding them.

Kasl (1983) suggests that causal–etiological interpretation of life events research is difficult because "Significant social problems come in uncomfortably large clusters and packages and the scientist is stymied in his efforts to unravel these and label some 'causes' and other 'effects'." (pp. 96–7). It does appear to be the case that life events are correlated with each other (Goldberg & Comstock, 1980; Lei & Skinner, 1980). Goldberg & Comstock, for example, administered a 41-item revised version of the SRRS to a general population sample and found that 15 of the events were moderately correlated to one another. Also a crude count of the number of life events is highly correlated with the weighted life change score (Lorimer *et al.*, 1979; Skinner & Lei, 1980). This suggests that differences in LCU scores may be caused by the infrequent occurrence of major events and the frequent occurrence of minor ones (see Table 2.1). The latter events will tend to show the greatest inter-respondent variation in reporting, are themselves most susceptible to respondent bias, and possibly occur in orchestration with other events. For example, Goldberg & Comstock found that 23.4% of their 2780 respondents reported no life events in the preceding year (excluding 'vacation') and only 11 of the 41 events were reported by at least 10% of the people. Moreover, those reporting five or more events tended to have distinct biographical characteristics.

Life Events as Mirrors of 'Lifestyle'

Kasl (1983) has argued that life events cannot be considered independent of the person to whom they occur because they

> are intimately bound up with a person's life style and reflect, furthermore, the person's stage in the life style. It is an intimate and indissoluble concurrent part of being an alcoholic or a heroin addict to experience many life changes. It is part of getting old to experience fewer and fewer life changes. To attempt to argue that SLEs (stressful life events) are causally antecedent to heroin use would certainly be foolish.... SLEs are not random happenings which follow a Gaussian or Poisson distribution; they are intimately embedded in life style and lifestyle dynamics, and they are not part of some separate causal matrix with its own dynamics (pp. 85–6).

Whilst this may be true to some extent, it does seem to be the role of science to disentangle the 'holistic', and one tool it has at its disposal is the theoretical axe. Theories are simplifications of reality, not isomorphic representations of it. If they are useful (and causal models are, at least in principle) the job should be attempted unless there is *a priori* reason to suggest otherwise. Kasl is effectively offering a criticism of all life events research techniques. Other techniques (e.g. Brown's contextual approach, below) attempt to examine the whole canvas of lifestyle and individual perceptions whilst at the same time making causal attributions.

Estimating Life Event Weightings

There has been considerable debate concerning the weighting of life events and the final derivation of the LCU score. Three aspects of this criticism can be discerned: the cognitive difficulty of assigning relative weightings to the list of events using magnitude estimation, the crudeness of scale weightings derived from consensus judgments, and the superiority of different scaling weights.

The techniques used to derive the SRRS have already been outlined in detail. Essentially, a number of judges are asked to 'use all your experience' to assign a specific number to the range of events, assuming that one such event (marriage) required 500 units of readjustment. The magnitude estimation weightings provided by the judges are then pooled to derive average life change scores for each of the events.

Brown (e.g. 1974) has argued that the judges' task is too *vague*, because the rater is not provided with sufficient detail concerning the situation to be rated. Different raters (and different subjects given the SRE or a similar instrument) will interpret the brief account of the event in different ways. Moreover, there is evidence that raters find the task rather abstract and cognitively difficult, especially if they have below-average educational attainment (Dohrenwend *et al.*, 1978). Thus, the weightings derived for the SRE are of little value. Moreover, Brown argues that averaging judges' weightings is too crude an instrument because the variability of the perceptions of the different judges is lost. The statistical end-result may well—like a 'committee decision'—not reflect any meaningful consensus. As Brown also points out, the fact that high correlations are obtained for the life event estimates in different studies is irrelevant, because each may be averaging nonsense, or to put it more kindly "assigning a standard weight by agreement must be a blunt tool" (Paykel & Rao, 1984, p. 80).

Shrout (1984) has also criticised the use of the derived weightings in the SRE because they fail to satisfy several necessary assumptions for the use of such a technique:

1. Readjustment is not necessarily the salient and unambiguous dimension which underlies all the life events to the same degree.
2. Readjustment is not the *only* salient dimension in such life events.

3. The list of events is likely to be incomplete. It is unreasonable to *sample* life events in this way (especially if the events are presumed to be independent of each other) because this will give an inaccurate estimate of stress for those who experience other events.

4. Holmes & Rahe use the magnitude estimation method to scale events based on the original ratio method of Stevens (1966) in the auditory perception field, but "since there are group differences in scale scores, it is clear that the 'change' dimension is not analogous to a dimension such as pitch, which is indeed universal. Because magnitude estimation is designed for unambiguous universal dimensions, it makes allowances for neither group nor individual difference" (Shrout, 1984, p. 39).

Dohrenwend & Dohrenwend (1984) have suggested that one reason to expect significant group differences in the perception of life events is that we use group-dependent social context norms in the absence of direct experience. In general, raters have to assess the impact of events they have not actually experienced, and thus substitute socially communicated expectancies.

It should be reiterated that using different statistical weightings on the data derived from instruments such as the SRE (e.g. regression weights rather than LCU weights) cannot remove these underlying difficulties even if they change the pattern of results. It is also meaningless directly to compare the results of life event research which utilise ratio scales (e.g. the SRE) with those which use categorical interval scales (e.g. Paykel *et al.*, 1971).

Dictionaries are not True Stories

To improve etiological interpretation in life event research Brown (1981) believes that "the most important need is to improve the general quality of measurement" (p. 470). He has been very critical of what he calls the 'dictionary' approach of instruments such as the SRE (e.g. Brown, 1974, 1981, 1984; Brown & Harris, 1978; Craig & Brown, 1984). According to Brown (1984) "Most life-event research has been based on a dictionary approach to meaning. A birth is considered a birth and no more.... They basically deal with events as would a dictionary" (p. 187). This results in the problems of vagueness, bias, inaccuracy, insensitivity, low correlations between events and illness and, at worst, inconsistency.

In very influential work Brown and his colleagues have developed the Bedford College instrument, which attempts to overcome some of the aforementioned problems by taking account of the specific *context* in which the life events occur. The technique enables judgments to be made about the meanings of events that individuals experience, *while ignoring what the respondents actually said they felt*, thus bypassing some of the problems of self-reporting (see below).

A full description of the technique is provided by Brown & Harris (1978). Essentially, the approach consists of two stages. First, 'provoking agents' are investigated at an interview using a Life Events and Difficulties Schedule, which measures 38 events falling into eight different categories (role changes for self, role changes for significant others, major health changes for self, and for significant others, residence changes and contact changes with significant others, forecasts of change, valued goal fulfilment and disappointment, other dramatic events occurring to self and significant others). The interviewer is very closely guided by a detailed manual so as to rule out subjective inaccuracies. The inclusion of an event is controlled by strict criteria. A very full account is collected about each event and its timing, with interviewers having a whole range of rating scales to assess the general characteristics of the event, the subjects' prior circumstances and preparedness, their immediate reactions, and the experienced consequences and implications. These scales do not take account of either the subjects' clinical condition or feelings about the event: they provide the 'objective' contextual information to supplement the exhaustive sampling of life events.

The second stage requires that the events isolated in the structured interview are presented to independent judges, together with the ratings of the circumstances of the subject and his or her biographical information. The judges are not made aware of the subjects' feelings or diagnosis. The judges then rate the degree or 'severity' of contextual threat. That is, they assess how threatening the events would be for a subject of that type living under those circumstances. Various qualities of the life events can be categorised using this technique. For example, Brown & Harris (1978) distinguish between two types of provoking agent: severe acute events and major chronic problems of more than two years' duration.

The Bedford College instrument has been used primarily to investigate the role of life events in psychiatric disorders such as depression and schizophrenia. In Brown & Harris's study, for example, 458 women were randomly selected from the electoral register in Camberwell, England. Of those who had become depressed in a 38-week period prior to the interviews (8% of the sample), 89% were observed to have suffered a severe event or difficulty. This compared to a figure of 30% for the non-depressed women. (The women suffering from chronic depression [9%] were excluded.) Moreover, there were 3.7 times the number of severe compared to non-severe events for the onset cases, with slightly fewer non-severe events occurring in the cases than the non-cases Thus, the context of the events is of paramount importance. Oatley & Bolton (1985) provide a discussion and review of the instrument as it has been used to investigate depression.

The Life Events and Difficulties test has been shown to be a very reliable instrument (Tennant *et al.*, 1981; Parry, Shapiro & Davies, 1981) although it does require considerable and skilful training to be used successfully (Schmid, Scharfetter & Binder, 1981, for example, report less than acceptable data using Brown's technique, but were not trained by Brown and have been so criticised by Brown &

Harris, 1982). The technique is also very time-consuming, when compared to administering 'dictionary-type' questionnaires, and it is not clear whether it is the extra time spent collecting and classifying information that makes it a superior technique, rather than some inherent quality of the technique itself.

GENERAL ISSUES

There are a number of more general issues of relevance in attempts to link life events with the onset of illness. These issues need to be considered whatever instruments of measurement are utilised.

Mediators and Confounding Factors in the Life Event–Illness Relationship

The relationship between stressors and strains is affected by *mediating and moderating factors*. These terms refer to factors which may alter the life events–illness relationship, or affect the translation of stressors into strains. Alternative terms would include 'vulnerability' (Brown & Harris, 1978), 'stress buffering' (Dean & Lin, 1977; Cohen & McKay, 1984), 'context' (McClean, 1979), and 'synergenics' (Cobb, 1976). An alternative, and more theoretically neutral, description of such factors is to call them 'confounding variables', inasmuch as failure to account for them adequately in empirical studies of life events and illness will diminish the likelihood of obtaining useful interpretable results.

Each of the variables below have been shown to affect life event scores. Undoubtedly the variables are confounded with each other, although there is insufficient evidence to give any picture of the interactions between them. No attempt is made to distinguish between *moderators* and *independent predictors* (Denney & Frisch, 1981) since most studies do not allow an evaluation of the necessary main and interactive effects in their statistical analyses.

Age

Younger people report more life events than older people (e.g. Holmes & Masuda, 1974; Masuda & Holmes, 1978). Using a 41-item version of the SRE, Goldberg & Comstock (1980) report that those aged 65+ were more than 11 times more likely to report no events in the preceding year compared to 18–24-year-olds, with the latter 23 times more likely to report in excess of four events than the former, even when the percentages were adjusted for all other independent variables. It does not follow, however, that they suffer more stress. Most life event measures are heavily biased towards life events that occur earlier in life and, therefore, sample a greater proportion of the event universe. Paykel & Rao (1984) have suggested that the more threatening events (e.g. death of a spouse) are also principally confined to later life. Moreover, Kellam (1984) has argued that the same event can have different strain-inducing properties at different points in life. This suggests that age-specific event lists are desirable (e.g. Bourque & Back, 1977), or that, at minimum, age should be carefully controlled or partialled out.

Socioeconomic status and social support

It is well known that morbidity and mortality risk is related to social class (e.g. Fletcher, 1988a). Liem & Liem (1984) provide a discussion of the relevance of life events to social class and mental illness. They suggest that those of lower social status experience more direct exposure to life events, and that the events have greater impact because the context in which they occur is less supportive. The more socially disadvantaged also avail themselves less of preventative medicine (Marsh, 1986), have fewer common surgical operations (Coulter & McPherson, 1985), and are more obese, smoke more, drink more, and take less exercise (Caplan *et al.*, 1975) than those in higher social classes.

Gore (1984) outlines a 'stress-vulnerability' model in which social support and other social resources play a mediating role between life events and illness, effectively reducing the burden of life events. Medalie & Goldbourt (1976), for example, found that the wife's lack of love was an important predictor of angina pectoris onset in a prospective study of more than 7000 men. Low social support has been shown to increase illness vulnerability in many studies (see Cohen & Wills, 1985; LaRocco, House & French, 1980; Winnubst, Marcelissen & Kleber, 1982; Sarason & Sarason, 1985). In a study of combat stress suffered by Israeli soldiers during the Lebanon War of 1982, Solomon, Mikulincer & Habershaim (1990) report that perceived social support was the most important variable that contributed to somatic complaints: life events and coping strategies being dependent upon social support levels. Payne (1979; Payne & Fletcher, 1983) also outlined a model of stress in which the effects of demand are moderated by the level of support (see Chapter 1).

It is likely that social support and socioeconomic class are intimately linked, even though they have also been shown to have independent effects on health (Berkman & Syme, 1979). Undoubtedly social class is an important variable in life events research. In their examination of a number of possible factors affecting SRRS scoring, Masuda & Holmes (1978) found that those with less than college degrees gave significantly higher scores to 24 life event items and a lower score to only one (spouse's death). Dohrenwend (1973b) found that lower-class people experience more undesirable life events than those of higher classes. Myers, Lindenthal & Pepper (1974) report a longitudinal study in which lower-class people experienced more unpleasant events in a two-year period, which were also shown to be related to changes in psychiatric symptomatology. It must be said, however, that there is contradictory evidence (see Goldberg & Comstock, 1980) which is probably a result of the use of different measures of socioeconomic status, poor sampling procedures, and failure to take account of other confounding variables.

Sex

If anything, women appear to report more life events than men (Masuda &
Holmes, 1978) although the literature has produced conflicting studies (see Goldberg
& Comstock, 1980) without any apparent reason to explain the contradictions.
However, a more important sex difference has been reported by Rahe (1984) in his
Vietnamese refugee study. He found that subjectively determined LCU scores were
significantly correlated with physical and mental health indices in women, although
for men a simple count of the number of events was a better predictor. Women also
have higher mean scores on some aspects of minor morbidity (e.g. on some subscales of the Crown–Crisp Experiential Index) and are more frequent users of
medical services than men. Sex-specific diseases are also major causes of death.
Therefore, it may be more important to consider sex differences in the relationship between life events and illness than to look for differences in life event scores.

Personality

It appears that there may well be personality traits which "promote resistance to
health breakdown after exposure to life changes" (Garrity, Somes & Marx, 1977,
p. 24). Garrity *et al.*, for example, found that three personality factors—emotional
sensitivity, liberal intellectualism and social conformity—added significantly to
the predictability of life stress measures in accounting for reports of student health.
Denney & Frisch (1981) report that Eysenck's neuroticism scale was also a significant predictor of reported health status, and Watson & Pennebaker (1989) have
shown that negative affectivity is a crucial factor in the relationship between
stressor and strain outcomes, including life event measures.

The actual strain-producing qualities of life events (as well as their perceived
stressfulness) is also affected by a person's *locus of control*, which is a measure
of how much people feel in control of their lives. 'Externals' are those who perceive
that life is largely outside their control and determined by outside factors. 'Internals'
perceive that they have a greater degree of control. Lefcourt (1984) describes a
study of 59 subjects who recorded their moods for four weeks. Locus of control,
as measured by Rotter's scale, was a significant moderator of the relationship
between negative life events and mood disturbance. Those subjects who were more
external were also more likely to exhibit distress in mood disturbance. Johnson &
Sarason (1978) report that negative life events were significantly related to measured
depression and anxiety in externals but not internals.

Matthews & Glass (1984) have suggested that *type A* personalities (see Chapter 5)
who are more thrusting, competitive and aggressive than their type B counterparts,
have a distinctive style in how they react to life events. They initially exhibit greater
attempts to control their environment than type Bs, but repeated failure to control
what is outside their influence leads them to blame themselves. These different

patterns of behaviour to life events are claimed to produce, to some extent, the different rates of heart disease observed in such personality types (Friedman & Rosenman, 1974).

Finally, *sensation-seeking* behaviour appears to moderate the effect of life events on health. People who score low on sensation-seeking scales are affected more by life events than those who score high (Johnson, Sarason & Siegel, unpublished, reported in Sarason & Sarason, 1985). Furthermore, subjects who score high on negative life changes experience psychological distress if they also exhibit low sensation-seeking, but not if they are high sensation-seekers (Smith, Johnson & Sarason, 1978).

Therefore, there is considerable reason to expect that the effect of life events on health will be partly determined by how different types of people react to their environment.

Cultural factors

There has been debate about whether cross-cultural factors affect the relationship between life events and illness. In the original work of Holmes & Rahe (1967) on the SRRS, the correlation between the ratings of readjustment between whites and Negroes was 0.82, and between whites and orientals 0.94, which led them to propose that there was universal cross-cultural agreement (p. 217). The sample sizes for the non-white groups were, however, very small (19 and 12) and all were middle-class Americans. Masuda & Holmes (1978) provide data for eight subcultural/ cross-national comparisons (middle-class Americans, black Americans, Mexican Americans, Western Europeans, Spanish, Salvadorians, Japanese and Malaysians), which supports the view that there are marked (albeit unfathomable) differences between different cultures. Other studies support the existence of cultural differences in the perception of, and likelihood of experiencing, life events (e.g. Goldberg & Comstock, 1980, Dohrenwend, 1973a). However, as Fairbank & Hough (1984) have discussed, it is difficult to translate similar meanings across cultures and cultural differences tend to be specific in nature. Not only do these factors reduce the probability of detecting differences which are present (because the measurement will be imprecise and error variance greater), but they also make the enterprise of cross-cultural comparisons using a common technique or measuring instrument of little theoretical or practical value. Only theoretical exercises which transcend specific cultural variations can usefully be done.

Data Collection Method

The SRE utilised a pencil-and-paper method for the collection of information about life changes. It is, therefore, primarily a *self-report or respondent-based* instrument. This method of data collection has a number of drawbacks compared to *interview or investigator-based* techniques such as the Bedford College instrument which was outlined above, or Paykel's Interview for Recent Life Events (e.g. Jacobs, Prusoff & Paykel, 1974; Paykel, Prusoff & Myers, 1975), which is discussed below:

Reliability

Reliability of self-report questionnaires is considerably lower than for interview techniques. For example, in reviews by Neugebauer (1984) and Paykel (1983) the test–retest reliability correlations for the SRE ranged from 0.07 to 0.90, with an average of about 0.52 across the whole range of test–retest intervals (2–104 weeks). Given that these reliability coefficients are simply the correlations between *total* life event scores taken on two separate occasions, it is possible that the actual events reported on each occasion were totally different. Thus, even with a very weak measure of reliability the SRE does poorly. Using a stringent measure with inter-viewer-based collection methods—the concordance between different judges on specific events or items—reliability coefficients are generally in excess of 0.80. Steele, Henderson & Duncan-Jones (1980) report 10-day test–retest reliabilities in excess of 0.90 for the quasi-interview technique of Tennant & Andrews (1976).

Event-report fall-off

With the passing of time there is some fall-off in the reporting of events. Paykel (1983) reviews a number of studies assessing the degree of fall-off in self-report and inter-view studies. On the assumption that fall-off is linear over time (which Paykel accepts is unlikely) self-report studies show a rate of 4–5% per month. In a study by Uhlenhuth *et al.* (1977) there was a 66% fall-off over an 18-month period. Studies using well-trained interviewers, on the other hand, show a much lower rate of between 1% and 3% per month.

It is not clear what accounts for the above differences, nor is it necessarily the case that the apparently superior results obtained by the interview methods are a reflection of a generally superior technique. Indeed, it is possible that poor test–retest reliabilities and some proportion of the fall-off obtained with questionnaire measures are a reflection of actual changes (rather than errors) in the criteria adopted by the subjects. This does, of course, imply that self-reporting of 'environmental' events is partly dependent on the subjects' judgments of the events changing over time. This would not be a surprise to any psychologist. Interview techniques may well mask these subtle judgmental changes, despite the belief that they are better able to extract contextual information.

Validity

In order to be sure that subjects actually experienced events which they report occurred, some objective check is required. One such check is to ask close friends or relatives (e.g. spouse) to report the events the subjects experienced. A study by Rahe (1974), for example, found that wives' reports of their husbands' life events correlated 0.5–0.75 with their husbands' self-reports. However, correlations between LCU totals provide a crude measure of validity because they are not event-specific, informants may guess without direct knowledge, and there is a pure statistical chance of agreement too. A study by Yager *et al.* (1981) showed that subject–spouse agreements concerning the occurrence of particular events, using a statistic which accounts for chance agreements, was a low 35%. Given that the investigators were asking only about the previous two months (when the previous 12 months is more common in the investigation of life events and illness), and the agreement for unambiguous or clear events was little more than 40%, some doubt about the validity of respondent-based instruments is warranted. The investigator-based measures produce considerably better performance, with subject–informant concordance for particular events being around 80% in Brown's work, for example (Brown & Harris, 1982; Brown *et al.*, 1973).

Meaning and context

Brown (1974, 1981, 1984; Craig & Brown, 1984) suggested that it is the vagueness of questionnaire instruments which makes them inherently unreliable: subjects cannot adequately clarify necessary issues for themselves. The Bedford College instrument does have the advantage that the independent raters, when making their judgments of contextual threat, can also account for many factors which would normally contribute to the unreliability of 'universal' questionnaires such as subject characteristics (cognitive ability, age, sex, ethnic status, socioeconomic status, etc.). The Bedford technique is of particular value in some contexts because it allows an evaluation of the *specific meaning* (Craig & Brown, 1984) of each event. Other measuring instruments have been developed to provide the researcher with a fuller understanding and greater precision in the measurement of the circumstances surrounding life events without providing the specificity of detail of this approach. One of the best-known techniques, which utilises a semi-structured interview procedure, is Paykel's *Interview for Recent Life Events* (ILRE) (Paykel, 1983, Paykel & Rao, 1984). Interviewers are provided with a list of definitions of up to 64 life events which cover 10 areas (work, education, finance, health, bereavement, migration, courtship, family and social relationships, marital, and legal matters). Subjects are also questioned about other events which they may have experienced which are not included in the list. Interviewers are provided with guide notes for what constitutes each event. For example, 'serious argument with spouse' is defined as "a one-way or interactive altercation adversely affecting behaviour of one or both parties for a minimum of five days" (Paykel & Rao, 1984, p. 17). If the subject has experienced an event the interviewer delves further for details of circumstances and timings. The instrument allows results to be collected for a number of dimensions:

- *Total number of events*—a count of total number of events experienced in the specified period.
- *Time pattern of events*—the event rate for specific time chunks, e.g. month by month. For example, suicide attempters showed an increased rate in all months prior to attempt; depressives showed a peak in the month prior to onset; healthy subjects had a constant rate (Paykel *et al.*, 1975).
- *Individual events*—the frequency of specific events themselves can be compared for group differences. For example, depressives were significantly more likely than schizophrenics to have had serious arguments with both a fiancé or steady date and non-resident family member. No other events produced significant differences (Jacobs, Prusoff & Paykel, 1974).
- *Desirability of events*—whether the events are desirable or undesirable. Suicide attempters report more undesirable events than either depressives or healthy controls, although no effects were present for desirable events (Paykel *et al.*, 1975).
- *Exits and entrances*—the exit or introduction of a significant person into the subject's social field. Depressives and suicide attempters report more exits than healthy controls, but suicide attempters report more entrances than the other two groups (Paykel *et al.*, 1975).
- *Area of activity*—the events categorised according to their area of activity. For example, depressives are more likely to have reported at least one event in both the 'financial' and 'health' categories than schizophrenics (Jacobs *et al.*, 1974).

It seems that the extra information provided by the IRLE has predictive power superior to that of the SRE. Its particular usefulness is that it is likely to reveal differences between groups on some of the dimensions, without the necessity that there is an overall difference in total life events. It also provides a profile on at least six dimensions to discriminate between different groups. The interview schedule only takes 30–75 minutes and has good reliability and validity (Paykel, 1983).

Two other instruments which have been used with success are the *Psychiatric Epidemiology Research Interview (PERI)* (Dohrenwend *et al.*, 1978) and the Tennant & Andrews Scale (1976, 1977). The former samples 102 events and is useful in epidemiological research in the USA rather than clinical work. Monroe (1982) has used it for self-report, although it has a high fall-off rate in reporting of events when so used. The latter covers some 67 events with only brief descriptions, but can distinguish different dimensions of life events such as the degrees of distress and change, and can be used as a self-report measure (Tennant & Andrews, 1978) or supplemented with interview investigations (Steele, Henderson & Duncan-Jones, 1982).

Isolating causes from consequences

We saw in Chapter 1 that it is necessary to distinguish between primary stressors, the causes of strain, and secondary stressors, the consequences of being under strain. For example, having to work to a tight deadline may make previously pleasant social interactions stressful; having a child may bring financial pressures which in turn may cause role conflicts not previously present. Each stressor may indeed be a cause of strain (i.e. primary stressors), but some stressors may be stressors only because the person's threshold for coping with stressors has been lowered (i.e. secondary stressors). Fletcher & Payne (1980b) suggest that both types of stressors will show correlational associations with the measures of strain being considered. Indeed, since the secondary stressors will be the most recently experienced stressors, they may show stronger associations with the health criteria. They are not, however, the causes of strain and their removal will not change the level of strain. This creates two problems. First, it implies that the primary stressors are likely to be difficult to distinguish from these secondary stressors. Second, the temporal appearance of stressors, as well as their presence, is of critical importance in looking for the causes of illness.

A consequence of the foregoing points is that dictionary instruments for measuring life events such as the SRE are totally insensitive to such problems. Prospective studies utilising such instruments will fare no better either, because the life events themselves are *a priori* deemed independent; yet it is the interrelationships between them, and how these factors change over time, that is crucial to understanding the *causes* of illness and the relationship between life events and ill-health. It is questionable that interview instruments will do much better. In the sense that we are dealing with contextual factors, however, they are, in principle, more suited to this role. One factor to be borne in mind is that the measurement of stressors (and not just the temporal appearance of illness) needs to be monitored on several occasions. It is probable that inconsistencies in the literature are a result of confusing primary and secondary events.

Prospective and Retrospective Studies

There are a number of possible research designs for investigating the relationship between life events and illness. Although there are many variations (see Kasl, 1983; Temoshok & Heller, 1984) the two major classes of design are *retrospective or cross-sectional* and *prospective or longitudinal*, with or without control or comparison groups. In retrospective studies one time slice of data is collected and the relationships between life events and health criteria are investigated by attempting to partition (e.g. healthy vs. disease groups) or correlate the variables considered important. This approach could be considered 'fishing for stressors' because the subject's present state is presumed to provide a causal and undistorted window into the past. This approach encompasses the majority of epidemiological and psychomedical research. Prospective designs, on the other hand, begin with only healthy subjects who provide a range of biographical, medical and psychological data at the outset of the study. These subjects are followed for a period of time. After a specific period of time, or when a number of them have developed symptoms or disease, the factors (taken from the original measures) which discriminate the healthy from the ill are investigated.

Although expensive, time-consuming, requiring massive samples or risky sample targeting, and often ending up with small case numbers, prospective designs are almost universally considered to provide a more scientific insight into the causal mechanisms between life events (or stressors) and illness (or strains). This belief should be tempered. Just as high correlation does not imply cause, low correlation does not imply lack of cause, cross-lagged correlations are suspect (Cook & Campbell, 1979), and health/disease discriminants are still open to many interpretations, whether retrospectively or prospectively obtained. Prospective studies should be done but they do not provide all the answers and are open to a number of criticisms. Brown (1981), for example, considers that it is the measurement of life events and disease that needs to be improved, not that studies need to be prospective in design. He outlines six reasons why prospective studies utilising the SRE are weak, which serve to summarize a number of points we have covered in detail above:

1. The desire to keep the study truly prospective has meant that there has been little attempt to use information about events occurring in the period immediately preceding the follow-up interview. Thus, the period during which any onset occurs is not covered.
2. Low reliability and validity of the SRE.
3. Vagueness of the SRE items.
4. Insensitivity due to using a non-contextual approach.
5. Unwarranted assumption of additivity of life events.
6. Not all events are relevant to all diseases.

Brown (1981) writes:

> Without wishing to question the value of prospective designs, I think that just what they can and cannot achieve is often misunderstood. If we are to study a wide range of events, research must deal with the past in the sense that the investigator has to question about events after their occurrence. The choice is therefore not whether to collect events retrospectively but only at an interview before onset (prospective design) or after onset has occurred (retrospective design) (p. 470).

In addition, Brown (1974) adds that 'indirect contamination' may occur in prospective studies. For example, a high level of anxiety may be the cause of a subsequent illness and a greater tendency to report life events.

Kasl (1983) outlines a number of general difficulties when interpreting the results of prospective investigations, even those which collect information on potential stressors and actual strains at each measuring time. He suggests that the payoff is small if the time interval is brief, because nothing much will happen. Moreover, the 'cause' may already have occurred, and will be confused by intervening variables. Frequent measurement to pin down the temporal sequence of events (e.g. every two weeks in Meyer & Haggerty's, 1962, study) may provide its own contaminants for some illnesses. One should also add in this context that if data on many variables are collected the results will be very difficult to interpret, and large numbers of cases will be required to do meaningful analyses (which has proved a problem particularly in cancer studies—see Chapter 4). Because of the assumptions of many parametric tests, many discriminant analyses and controlled multivariate comparisons should not be performed; nonparametric alternatives are less powerful and often unavailable. However, multivariate aspects are almost always important in the onset of disease (not least because there are many traditional risk factors, as well as many potential psychological stressors). Kasl (1983) also suggests that there are self-selection and reactive effects in some conditions (e.g. those that have many life events, or when clinical signs of illness are being monitored) which add further contaminants. Finally, if the researcher is using a doubly prospective design in which the cohort shows neither disease onset nor risk factors, there is the problem of deciding what constitutes a baseline value on the life events measure. Life events are precisely events that normally happen. Besides the problems for using statistical regression techniques, a score of zero would be unusual and non-representative. But what score might we use?

Models, Models, Models

When determining the role of life events in the onset of disease one can begin from different theoretical perspectives. What perspective one begins with will determine to a large degree what one needs to measure, and the type of design that should be employed. At an abstract level, for example, Dohrenwend & Dohrenwend (1984) distinguish between six different models, each of which proposes different roles for life events:

1. *Victimisation model.* This is the simplest model, which suggests that life events directly cause illness. Although Dohrenwend & Dohrenwend note that it is derived from the observations of the effects of extreme circumstances, it is applicable to ordinary events if one does not make the assumption that events must be consciously perceived as being stressful. The context in which the events occur, and the personality of the individual, play little, if any, role in the translation of the event into the illness: if they occur, it occurs.
2. *Stress–strain model.* Similar to Kagan & Levi's (1974) model of stress, in which the relationship between life events and illness is wholly mediated by psycho-physiological strain and other non-pathological responses.
3. *Vulnerability model,* in which it is proposed that the social setting of the event, and the dispositions of the person who experiences the event, attenuate or otherwise modify the direct consequence of life events on health.
4. *Additive burden model,* in which the social setting and personal dispositions do not modify the effects of life events on illness, but each has its own additive effect on the likelihood of ill-health.
5. *Chronic burden model,* in which the life events play no role in the onset of illness.

Instead the chronic state of the social situation and personal dispositions are the sole determinants of illness risk. This model proposes that contextual factors are the prime determinants of ill-health.

6. *Event proneness*. This suggests that the symptoms of health change (not necessarily consciously perceived) themselves directly affect the experiencing or reporting of the life events which in turn cause ill-health.

RESEARCH REQUIREMENTS

A number of themes emerge from this discussion which inform us about what requirements should be borne in mind when evaluating previous work or embarking on new investigations:

1. There is a need to define the theoretical perspective of the work, in order to delimit the range of measures and delimit the design of the study. It was suggested in Chapter 1 that the configural model could provide a backcloth for this purpose. Clearly, the model makes a number of predictions which have been borne out by some of the criticisms of previous life events research (e.g. that life events should be considered as clustered, that life events should be considered in terms of their impact in a given context, rather than as an invariant objective measure of required change, etc.).

2. Interview techniques are more valid and reliable than questionnaire instruments, and can reveal better insight into causal relationships and contextual issues. They can also measure the impact of events independently of the subject's perceptions of those events, although careful training and guidelines are required. Well-validated questionnaire instruments, however, are available and can be usefully and more economically used to investigate a certain range of issues, especially those requiring large samples or a consideration of the interactions between many variables.

3. Life events should not be considered as purely environmental in origin, as is implicit in the configural model. Personal dispositions and states affect their perception. In addition, many factors are likely to confound and mediate the relationship between life events and their effect on health.

4. Careful dating is required of the onset of the illness or its precursors, and of the events that occur. Careful examination of the interrelationships between events, and between events and health criteria, is necessary if causal interpretations are required.

5. Cause is a relative term. Neither prospective nor retrospective studies will provide unambiguous causal data because each type of study has its own peculiar limitations. Nor are these designs mutually exclusive. If causal interpretation is the primary goal of the study both prospective and retrospective aspects should be incorporated with aspects of the former providing validations for data obtained by the latter techniques, and vice-versa.

6. What people say (either in an interview or on a questionnaire) is not necessarily what they do or think, even if they (and you) are sure they are telling the truth. Causal relationships and other interrelationships are more complicated than people think (as is shown by the configural model of stress).
7. Psychologically causal factors in disease are not confined to emotional affects. Such a view admits of only a very limited range of models describing the relationships between life events and illness.
8. Different diseases are probably influenced by different categories of life events, and different life events probably have different kinds of effects (emotionally and physically). Different diseases and life events may also be affected by different mediating and moderating factors and their relationships confounded by different factors too.

To this list can be added other requirements mentioned consistently (e.g. Dohrenwend & Dohrenwend, 1974; Hugdens, 1974; Temoshok & Heller, 1984):

9. There is a greater need for more adequate operational definitions of the independent variables or life events and of the dependent variables or ill-health criteria.
10. A great deal is to be gained by the use of standardised replicable techniques and measures.
11. Suitable (and preferably multiple) control groups are required, and each group should be diagnostically cohesive.
12. Every attempt should be made to distinguish different levels of causal interpretation. At minimum, one should distinguish between events that may be caused by the illness.
13. Larger numbers of potential causal variables, mediating variables, and outcome variables should be measured, and their interrelationships considered.
14. Controlled comparisons of the relative contributions of life events and other risk factors are required, although statistical measures other than those providing information on "percentage of predictable variance explained" will, perhaps, be less misunderstood.

Clearly the problems are complex. One thing only appears certain: the task of establishing causal links between life events and illness is inherently difficult and different kinds of approaches have different contributions to make. The work of Holmes & Rahe is by no means exempt from criticism. On the contrary. The criticisms cannot, however, outweigh the contribution they made to this area. The contribution has been invaluable precisely because it has raised these important issues.

Chapter 3

Stress and the Immune System

This chapter begins with a simple outline of how the immune system works, in order to provide an understanding of the literature to be discussed. The chapter proceeds with a discussion of the role of stress in immune system functioning, considering such aspects as conditioning of the immune system and stressors which affect the competence with which it deals with assaults on it.

THE IMMUNE SYSTEM

The function of the immune system is to protect the organism against the infection of pathogens (things that do not belong to the body) of all sizes and types such as metazoa or *worms* (e.g. tapeworm), *protozoa* (e.g. malaria), *fungi* (e.g. candida), *bacteria* (e.g. streptococci, salmonella) and *viruses* (e.g. rabies, influenza, glandular fever). The range of diseases in which the immune system plays a central role is extremely large (colds to cancer).

Essentially there are two types of immune response to a pathogen.

The first, *nonspecific or innate immunity*, is present in all vertebrates and invertebrates. It is a general response to the pathogen and is affected by species and genetic susceptibility; physical barriers such as skin and the ciliated epithelium of the mucous membranes; biochemical reactions such as the cellular synthesis of interferon and its secretion into extracellular fluids, the widespread lysozyme present in tears, hydrochloric acid in the stomach and the serum complement–properdin system; and cellular mechanisms involving the phagocytic activity of the monocytic macrophages and the granulocytic neutrophils. Factors such as age and neuroendocrine status also affect innate immune function.

Polymorphonuclear granulocytes represent one type of immune system cell involved in innate immunity. These cells mature in the bone marrow and are released into the blood stream where they stay for about six hours. They adhere to, and emigrate between (by a process known as chemotaxis), the endothelial cells of the blood vessels where they have their action. Their defence is effected by phagocytosis (or engulfment) or bactericidal killing of the pathogen. Defective phagocytosis leads to an increased susceptibility to bacterial and fungal infections, but not the smaller cellular acting viruses.

Monocytic macrophages are of the same bone marrow 'family' as the granulo-cytes, but are less important in local defence. They too respond to chemotactic stimuli and phagocytose. They monitor blood entering the reticuloendothelial system (the main sites of which are the bone marrow, spleen, liver and lymphoid system) which plays a major role in immunity. In this sense they are 'self defenders' although they also play a role in the second type of immune reaction.

The second, *adaptive or acquired immune response*, is present only in vertebrates. It is an active bodily response (although it can be passively acquired for a short duration by injection for some diseases). Acquired immunity has three essential characteristics: recognition of 'non-self', specificity and memory.

The production of *antibodies,* which forms the basis of one type of acquired immune response (see the B lymphocytes below), is contingent upon the recognition of an *antigen* or 'non-self' (an antigen is a foreign agent that elicits an immune system response). Upon recognition the antibodies combine with the antigens to eliminate them. The initial antibody response to the antigen is known as the *primary response* and is characterised by delayed production of antibodies whose level of concentration in serum is relatively low. Upon reintroducion of an antigen, however, the *secondary response* is very rapid and more intense. The basis of vaccination is precisely to prime the individual to produce the more powerful secondary response upon infection. Autoimmune diseases are a consequence of a failure of the immune system to recognise 'self' from 'non-self' which leads to the synthesis of autoantibodies which become directed to the individual's own body.

The recognition of antigen is relatively specific. This specificity is fundamental to the acquired immune response and is not confined to the simple recognition of 'non-self'. The acquisition of immunity to one antigen does not confer immunity from other diseases because the system is able to differentiate the different organisms. The antigen–antibody reaction is specific, rather like a key is specific to a lock (although weaker cross-reactions occur if there is sufficient similarity between the receptors of different antigens).

One major distinction between innate and acquired immunity is that the latter demonstrates memory to the foreign-body infection. This is clearly shown by the secondary immune response.

There are two major forms of acquired immune response: *humoral and cell-mediated immunity.*

Humoral immunity involves the synthesis and release of antibodies into the blood, lymph and other body fluids. These are said to be *free* antibodies. The cells in the body which recognise the antigens are the immunocompetent small *lymphocytes.* These are produced in the bone marrow. The *B lymphocytes*, one of two classes of lymphocytes, are responsible for humoral immunity. Following antigen challenge the B lymphocytes undergo morphological change into plasma cells and memory cells which resemble the B cells. The plasma cells synthesise and secrete antibodies for their 18–48 hour life span. *Immunoglobulin* (Ig) molecules, which we will see are important in the immune response, have been shown to be present on the surface of B cells. Each lymphocyte will produce only specific immunoglobulins, and the specificity of the surface immunoglobulins provides the specific receptor for the antigen. Structurally, all antibodies are immunoglobulins. There are species differences in the structure of immunoglobulins, but in the human there are five major structural classes: IgG, IgA, IgM, IgD and IgE. Of these IgG is the most abundant; it accounts for about 75% of serum Ig and it has important extravascular functions for combating microorganisms and their toxins. IgG (and IgM) antibodies are valuable activators of the classical (C1) complement system and promote phagocytosis. IgA is present in serum and the seromucous secretions of the gastro-intestinal and respiratory tracts, genitourinary surface membrane secretions, and other secretions such as sweat, colostrum, nasal fluids, and saliva. For example, about 80% of gastric juice immunoglobulin is IgA. It functions by coating the pathogens and inhibiting their adherence to the mucosal cells. Its serum role is uncertain. IgM is the largest immunoglobulin and is the earliest line of immune defence, but it is short-lived, and its presence indicates recent infection. It is functionally limited to the blood stream. It is a very effective agglutinator (clumping of bacteria or erythrocytes) and has powerful classical complement-fixing cytolytic capacity. IgD is primarily to be found in the blood stream on the surface of lymphocytes, but it is present only in small amounts (on about 3% of lymphocytes in adults). It has no complement function. It may act together with IgM as an antigen receptor for the control of lymphocyte suppression and activation. IgE is mainly found in the perivascular mast cells. It has extended life. It is not clear what defensive role IgE plays. It may help in helminthic (worm) infestations. It plays a pathogenic role in the degranulation of mast cells and the subsequent release of vasoactive amines (e.g. histamine) in certain atopic allergic reactions (e.g. hay fever, extrinsic asthma). Plasma levels of immunoglobulins are very stable even under quite severe changes (e.g. starvation for 10 days) and some researchers (e.g. Palmblad, 1981) doubt that everyday stressors are likely to have demonstrable effects, although the evidence for this view will be considered later.

The second type of immune response is known as *cell-mediated immunity*. This type of immunity is utilised against bacteria and viruses which live and replicate *within* the host cells. It is the final line of defence against infection. Thus cell-mediated immunity is the prime protection against slow-growing intracellular pathogens. Cell-mediated immunity is achieved through the second category of lymphocytes known as *T lymphocytes*. These T cells are derived from the bone marrow too, but they are somehow dependent on the thymus. Upon antigen invasion the T cells undergo morphological change to lymphoblasts. The term 'delayed hypersensitivity' is often used to refer to cell-mediated immunity. This is evidenced by tissue damage a day or two after contact with an antigen to which the individual has become specifically sensitised (e.g. the Mantoux reaction in individuals immune to tubercule infection). The primed individual shows a secondary boosting of the immune response when presented to the pathogen. Transplant tissue rejection, atopic allergic states, and some autoimmune diseases are in the same category. In the initial cell-mediated response, recognition of the antigen causes the T cell to interact with the macrophage-presenting antigen. This activates the T cell through the synergistic mediator interleukin-1 from the macrophage. A new synthesis of RNA and protein occurs as a result of the increase in intracellular cGMP and calcium ions. This produces blast-like cells which have surface receptors for a T cell growth factor, interleukin-2, producing proliferation into one of the subpopulations of T cells (e.g. T-helper cells, killer T cells, T-suppressor cells—see below).

Cytotoxic T cells or killer cells which have been generated as a result of a pathogen (e.g. a virus, an allogenic graft) are specifically cytotoxic to that pathogen. The killer cells are, like plasma cells, 'end cells' and die when their function is complete. Their killing action is thought to be direct, but because of the large numbers required, not very efficient. They are effective against a few neoplastic cells, histocompatible transplant tissue, and virally invaded cells with cell membrane viral antigens.

The other method of T cell-mediated immunity involves macrophages which are stimulated by lymphokines which are biologically active proteins (e.g. interferon) secreted during the process of T cell proliferation. Activated T cells draw lymphocytes to the antigen site, stimulate them to divide and differentiate, which in turn releases more lymphokines which facilitate the inflammatory reaction. The macrophages from the blood stream (and some polymorphonuclear granulocytes) are attracted to the site of the inflammation where they accelerate phagocytosis of the pathogen. A migration-inhibition factor is involved in keeping the macrophages on site.

T-helper cells are essential to humoral immunity inasmuch as they are necessary to activate B cells to produce antibody to all but a few antigens. Although immunoglobulins are not readily identifiable on the surface of T cells the presence of T cells stimulates antibody synthesis considerably. Immunoglobulins also play a role in cellular immunity. For example, IgG helps induce killer cell destruction which is important in transplant rejection and autoimmune disorders.

As can be seen, therefore, there are many possible measures of the immune system which can be assessed to determine likely immunocompetence, including simple leucocyte counts, the percentage of T-helper cells, T-suppressor cells, NK cells, immunoglobulins, etc., antibody titres to viruses (e.g. the Epstein–Barr virus involved in infectious mononucleosis or glandular fever), the amount of chemotactic activity, and blastogenesis (or a functional assay to determine lymphocyte proliferation in response to *in vitro* mitogens such as concanavalinA [ConA] and phytohaemagglutinin [PHA]).

PSYCHOIMMUNOLOGY: ILL-CONCEIVED, STILLBORN, IN ITS INFANCY OR BEFORE ITS TIME?

The relationship between the central nervous system (the physical embodiment of the psyche?) and the functioning of the immune system is poorly understood, as is their interaction with the endocrine system. This is not surprising. Nor should it be assumed that the former plays little role in the functioning of the latter unless gross psychological factors can be demonstrated to have very marked (crude?) direct effects on measures of immunocompetence in humans. It is certainly true that simply observing that psychological factors are correlated with immune *diseases* is no proof of any significant causal relationship. It must be borne in mind that we are dealing with a relationship at the forefront of our understanding. Complex systems do not admit of simplistic answers or theories, but we are not at the stage of being able to offer sufficiently detailed theories. That is the dilemma. Certainly science does not cease in the face of such dilemmas, nor does it assume there is no case to answer. The search for connections between the CNS and the immune system at the functional level is difficult, but the dilemma is surmountable because the probability of a significant link is easily accepted. As John Maddox put it in an editorial in *Nature* in 1984, "The doubt is whether enough is yet known to sustain people's hopes of explanation.... In short, the explanation is likely to be part of a more complicated tale" (p. 400).

The Link Between the CNS, Hormones and Immune Function

We are not in a state of ignorance. We know that some types of lymphocytes have receptors for simple peptide hormones also found in the brain. It has been hypothesised that the hypothalamic–pituitary axis has direct influence on immune functioning via its effects on the thymus (and, therefore, T cells) and indirect effects via the adrenal cortex hormones such as adrenocorticotrophin (Maclean & Reichlin, 1981; Ader & Cohen 1985; Krug, Krug & Cuatrecasas, 1974). Peptide hormones may well control the circulating lymphocytes through the second messenger system, intracellular cAMP and cGMP (Bourne *et al.*, 1974). The existence of cholinergic and beta-adrenergic receptor sites on certain lymphocytes provides a route for understanding how the CNS may exert an influence on immune functioning. We know that psychological factors such as bereavement can have effects on lymphocyte responsiveness to mitogens (Schleifer *et al.*, 1983). We know that immunosuppression can be conditioned to occur to a previously neutral substance for both cell-mediated (Ader, Cohen & Bovbjerg, 1982) and humoral immunity (Gorczynski, Macrae & Kennedy, 1984). We know that the delayed hypersensitivity reaction in individuals who show positive tuberculin skin tests can be diminished by subjective knowledge or expectancy effects (Smith & McDaniel, 1983). We know that benzodiazepines, which are among the most widely prescribed drugs with antianxiety effects, are potent stimulators of human monocyte chemotaxis (Ruff *et al.*, 1985). Whilst we may not be able to go as far as saying that there is no psychological factor which is not reflected in the state of the human immune system, or that the immune system may be considered as a functional sense organ (Blalock, 1984), we can make some good guesses from the accumulating evidence about what psychological factors may affect immunological functioning and how these effects are operationalised.

Recent years have certainly seen rapid advances in our understanding of the interaction between immunology and various psychological states, usually termed 'stress'.

The importance of this research is its attempt to show that the psychological states that are caused by stress increase the person's vulnerability to certain diseases because they have an immunosuppressive effect. Thus, diseases which are directly linked with immunological function (e.g. infectious diseases and allergies, cancers, autoimmune disorders) may be affected by the psychological state of the host. As we have discussed earlier, however, it is a mistake to equate 'psychological' with 'attentionally mediated' or 'affective' or 'emotional' (depending on whether the work is done on humans or other animals). The belief that heeded factors may exert a more power-ful influence on the immune system than non-heeded factors is not based on research. There are probably three reasons why this bias has occurred. The first is that it is difficult to study non-heeded psychological factors because one cannot rely on subjec-tive reports. Second, research on chronic stressors, which may be a characteristic of many non-heeded factors, is inherently more difficult to control and interpret. Finally, these 'unconscious' psychological factors may be primarily *Homo sapiens*: they may even be culturally specific and influenced by many other factors (e.g. sex, social status, occupation) and this makes their study in non-human animals impossible.

From what has been said so far it should be clear that recent work does not support the view that the regulation of the immune response is governed only by the immune system itself (i.e. that it is a closed-loop system, as far as the psyche is concerned). The hypothalamus seems to play a major role in cell-mediated and humoral immunity (e.g. Stein, Schleifer & Keller, 1981; Roszman *et al.*, 1982) as well as in neuroendocrine and autonomic nervous system function, there is evidence of dual innervation of lymphoid tissue in a number of animals (e.g. Bulloch & Moore, 1981), both lymphocytes and macrophages have receptors for hormones and neurotransmitters (e.g. Hilderman & Strom, 1978), antigenic stimulation affects hormone levels (e.g. Shek & Sabiston, 1983) and the immunoresponse to an antigen is affected by hormones (e.g. Comsa, Leonhardt & Wekerle, 1982).

In a commentary entitled 'The emerging field of psychoneuroimmunology' George Solomon lists 14 different hypotheses, for which there is evidence, to link the immune system with the CNS: "a far cry from the single 'stress should be immunosuppressive' I set out to verify 15 years ago" (Solomon, 1985, p. 411). These hypotheses included:

1. *Individual differences* (personality, genetic make-up) influence the effects of natural and experimental exogenous factors on the functioning of the immune system.
2. *Emotional factors* alter the likelihood or course of diseases which are affected by immunological resistance (infections and neoplasia) and aberrant functioning (allergic, autoimmune, acquired immune deficiency).
3. Mental or emotional *dysfunction* should be associated with immunological abnormalities.
4. Immunological abnormalities are sometimes accompanied by psychoneuro-logical symptoms.

5. *Substances* with a CNS control (e.g. hormones) affect the immune system.
6. The immunologically competent cells have *receptors* for these substances or their precursors.
7. *Manipulations and interventions of a psychological* or behavioural nature (e.g. stress, conditioning, psychotherapy, biofeedback, hypnosis) have immune system consequences.
8. Manipulation of *relevant CNS components* has immune system consequences.
9. Changes in the immune system (e.g. immunisation) are *accompanied by changes in CNS functions*.

One area in which the link between the immune system and psychological mechanisms has been investigated is in how the immune system can be taught to *learn*. If it can be shown that non-physical environmental factors can directly influence immunocompetence, the link between psyche and disease processes is firmly established. One of the most promising factors established in this connection is that of immune system conditioning.

Conditioning and the CNS–Immune System Interaction

The outstanding work of Ader & Cohen (e.g. 1975, 1981, 1984, 1985) attempts to enlarge the simplistic classical biomedical model of immunology by examining conditioning phenomena in relation to immune system functioning. They take it as axiomatic that etiologically multifactorial diseases need to be researched from a wide perspective which includes the influence of psychologically important factors such as behavioural conditioning and stress. Moreover, they "believe that conditioning, as a potent immunoregulatory mechanism, should be considered apart from the immunomodulating effects of stress" (1985, p. 380). Ader & Cohen (1985) suggest that there is no body of evidence to support the view that conditioned immunity is mediated by conditioned or nonspecific adrenocortical steroids (although growth hormone, insulin and thyroxine potentiate, and glucocorticoids, androgens, oestrogen and progesterone suppress, immune responses). This view is not without its critics (e.g. Ballieux & Heijnen, 1985; Cunningham, 1985) whilst others take the view that "in a causal world nonspecificity is a meaningless notion" (Engel, 1985, p. 399).

Influenced by a number of Russian studies, and by serendipitous observations of rat mortality in taste aversion experiments, Ader & Cohen (1975) did a carefully controlled experimental examination of behaviourally conditioned immunosuppression. Experimental rats drank sodium saccharin (the conditioned stimulus) and were immediately given an intraperitoneal injection of cyclophosphamide (the unconditioned stimulus, which is a powerful immunosuppressant and gastrointestinal aggravant). Control rats were given plain water instead of saccharin. Note that, in contrast to the earlier work, animals receive only a single conditioning trial. After 72 hours some rats were given an intraperitoneal injection of sheep erythrocytes as an antigen or a simple saline injection, followed 15 minutes later by a drinking bottle containing saccharin or one containing plain water. After six days blood samples were titrated for haemagglutinating antibody activity. Ader & Cohen found that the rats who had not been exposed to any immunosuppressive substance had high antibody titres, whilst the conditioned rats with cyclophosphamide immunisation showed the lowest antibody titres. Rats showed a clear effect of classical conditioning to sodium saccharin in the absence of re-exposure to cyclophosphamide. This was an elegant demonstration of conditioned humoral immunosuppression which has generated a considerable amount of subsequent research employing different controls, immunosuppressors and dose levels, different antigens and different measures of immunocompetence. The evidence supports the general conclusion that humoral immunity conditioning effects exist, are powerful, occur for B and T-helper lymphocytes, are dose-related to the immunosuppressor, are not confined to the peculiar effects of cyclophosphamide as an immunomodulating substance, or of saccharin as the novel conditioned stimulus (see Ader & Cohen, 1985). Almost all these findings have, however, been derived from experiments on rats and mice.

In addition to humoral immunoconditioning, a number of researchers have demonstrated T-lymphocyte-mediated cellular conditioning. For example, Bovbjerg, Ader & Cohen (1982) observed a marked reduction (compared to placebo and non-conditioned rats) of popliteal lymph node weights after subdermal grafts of splenic leucocytes in rats given saccharin (which had 48 days previously been paired with cyclophosphamide) and a saline injection, followed by a one-fifth dose of cyclophosphamide, and a re-exposure to just the saccharin on successive days. Gorczynski, Macrea & Kennedy (1982) have also reported a conditioned enhancement of cell-mediated immunocompetence in which the grafted tissue antigen itself served as the unconditioned stimulus. Whilst this work too is on rodents, in an experiment using human subjects Smith & McDaniel (1983) have shown that conditioning (or expectancy) can diminish the delayed hypersensitivity reaction. Seven individuals who showed positive tuberculin skin tests were given the scratch test for five months on one arm and a saline test on the other. Without knowledge on the sixth month the tests were done on different arms. Whilst saline did not produce a positive reaction, the erythema and induration of the new treatment arm was markedly diminished compared to previous levels, and the immune reactions returned to normal levels on a subsequent control trial (see Figure 3.1, which shows the lump sizes for each subject separately on Trial 5, the experimental trial, and a subsequent control trial). The results, therefore, supported the hypothesis that the immune response could be significantly diminished by psychological mediation.

Whilst the disease-related implications of these conditioning studies are somewhat removed, they are important inasmuch as they clearly demonstrate the impact that previously neutral stimuli may have on the immune response and the potentially 'accidental' nature of an organism's immunocompetence at any particular time. They should also serve as a reminder to those who all too easily equate 'psychological' with 'emotional' or 'attentionally heeded'. Whether conditioning phenomena have a very much broader role to play in human immunocompetence is yet to be established (although Kimmel, 1985, has commented that in transplant

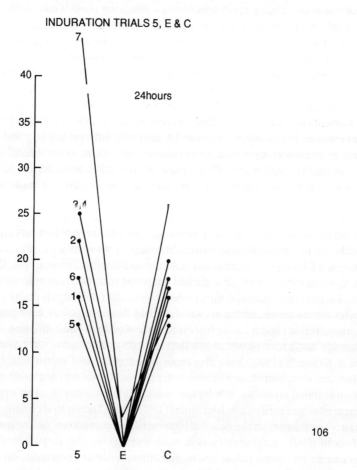

Figure 3.1   Millimetres of induration at 24 h for Trial 5, experimental (E) and control (C), for each of the seven subjects (reproduced by permission from Smith & McDaniel 1983)

surgery—the baboon–human heart transplant in 'Baby Fae', for example—one should be able to condition antirejection in advance of transplant surgery). Moreover, whether non-Pavlovian conditioning can affect the immune system in a significant manner is a moot question.

Is there a Need to Consider Psychological Influences in Immune System Functioning?

Colonisation of an organism by a pathogen does not necessarily result in the symptoms of clinical illness. This alone is sufficient to require the abandonment of the autonomous biomedical model of disease paraphrased by "one germ, one disease, one therapy". It is, perhaps, the extent of the abandonment that is most in question. One consequence of the shifted perspective is the concept of multiple causation of disease which admits of psychological factors as having etiological significance. There is now a considerable literature on the effects of certain psychological factors on direct indices of immunological functioning. Undoubtedly, however, it is not generally accepted that psychological factors play a major role in affecting measurable indices of immune functioning. Some of this reluctance is due to methodological difficulties in studying the relevant processes: the "in-field" simpler measures of immunocompetence are crude reflections of a complex and little-understood system. Stressors do not necessarily, if at all, produce marked changes in total blood cell counts, phagocytic activity, or antigen–antibody response. Some researchers have suggested that changes in the functional capacity of the human immune system should be assessed by more sensitive measures such as the rate of lymphoblast transformation, or specific lymphocyte effects (Irwin & Anisman, 1984). Added to this is the difficulty of pinpointing and conceptualising the psychological stressors. Definitions of these factors are not precise or universal (McQueen & Siegrist, 1982). The potential maximal impact of psychological stressors is often perceived as relatively minor even by sympathetic researchers. Palmblad (1981), for example, suggests that as plasma levels of immunoglobulins, lymphokine production, and delayed hypersensitivity effects are little affected by quite severe physical stressors (e.g. 10 days' starvation) everyday psychological stressors are unlikely to have any effects. In the same volume Fox (1981), in his discussion of the effects of stress on cancer, produces a number of cogent arguments to support the view that "stress is likely to have a relatively small effect on carcinogenesis when placed beside other factors that tend to induce cancer" (p. 143).

What are the arguments against this view? The first is based on the widespread intuitive view that psychological stressors do contribute to disease through their action via the CNS, but as Anisman & Zacharko (1985) have put it, "hard data are often greeted with skepticism. It seems that data may sometimes be less compelling than our intuitions!" (p. 395). One reason for this less-than-compelling evidence is probably that psychoimmunology is a relatively new discipline, and its contribution will have to be measured by the gradual accumulation of more evidence using ever more sophisticated techniques and conceptualisations: the tests of our intuitions have not been completed. Ader & Cohen (1984), in a review of behavioural influences on the immune system, observed: "the effects of experimental factors on immunological reactivity are frequently small and, superficially at least, inconsistent. This, we believe, reflects upon our incomplete understanding of the mechanisms involved, rather than upon the phenomenon itself" (p. 139).

The second reason for pursuing psychological influences on the immune system is that much of the variance of individual reaction to pathogens remains to be explained. We should abandon psychological explanations only if we have something more adequate to replace them with: it is my guess that psychological factors will prove to have major etiological significance in immune system functioning and that the closed-system approach in immunology is untenable to explain disease occurrence in normal human functioning. Third, real-life immunofunctioning must be explored more fully: the majority of studies which have examined human psychological stressors and immune function have concentrated on major acute stressors. One reason for this is that they are unambiguous—the death of a spouse or taking part in a space flight are incontrovertible occurrences. Such events are not, however, part of everyday living, and I would question the assumption that if the effects of such stressors on immunocompetence are small the effects of more everyday events will be even less clear. The cumulative effects of many minor everyday events may well overwhelm the adaptive capacities of individuals, especially when these events are unpredicted and outside the control of the individual. Such a contention is supported by a range of evidence in other fields (e.g. Weiss, 1970; Broadbent & Gath, 1979; Karasek, 1979). The problem in testing such a contention in the field of immunology is not a minor one, however. Crude measures and lack of adequate baseline controls are major obstacles to advanced understanding and investigation.

Fourth, whilst it is necessary to study the effects of chronic stressors in longitudinal studies it is not at all clear that non-human research can contribute to our understanding of psychological factors on immune system functioning. There are two problematic issues. With humans a minor acute stressor may have significant chronic effects because attentional mediation can reinforce and distort it. In contrast, a major stressor can be diminished by reasoning and resignation. In addition, there are many reasons for believing that the effects of psychological stressors will be differentially important for mice and humans even if some of their structural mechanics and biological responses are equivalent. Fox (1981), for example, outlines a number of important points in relation to stress and cancer. Whilst he concludes that equivalent levels of stress on mice and humans should contribute a greater relative proportion of influence in mice than humans he is careful to add the rider "I did *not* say that stress has a more powerful effect in mouse than in man" (p. 147). People can create their own stressors.

PSYCHOLOGICAL FACTORS IN DIRECT MEASURES OF IMMUNOCOMPETENCE

Non-human Studies

The majority of studies investigating the effects of psychological factors on the immunological functioning of animals have utilised avoidance training paradigms with aversive stimuli, daily exposure to loud noises, electric footshock, physical restraint, surgical trauma, whole-body irradiation, isolation, crowding, proximity to predators and so on. Such stimuli have been shown to have immunological consequences (see Ader, 1981; Ader & Cohen, 1984). For example, Solomon (1969) reported a marked reduction in both the primary and secondary responses to a bacterial antigen in crowded group-housed rats compared to individually housed controls. Hamilton (1974) showed that exposing mice to a cat increased tapeworm reinfection rates and was correlated with atrophy of the splenic corpuscular germinal centres with high lymphocyte counts. Pavlidis & Chirigos (1980) found that mice who were physically immobilised for more than 18 hours had lower *in vitro* interferon activation of peritoneal macrophages decreasing tumoricidal cytotoxicity. Even in animal work, however, where experimental controls can be rigorous, there is a marked degree of inconsistency in reported results. Whilst this could be taken as a sign that the effects of such psychological factors on immune functioning are not large, a more positive interpretation would suggest quite the contrary. A number of studies suggest that the effects of uncontrolled psychological factors can be revealingly significant (we will ignore individual differences for the present). Solomon, Levine & Kraft (1968), for example, have demonstrated that the early handling of animals enhances antibody responses when adult. The effects of such delayed immunocompetence reactions with factors other than handling could have significant effects on immunocompetence. Some studies also suggest that stressors may have protective as well as infective effects. Marsh *et al.* (1963) have shown that monkeys have decreased susceptibility to poliomyelitis after avoidance stress; Friedman, Ader & Grota (1973) have reported a protective effect of noxious stimulation in mice infected with rodent malaria; Rasmussen, Spencer & Marsh (1959) have shown that mice given daily avoidance conditioning do not exhibit as marked an immediate hypersensitive anaphylactic shock reaction compared to controls; and Fox (1981) believes there has been an underestimate of the beneficial effects of stress in cancer because no cancer occurs as a result of the protective effect. Whilst these effects may simply serve to illustrate a conceptual confusion about what stress is (see Chapter 1), they do suggest the influence of psychologically relevant factors.

The picture is complicated further by the qualitative changes in immunoreaction over time to a specific stimulus. Monjan & Collector (1977), for example, subjected mice to five second bursts of noise for up to three hours over 39 days. Lymphocyte proliferation to mitogenic stimulation of lipopolysaccharide and ConA (reflecting B- and T-lymphocyte function respectively) was depressed to below 50% of control values initially, with depressed function remaining for mice exposed for 20 days of sound stress. After 25 days, however, the lymphocyte reactivity became considerably enhanced (showing up to 240% of control values) before returning to control levels at 39 days. T-lymphocyte cytoxicity showed a similar biphasic change over time.

Human Studies

In 1981 Jan Palmblad wrote "So far the evidence for a link between mind and immunity in man rests only on approximately a dozen well-controlled studies" (p. 248). Whilst the situation has improved somewhat in more recent years, and the weight of evidence increased, several of the earlier studies have been influential and require description.

One advantage of the human studies is that they make possible the careful investigation of personality and other individual differences (e.g. suppressed anger, coping ability, inhibited power motivation) on immune system functioning. The studies which have considered the role of such factors will be reviewed in Chapters 4 and 5.

Life Events

The literature relating life events to disease risk was discussed in the previous chapter. Some studies, however, have concentrated on the relationship between major life events, everyday minor hassles and immunocompetence. The evidence that the number of significant life events and their magnitude can affect direct measures of immunological function is limited, but generally supportive of a relationship. Greene *et al.* (1978), for example, reported that those subjects experiencing more life changes in the previous year showed reduced lymphocyte cytotoxicity to inoculation with virus A/Victoria/75H3N2, as well as lower mitogenic responses. This study, along with a number of others, however, failed to find any main effect of life event change and haemagglutinin antibody titre (see Jemmott & Locke, 1984). Kiecolt-Glaser *et al.* (1984a) report that subjects scoring high on the Holmes–Rahe life events scale had lower levels of natural killer (NK) cells, which are probably involved in antitumour surveillance, in both baseline and examination period blood tests. A similar reduction of NK activity was observed in those scoring high on a measure of loneliness. Because of technical problems, however, it was not possible for the investigators to consider the relationship between life events and plasma immunoglobulins, salivary IgA, and C-reactive protein.

Kemeny *et al.* (1989) examined 36 subjects with genital herpes in a prospectively designed study over a number of months. The herpes simplex virus remains in the body after the primary infection and is prone to reveal itself by recurrent clinical manifestation from time to time. The question Kemeny *et al.* considered was whether or not life events were the cause of recurrence. As predicted, the amount of life event changes, and the psychological moods of the participants, were significantly related to the proportions of T lymphocytes (both helper and suppressor cells). Those people with higher negative affect, and those with more life events, showed lowered immunocompetence, and the immune system measures were also related to the likelihood of herpes recurrence. Whilst this study can be criticised on a number of points, and the actual recurrence measures were not associated with the life event scores, it does go some way towards showing that chronic stressors are related to immunocompetence.

Jemmott & Locke (1984) have outlined a number of possible reasons for the lack of observed effects of life events on antibody titre. In addition to methodological problems with using life event measures (see Chapter 2), they suggest that antibody titre may be a state-dependent measure of immunological functioning which is more susceptible to acute, rather than chronic, stressors. Finally, previous research which has studied life change and antibody response to experimentally controlled viral exposure, has not considered dose–response effects. It may be that the doses used in these studies "have been so potent that little room was left for the effects of stress; if smaller doses were used, the effects of stress might become apparent" (p. 92).

Bereavement

Bartrop *et al.* (1977) conducted a detailed prospective study of the effects of bereavement on the immune functioning of 26 spouses. Their study utilised well-matched control subjects who were hospital staff members. Blood samples were taken at one to three weeks following bereavement and six weeks later. The serum was assessed for a number of immunological and endocrinal indices. They found that the bereaved subjects showed lower lymphocyte responsiveness, principally in the second blood sample, to *in vitro* mitogenic stimulation by the plant lectins phytohaemagglutinin (PHA) and concanavalin A (ConA), suggesting a diminished T-cell function. There were no effects of bereavement on a whole array of other indices including T- and B-cell numbers, autoantibodies, delayed hypersensitivity tests, IgG, IgA and IgM immunoglobulins, T3 and T4 thyroid hormones, cortisol, growth hormone and prolactin. This was a significant study because it was the first time a psychological stressor had been observed to have a measurable effect on a direct measure of immune system functioning which could not be attributed to hormonal changes. The apparent *selectivity* of immunodepression was also important because it suggests that adequate controls had been employed, and that the effects of bereavement should be reflected only in enhanced susceptibility to *some* illnesses.

A study by Schleifer *et al.* (1983) largely replicated the work of Bartrop *et al.* (1977), although it does not use non-bereaved controls. This weakness is outweighed, however, by a prospective design which permitted the determination of whether the depressed lymphocyte responsiveness of the bereaved was a direct consequence of bereavement or some pre-existing alteration of state. Schleifer *et al.* took pre-bereavement measures of immune functioning of the spouses of 15 women with advanced metastatic breast cancer every six to eight weeks, and post-bereavement measures at different stages up to 14 months. The partners had been married for between five and 43 years (median 30). They found no pre–post-bereavement differences in leucocyte count or T- and B-cell count, but there were significantly lower mitogenic responses to the T-cell indicators PHA and ConA, and the B-cell mitogen pokeweed (PWM). The suppressed lymphocyte reactivity was most marked in the early months following bereavement (a highly significant suppression being recorded as early as one month after bereavement), but was still present to a lesser degree at the later follow-up period of up to 14 months.

These two studies provide the best evidence of immunodepression following bereavement. Even so a good deal of further work is desperately needed. The studies employ only a few subjects (26 and 15), there are inconsistencies between them (for example, Bartrop *et al.* found no differences in mitogenic responsivity until eight weeks after bereavement), it is difficult to generalise their findings to those who suffer a sudden bereavement (although the Bartrop *et al.* study included such subjects no data are specifically presented about them). This makes it difficult to extract the immune consequences of an acute stressor independently of chronic conditions (it is possible that suppression occurs only in those suffering chronic stress) which makes generalisation to other stressors difficult. A major constraint on the usefulness of studying bereavement effects of this kind, however, is that the subjects are not very young (the median in Schleifer *et al.*'s study was 57 years). It may be that younger subjects exhibit a different immune response for a whole range of biological and psychological reasons.

Such difficulties should not be taken as casting doubt on the effects of psychological factors on immune functioning: rather, they suggest that the nature and subtlety of the effects requires elaboration.

Spaceflight

Studies of the NASA astronauts have provided useful data, if limited in generalisability! The work was of particular value at a stage when any evidence of a link between psychological stress and immune function was useful. Spaceflight is a major life event which only a few specially selected personnel experience. Like most bereavements, the actual acute stress of the flight takes place against a backcloth of unusual expectancies and uncertainties. This may have marked effects on the immune system independently of the actual flight. For example, an early study by Fischer *et al.* (1972) found no pre-flight/splashdown differences in lymphocyte response to PHA, although splashdown lymphocyte count was higher. Kimzey *et al.* (1976) also reported higher post-flight levels of leucocytes which, on differential counts, were due to an increase in polymorphonuclear leucocytes. The T-cell count was depressed, whereas serum immunoglobulins and C3 complement were unchanged. The probable effects of anticipation were also reflected in T-cell mitogenic response to PHA, which was slightly depressed before the launch. Mitogenic responsivity was again depressed at splashdown, which could be attributed to a number of factors including the physical stressors of the exercise itself. Studies of such unusual and extreme events are difficult to interpret, not least because of inconsistencies between different data from the same investigators and the multiple indicators of immune functioning. One major obstacle to demonstrating a specific immunological effect of some of the psychological stressors involved in spaceflight, however, is that such events have been shown to elevate adrenal–cortical and adrenal–medullary hormones (Leach & Rambaut, 1974) which themselves have immunosuppressive effects.

Long Vigils

Palmblad and his co-workers have done a number of studies of the effects of stressful vigils and sleep deprivation on immune functioning. Palmblad *et al.* (1976) required subjects to take part in a number of $2\frac{3}{4}$-hour simulated battle sessions over a 77-hour period in which they were sleep deprived. *In vitro* lymphocyte production of interferon to the Sendai virus was increased during the vigil and remained elevated five days later, but the phagocytic capacity of polymorphonuclear leucocytes (to *Staphylococcus aureus*) was depressed during the vigil compared to the pre- and post-vigil measures. In fact there was a greater post-vigil enhancement of phagocytosis of neutrophils five days later than there was an inhibition during the vigil. This suggests a dynamic response of the immune system to the stressors imposed. Although urinary catecholamines and serum cortisol levels were also elevated by the vigil they demonstrated some independence from the immune function measures, and in a further study (Palmblad *et al.*, 1979b) were lower during vigil, whilst mitogenic response to PHA was reduced. Taken together these findings suggest that the hormones were not mediators of the immune response. Indeed, in a review of the role of psychological factors in infectious diseases Jemmott & Locke (1984) also conclude that the evidence "makes plausible the assertion that the autonomic nervous system plays a role in immunomodulation, one that does not entirely depend on mediation by the neurohormones of either the pituitary–adrenal axis or the sympathetic–adrenal medullary axis" (p. 98).

There are difficulties in interpreting what the observed immunological responses from these studies imply. As Jemmott & Locke (1984) have pointed out, these studies do not include control groups who were deprived of sleep but not exposed to the various 'psychologically stressful' tasks. Thus it is difficult to disentangle precisely what is affecting the immune system indicators. The failure to detect differences in neutrophil adherence after only a 48 hour vigil (Palmblad *et al.*, 1979b) makes interpretation of the body of evidence more difficult, especially since different techniques have been employed in these studies to measure phagocytosis (Irwin & Anisman, 1984). Nonetheless, it does appear incontrovertible that stress of some kind is affecting the immune system. The situations used in the experiments have been perceived as being stressful by the subjects (Palmblad, 1981), as well as generally producing some hormonal evidence to support this view. In addition, Palmblad *et al.* (1979a) have shown that a decrease in the erythrocyte sedimentation rate (ESR) (which is associated with, amongst other things, increased serum corticosteroids) occurs in response to shooting range battle-simulation stress in army officers subjected to 75 hours' sleep deprivation.

Surgical Stress

Healthy individuals who have to undergo minor surgery appear to show immune system changes to the stress, as shown in the work of Linn & Jensen (1983). They observed that the phagocytosis of neutrophils was diminished one day after surgery, compared to presurgical levels, although adherence returned to normal levels within five days. T-cell transformation of the group of patients over 60 years old showed depressed levels, which reinforces the possibility that studies of bereavement should not be generalised to the effects of psychological stressors on younger patients.

Examination Taking

Dorian *et al.* (1982) examined the immune system consequences of psychiatrist residents taking an oral fellowship exam. The researchers employed a sample of age- and sex-matched controls. They found that, compared to the controls, the examination subjects exhibited lower B-cell lymphoblast transformation as well as lower T-cell mitogenic response to ConA and PHA, from samples taken two weeks prior to the examination. The examination group also showed elevated leucocyte and B- and T-cell counts. Samples were taken two weeks after the examination and showed that the differences between the groups had largely disappeared except that the examination subjects now exhibited an enhanced PHA 'rebound' response. It should be noted that this study reports lower cortisol levels in the examination subjects, which adds further weight to the view that the observed immunological differences were not hormone-mediated.

Kiecolt-Glaser and her colleagues have published two studies of examination stress in medical students. In the first study Kiecolt-Glaser *et al.* (1984a) took blood samples from 75 first-year students one month before examinations and again on the final day of examinations. They examined one indicator of cellular immunity, natural killer (NK) cell activity, a possible key in antitumour surveillance, and a number of indicators of humoral immunity (total plasma IgG, IgA, IgM, C-reactive protein, and salivary IgA). They found significantly less NK activity, and greater total plasma IgA, in the second blood sample. None of the other measures produced effects. In some ways the observed effect on plasma IgA was surprising, since previous studies using apparently more extreme stressors have failed to show effects on IgA (for example, Palmblad *et al.*, 1979, using 48 hours' sleep deprivation). However, as the investigators point out, plasma IgA has a half-life of six to eight days (compared to 25–35 days for IgG, and nine to 11 days for IgM) and one may expect to find effects with chronic stressors lasting a number of days rather than less than 48 hours.

In the second study, Kiecolt-Glaser *et al.* (1984b) found that B-cell mitogenic response to the Epstein–Barr virus (an herpes virus involved in infectious mononucleosis or glandular fever) in seropositive students was lower on the first day of examinations than one month beforehand.

Jemmott *et al.* (1983) observed the effects of low and high levels of academic stress at five different times of the academic year (before examinations, during three periods of major examinations from November to June, and at a final stage in July) on the salivary IgA secretion rates of 64 first-year dental students. They found that secretion levels were depressed during the high stress periods. Secretion rates also showed sensitivity to personality variables. For example, those with high inhibited need for power showed a continual decline in salivary IgA rates in the final low stress period, compared to the return to baseline results of the other groups. This study is also significant in that it enabled an examination of within-student perceptions of stressfulness (varying along a scale of six specified adjectives) and IgA levels for the five time epochs. A significant correlational relationship was observed. Given these results, it is unclear why the first Kiecolt-Glaser *et al.* study failed to find effects of the stressful examination period on salivary IgA levels. Given that the latter study did obtain serum IgA effects, the explanation may well lie in technical differences. Kiecolt-Glaser *et al.* do point out that salivary IgA levels are dependent on flow rate, which is markedly affected by inadequate hydration. They did not have comparative flow rate data.

Loneliness and Interpersonal Factors

Loneliness suggests a misfit between the desired levels (or intensity) of interpersonal interaction and the actual levels experienced. It is a difficult concept to operationalise because it will undoubtedly be confounded by many other factors. For example, it may be more likely to occur in the transition from one social situation to another (e.g. going from home to university or polytechnic, which is stressful for a significant number of students (Fisher, 1990), and involves many changes some of which may result in temporary feelings of loneliness). Kennedy, Kiecolt-Glaser & Glaser (1988) report a number of studies suggesting that such interpersonal factors do impinge on the immune system. For example, Kiecolt-Glaser *et al.* (1984a) showed that students who were more lonely had poorer immune system responses as evidenced by lower NK cell levels and lower T-cell proliferation to PHA (as well as higher cortisol levels). In a comparative examination of 38 single/divorced women with matched controls who were married, the former showed poorer immunocompetence in terms of a lower percentage of NK cells (7.5% vs. 12.8%), lower blastogenic responsivity to the mitogens ConA and PHA, fewer helper T lymphocytes (26.4% vs. 32.9%), and higher antibody titres to the Epstein–Barr virus viral capsid antigen (520.5 vs 147.2). The single/divorced women also showed a relationship between the perceived attachment to the (ex)-spouse and immune system functioning as measured by mitogen responsivity to ConA and PHA (i.e. those who were more attached showed reduced proliferation responses). Similar effects of separation have also been reported for men and for different viruses, including herpes simplex (Kennedy *et al.*, 1988).

CONCLUSION

The literature does appear to warrant the definite conclusion that psychological factors can markedly affect the immune system, although a clear causal chain has not been established as yet. The mechanisms for understanding how stress has its effects are becoming clearer. A large array of psychological factors have been shown to influence the state of the immune system, although there is some degree of inconsistency across studies. This could be due to a failure to take adequate account of chronic or contextual factors, individual differences, the complexity of the factors involved in events, the relative lack of real longitudinal investigations, and the bias towards the study of major acute stressors. In view of these difficulties it may be that the important role stress plays in disease is better established by a consideration of the disease end-points themselves. The next chapter reviews the evidence that psychological factors do play a causal role in the development of one of the major killers in developed countries—cancer.

Chapter 4

Stress and Cancer

This chapter examines the evidence for the view that psychological factors play a role in the onset of cancer. After some preliminary remarks concerning general issues, the chapter briefly reviews animal evidence. It has only been in this research that adequate experimental controls have been employed. The animal research is characterised, however, by inconsistencies and the examination of a small range of psychologically relevant stressors. The bulk of the chapter discusses research showing what stressors have been linked to human cancer, and considers the concept of cancer-prone personality.

Cancer cells are characterised by their uncontrollable proliferation, invasion of normal tissue, and by their later metastasis. Cancer is the result of a mutational change in the genetic cellular substructures (e.g. DNA, RNA) which may be caused by a whole array of factors including radiation, chemical and inert carcinogens, viruses, hormonal actions, and tissue damage. Carcinogenesis is also moderated by such factors as genetic characteristics, age, the state of the immune system, and species weight (Fox, 1981).

Cancer is the second leading cause of death in developed countries, being responsible for one in five deaths (Fobair & Cordoba, 1982). In the UK the most common malignant cancers in men are trachea, bronchus and lung (ICD number 162); stomach (150); intestine, rectum and rectosigmoid junction (152–154); and pancreas (157) in ranked order. For women the common cancer causes of death are breast (174); intestine, etc., trachea, bronchus and lung, ovary, fallopian tube and broad ligament (183); and cervix uteri (180). For both men and women the most common lethal cancer accounts for around three times as many deaths as the second ranked (OPCS, 1978). Mortality rates for cancer are steadily increasing, particularly for lung cancer (Pollack & Horm, 1980), although there is fossil evidence of cancer in dinosaurs, and in the remains of Java man and Egyptian mummies (Fobair & Cordoba, 1982).

It is probably impossible to prove that stress causes cancer. We have seen that there are many definitions of stress. Cancer is not a single disease but a range of diseases each with its own constellation of multiple causes and therapies. The term is used for over 100 different conditions. Even for a single organ there are different types of disorder. For example, Kreyberg (1962) has shown that there are two histologically distinct types of lung cancer which presumably may have different sets of causal mechanisms. Neoplasms can also have prolonged latencies before clinical identification (see Fox, 1978, pp. 71–2) and it is difficult to identify the onset of malignancy partly because of biochemical ignorance about what universally differentiates cancer cells from normal cells.

Nonetheless, there is a wealth of anecdotal medical evidence dating from the earliest recorded medicine that cancer is related to stress and emotional factors which are inherent in civilised societies (see LeShan, 1959; and Rosch, 1984, for historical reviews).

Recent years have seen a remarkable growth in the weight of scientific evidence to reinforce the suspicion of such a causal relationship. There is widespread belief that psychological factors are unlikely to have major influences in cancer etiology, even among stress proponents working in the field. Solomon & Amkraut (1979), for example, have come to the conclusion that "stress-induced changes in the immune systems are generally small and determine the course of the disease chiefly by shifting the balance between toxic factors and defence mechanisms in disease processes" (p. 220). Bammer (1981) concluded in his review that "There is no known data to support the concept that stress will produce a primary tumour" (p. 154), and Fox (1981) suggests "the contribution of PF (psychological factors) to cancer incidence is probably relatively small...[and] if it exists, is almost certainly specific to certain organ sites, and depends on several things" (p. 148).

These authors may be right. They are certainly informed opinions. It is possible, however, that they underestimate the role of psychological factors in cancer etiology for a number of reasons:

1. The conclusions are based on an examination of a very restricted range of stressors and psychological factors. In animal research this includes such stress as physical restraint, electric shock, and restricted feeding regimes. In the human work the two major areas considered have been personality or emotional mediators and the experience of major life events such as the loss of a central person. This emphasis ignores most psychologically relevant aspects of every-day normal life (e.g. occupational factors). It also pays scant attention to psychological factors which an individual may not themselves perceive as important, including the non-heeded factors which do not command their attention or response. Thus, psychological factors can be 'hidden' in a number of different senses. They can also be theoretically constructed factors such as 'role conflict', or 'job complexity person–environment misfit' which have psychological referents and possible disease consequences but no personally recognised impact or reality. Most of the models outlined in Chapter 1 show how important such aspects are.

2. The animal research is necessarily restricted in the psychological factors it can investigate. Even if we presume that all the findings from animal research were applicable to humans (see Fox, 1981, for a debate relevant to cancer research) animals cannot be exposed to essentially human stressors. Humans may be

affected more by the psychological environment than other animals. It may also be the case that humans show additional strain consequences when exposed to stressors which other animals do not. For example, with humans, an acute stressor can have chronic effects because attentional mediation (and contemplation of it) may reinforce it chronically.

3. What would count as a demonstration that psychological factors cause primary cancer? Could we expect anything other than small effects and apparently contradictory findings from research measuring a few psychological factors measured over a relatively short period, when we are dealing with diseases which have a latent period of several years and where repeated exposure is probably required? Fox (1978) provides a good discussion of some of the difficulties associated with research in this field. It may be that the thrust of the work should consider fundamentally different types of approaches and assumptions. The potential role of psychological factors should not be devalued because their examination is fundamentally difficult. Failure to find consistent and significant relationships between specific psychological factors and cancer measures does not imply that psychological factors other than those observed are not of major importance. Apparently inconsistent findings (for example, that a stressor may enhance or inhibit tumour development in mice) become understandable when other factors are taken into account (e.g. timing of stressor). Subtle actions of this type should not be taken to imply that such factors are less significant or not major causes. On the contrary, the real environment is more complex than the controlled laboratory one.

4. Psychological factors may not be any different in status to physical carcinogens. Whilst a single cigarette may 'cause' lung cancer, research considers whether smoking behaviour in general increases cancer risks. Why should we expect a single life event (or several) to be related to cancer incidence? Perhaps research on environmental stressors should take more cognisance of factors which are not themselves major, but where their interactive and/or cumulative effects may have significant implications for cancer etiology. It is interesting to note that Horne & Picard (1979) observed that a composite psychological measure they generated was as good a predictor of lung cancer risk as smoking history. Eysenck (1988) also reports research showing that the link between lung cancer mortality and cigarette smoking is dramatically affected by the degree to which a person is rational or anti-emotional: the mortality risk associated with the number of cigarettes smoked (for those who smoke in excess of 20 cigarettes per day) is present only for those who score highly on rationality/anti-emotionality.

5. The majority of research on stress and psychological factors and cancer has considered factors which are additional to the general or everyday stresses of living. It may be, however, that psychological factors in our everyday environment produce primary cancers and that our relative failure to observe many other significant relationships is because those psychological factors are themselves major causative agents. In this context, for example, Riley (e.g. 1981) has shown

that removing mice from the stresses of normal housing conditions may reduce the likelihood of tumour growth. Riley's work suggests that basic living is ordinarily stressful enough!

6. Psychological factors might have protective as well as injurious effects. They may cause physiological changes that act as injurious carcinogens or beneficial anticarcinogens (Fox, 1981; Sklar & Anisman, 1981).

One may distinguish between three phases of cancer (Sklar & Anisman, 1981): tumour induction, tumour growth and metastasis. How much sense it makes to ask whether psychological factors can affect these different stages of induction, growth or metastasis, rather than just the clinical development of cancer, is unclear. First, most clinicians would be primarily concerned about clinical manifestations of cancer and whether or not psychological factors may play an important role in the cause of the presented case(s). Second, since it is possible that an animal or person has many non-clinical episodes of cancer which are successfully dealt with by defence systems (e.g. by natural killer cells), the distinction between induction and growth, for example, has fuzzy pragmatic consequences. Nonetheless, it does make sense to distinguish between those psychological factors or stressors which are environmentally based and measurable across a number of individuals (e.g. life events, temperature, electric shocks, social structures) and those which are intra-individual and reflect aspects of personality (e.g. inability to express negative emotions). Previous failure to distinguish between personality factors and situationally dependent factors has been thought to be responsible for apparently inconsistent and contradictory results. Cox & Mackay (1982), for example, end their review of the role of psychosocial factors in the etiology of cancer, by highlighting the "failure to discriminate adequately between fixed personality characteristics as measured, and situationally determined coping strategies as used, which may reflect different psychological processes" (p. 391). It will also be necessary to distinguish between acute and chronic stressors, since there is considerable evidence that they have separable and opposite effects on tumour development (e.g. Sklar & Anisman, 1981).

One difficult question concerns the role of transmitter and hormone responses in the development of cancer. Hormones may be direct carcinogens, as well as playing an important role in tumour growth and vascularisation of solid tumours. In particular, there is considerable evidence that hormones play a major role in breast cancer (e.g. Kirschner, 1977). However, since Marmorston and her colleagues (Marmorston, 1966; Marmorston, Geller & Weiner, 1969) have shown differences in the hormone profiles of lung, prostate and breast cancer, it may be that such hormone mechanisms are site-specific. The role of stress on cancer, as mediated by neuroendocrinal substances, thus becomes a more complex empirical problem to unravel. Fox (1981), for one, has called for differential site-specific stress investigations.

Investigations of the effects of psychological stressors on the etiology of cancer can be difficult to interpret due to the conceptual difficulties inherent when a response-based definition of stress is used. Some researchers, for example, have defined stress by its neuroendocrinal consequences (particularly on adrenal hormones—see Selye's work in Chapter 1) and discuss immunological and neoplastic responses as 'secondary manifestations' (Riley, 1981) of the stress reactions. Adrenal cortical hormones, as well as other hormones, have a marked immunosuppressive effect. Cox & Mackay (1982) provide a readable review of the relationship between hormones and various indices of immunological functioning relevant to cancer. This view logically excludes non-endocrinologically mediated stress effects on carcinogenesis. Some models of stress and cancer (e.g. Cox, 1984; Selye, 1979; Sklar & Anisman, 1981) specifically view the promotion of tumours as mediated by stress-sensitive hormones. There are, however, a number of reasons for hypothesising a direct link between psychological factors and immune function. First, Stein, Keller & Schleifer (1979) provide evidence that the hypothalamus may directly modulate the immune mechanisms. Second, Solomon & Amkraut (1979) report studies in which adrenocorticotrophic hormone (ACTH)-treated animals show no change in tumour size despite an increased production of corticosteroid. Solomon, Merigan & Levine (1967) have reported that the administration of neither ACTH nor corticosterone affected interferon production prior to inoculation with a NDV virus (Newcastle disease virus), although the electric shock stressor did enhance interferon levels if it preceded inoculation. There is also evidence that suffering the bereavement of a spouse has effects on T-cell response in the absence of changes in cortisol, prolactin, growth hormone, and thyroid hormone assays (see Chapter 3, and Bartrop *et al.*, 1977). Such evidence can only be suggestive of a direct metabolic effect of stress on immune function, because other neuroendocrinal systems may be involved. Finally, there is growing evidence of a direct link of the CNS with the immune system (see Chapter 3). Despite the suggestive nature of the evidence of direct influence, it does make it important to adopt a wider definition of 'stress' in order to ensure we do not incorrectly reject possible stress influences in cancer. The disease itself may have a time-course of development of many years, which makes the detection of effects of psychological stress difficult enough even in long-term prospective studies (Fox, 1981; Cox, 1984) without logically excluding them at the outset! This is particularly important in an examination of the role of stress in cancer because the sphere of possible influence should not be confined to virally caused cancers (e.g. cervix, hepatic, lymphatic, nasopharynx) which account for less than 3% of all cancers in human beings (Fox, 1981).

It is widely held that immunological factors substantially influence and control cancer, particularly once neoplastic cells are present. Whilst there is considerable uncertainty about the mechanisms of immunological control, the main cells active against cancer are various T lymphocytes, the T-derivative natural killer cells (and interferon which activates them), polymorphonuclear leucocytes, B lymphocytes (particularly in defence against metastasis) and their immunoglobulins, and macrophages (Castro, 1978). One view of the role of the immune system in the control of cancer is that it acts as a surveillance system which recognises and destroys tumour cells as they appear (Burnet, 1970, 1971; Keast, 1981). Thus, immunodeficiencies of whatever origin will increase the likelihood of the system missing a tumour cell. If psychological factors are immunosuppressive they may, therefore, be expected to be associated with tumour incidence. This 'immunological surveillance' view has been criticised, however, primarily because the immunosuppressed animals exhibit only a restricted range of neoplasms and do not develop spontaneous tumours which one would expect (Moller & Moller, 1978). Alternatively, it may be that psychological stressors interfere with the repair mechanisms which operate to correct errors in cell division. For example, in his analysis of the DNA damage caused by radiation, Little (1977) proposes that the body immediately effects a rapid but error-prone repair which is subsequently checked and corrected by slower mechanisms. If stressors interfere with this mechanism the errors (however caused) will remain, and may result in malignancy within a dozen divisions. It should be noted, however, that the relative importance of immunological factors in tumour development is likely to differ with the different tumour systems: studies by Jamasbi & Nettesheim (1977) and Peters & Kelly (1977) suggest that immunological changes are not very important in determining the effects of stress for some tumours.

Fox (1978) makes a distinction between two types of cancer-causing mechanisms. Cancer may be the direct result of "an agent or mechanism overcoming existing resistance of the body" or an indirect result of "lowered resistance to cancer, which permits a potential carcinogen normally insufficient to produce cancer to do so" (p. 51). It is conceivable at least that different categories of psychological factors can play both causal roles. We need to examine whether such factors can indeed have such effects. Do psychological stressors act as direct carcinogens (with concomitant neuroendocrinological effects)? Do they act simply to moderate the effects of other physical carcinogens? Do they do both?

Eysenck (1984) has pointed out that physical environmental agents do not provide either necessary or sufficient causes of cancer. He quotes the example of cigarette smoking and lung cancer: only 10% of heavy smokers die of lung cancer, and 10% of people who die of lung cancer are non-smokers. Genetic factors play a significant role in cancer (e.g. Lynch, 1981), in the maintenance of smoking behaviours (Eaves & Eysenck, 1980), and in personality variables (psychoticism, extroversion and neuroticism—see Fulker, 1981) which are related to smoking (Eysenck, 1980) and possibly to lung cancer risk (see, for example, the work of Kissen, discussed below). It is clearly not sensible to consider that specific cancers have single necessary and sufficient causes (e.g. cancer as being genetically determined, smoking causing lung cancer). Rather one needs to consider the constellation of relevant factors and the interrelationships between them. An examination of the literature supports the view that the two classes of psychological factors outlined above (personality and life or environmental stressors) play a significant part in cancer etiology. The purpose of the discussion below is to demonstrate that these are important variables in cancer research. They too are unlikely to be necessary or sufficient variables, but their influence on the disease is still of major significance. Before discussing the research on cancer in humans, however, a cursory review of the animal evidence is presented, because it is often in the laboratory that scientifically rigorous links between stress and cancer can be investigated.

PSYCHOLOGICAL STRESSORS

Animal Evidence

In discussing the animal evidence suggesting a link between psychological stressors and cancer, the reader may feel uneasy at labelling some of the stressors as 'psychological' since several of them involve physical assaults on the animals (e.g. electric shock, restraint, rotation). The actual levels of physical assault are, however, generally very minor (especially compared to the surgical or inoculation procedures involved for all animals including the non-stressed controls). For example, Riley's (1981) work on rotation stress involves less than $1g$ force even at the fastest revolution speeds; electric shocks in the work of Nieburgs *et al.* (1979) involved 2.8 mA for 2 s, and in Otis & Scholler (1967) 0.5 mA for 5 s; cold temperatures in Wallace, Wallace & Mills (1944) were 68 °F. These are random examples. Their labelling as 'psychological' is further justified if one bears in mind that their effects on neoplastic growth (if any) are largely determined by abstract properties such as whether the shock is escapable or not, or whether the stressors are predictable. Animals will choose shock up to three times more intense, and lasting up to nine times longer, when it is signalled rather than unpredictable (Harsh & Badia, 1975), for example. Nonetheless it is likely that some of the stressors do have direct metabolic consequences as well as psychologically mediated ones.

A number of stressors have been found to affect different aspects of tumorigenesis and growth. These have been discussed in greater detail by other writers (e.g. Newberry, 1981; Riley, 1979). There is considerable inconsistency in the literature, and it will be apparent that some have an enhancing effect on neoplasia, some an inhibitory effect, and some mixed effects. Some reasons for this are discussed below, but it is difficult to be precise in interpretations because there are not enough studies to allow orthogonal comparisons. Little is known, too, about how some of these variables interact with each other, although some of the explored interactions are mentioned. The major variables explored include:

1. *Early experience of the animals.* Handling young animals, or subjecting them to such stressors as intermittent separation, has been shown to both inhibit (Ader & Friedman, 1965; LaBarba & White, 1971; Newton, Bly & McCrary, 1962) or facilitate (Ader & Friedman, 1965; Levine & Cohen, 1959) tumour growth. It is

possible (Anisman & Sklar, 1984) that the type of effect these stressors have on transplanted cancer growth is determined by the stage of development the animal has reached, although the evidence for this is not strong (see, for example, Otis & Scholler, 1967).

2. *Social isolation.* Animals housed in isolation from very young show greater likelihood of developing spontaneous tumours (Muhlbock, 1951). Using transplanted tumours, Dechambre & Gosse (1968, 1971) report the opposite effects of the stressors. Individually caged mice survived for more than half as many days again compared to those in groups of 10. This difference is not due to the use of transplanted, rather than spontaneous tumours, since Sklar & Anisman (1980) show tumour growth of transplanted mastocytoma to be greater in isolated animals, and Riley (1981) reports the regression rate of implanted lympho-sarcoma was only 60% in isolated mice but ranged from 00% to 100% in other population densities. The previous housing history of the mice may be relevant, but it seems that the contradiction can partly be resolved by considering the effects of change in housing conditions (see (13), below). Sklar & Anisman (1980) also showed that the effects of isolation interact with the effects of acute electric shock. Singly housed mice did not show any effects of tumour enhancement from shock stress.

3. *Cage population density.* It seems that greater population density (up to a limit) is associated with lower cancer incidence. Albert (1967) reports Polish research in which the mice were housed either in pairs or groups of 25 from seven weeks. The latter group exhibited only 22% incidence of tumours, compared to 81% for the pairs. The pairs also had a greater incidence of multiple tumours. Muhlbock (1951) found that animals in groups of 50 had 29% tumour incidence compared to 56% for those housed five per cage, given at least as much floor space per animal. In dimethylbenzanthracene (DMBA)-induced rat tumours, Newberry (1981) reports that tumour latency was greater in animals caged in fours compared to one or eight per cage. However, using transplanted lympho-sarcomas Riley (1981) reports that mice cage densities between three and 20 per cage had no effect on regression rates, and the growth rate of a normally rapidly growing melanoma was not differentially affected by densities from one to 20 in animals housed in low stress conditions.

4. *Physical restraint.* Immobilisation or restraint (e.g animals placed in plastic holder with limbs tied) has been associated with marked inhibition of growth in induced rat tumours (Battacharyya & Pradhan, 1979; Newberry *et al.*, 1976; Pradhan & Ray, 1974). These studies represent a wide variation in the amount of restraint to which the animals are subjected, ranging from some 42 hours over four weeks to 720 hours over six weeks. The Newberry *et al.* (1976) study also suggests the amount of physical activity the animals engaged in is not itself a moderating variable.

5. *Temperature.* There is suggestive evidence that both 'cold' and 'hot' conditions can affect neoplasia. Wallace, Wallace & Mills (1944) report that mice kept

at 19 °C ('cold') who were carrying a mammary tumour virus produced significantly more spontaneous tumours (72%) than those kept at either 32 °C ('hot') or 25 °C (50%). The tumours of the cold mice were larger and appeared earlier. However, Young (1958) found that induced tumours appeared earlier in animals kept at 32 °C than those at 5 °C. Moreover, tumour incidence at 120 days was higher in the hot (67%) than the cold (42%) conditions. These apparently contradictory results could be a result of species or tumour system differences. Other studies using spontaneous tumours, for example, report relative inhibitory effects of 'hot' temperatures (Fuller, Brown & Mills, 1941), and others using induced tumours report inhibitory effects of cooler temperatures. Baker & Jahn (1976), for example, report that *post-carcinogen* cold stress (2 °C) inhibited radiation-induced tumours. Wallace, Wallace & Mills (1942) chemically induced sarcomas in mice and observed that hot conditions (33 °C) promoted sarcoma compared to cool conditions (18 °C). An alternative explanation is that these studies demonstrate that temperature can have protective and harmful effects, and that the actual effect exhibited depends on the interaction of a number of contextual factors including tumour system.

6. *Surgical trauma.* The acute stress of surgery itself has been shown to facilitate tumour growth. For example, pulmonary and liver cancers after intravenous injection of malignant cells are more evident in animals who have undergone the stress of surgery than in those who have not (Saba & Antikatzides, 1976). Such stress also increases the incidence of secondary metastasised tumours and decreases the effects of prior immunopotentiating drugs (Hattori *et al.*, 1982).

7. *Noise* seems to have protective effects in some circumstances. Pradhan & Ray (1974) found that sound stimulation for 90 minutes daily for four weeks resulted in lower final tumour weights in both induced and implanted tumours, compared to controls. In a later study Battacharyya & Pradhan (1979) observed that individually housed rats placed in a crowded cage and subjected to 100 db noise for a total of 72 hours over a six-week period had smaller and lighter DMBA-induced tumours than controls. The fact that there were plasma corticosterone differences between the groups might suggest the involvement of a hormonal axis.

8. *Electric shocks* also have some inhibitory effects on tumour development. In animals housed individually, Newberry *et al.* (1972) observed that chronic shock regimes lasting up to 24 hours consisting of 30 shocks lasting 0.5–1.5 minutes every 15–60 minutes, produced a significant reduction in the number of induced tumours without affecting latency to first tumour or their size. Nieburgs *et al.* (1979) also reported an inhibition of tumour induction with a 90-day shock regime, although the rate of growth was enhanced. A 150-day regime resulted in enhanced tumorigenesis, but smaller tumours. Reznikoff & Martin (1957), on the other hand, report no effects on spontaneous tumours of daily shocks administered for more than six months to mice who did not carry the mammary tumour virus. Moreover, infected shocked animals did not have a higher incidence

of tumours than non-stressed infected mice, although the tumours tended to appear earlier.

9. *Hormone invasion.* Riley (1981) reports that implantation of slow-release corticosterone pellets in female mice produced marked enhancement of the growth of virally induced tumours. Exogenous corticoids (e.g. dexamethasone) have also been shown to inhibit induced tumours (Slaga, Thomson & Smuckler, 1975) and facilitate transplanted tumours (Riley, 1981).

10. *Non-oncogenic viral invasion.* A slowly growing melanoma can develop into a rapidly growing one in mice injected with a non-oncogenic virus. The virus may also enhance the growth of implanted lymphocarcinoma in mice who would otherwise have shown complete regression (Riley, 1981).

11. *Unpredictability of stressor.* It is known that unpredictable shock produces greater hormonal stress reactions than predictable shock (Weiss, 1970) and that animals will choose predictable shock if given the option (Gliner, 1972). Newberry (1981) reports experiments to test the predictability hypothesis. Using either predictable or varied restraint daily for between 10 and 14 hours for mice from age 59 until 445 days, the varied stimulation produced significantly more tumours (42%) than the predictable restraint (7%). It is interesting to note than control mice showed a 13% incidence, and that the ratio of thymus weight to adrenal weight did not parallel the pattern of tumour development. In a study using rats, Newberry *et al.* (1972) found that chronic electric shock stress had a smaller *inhibitory* effect on induced tumours if the stressor was signalled than if it was not.

12. *Lack of control over stressor.* Inescapable shock, but not escapable shock, has been shown to increase the rejection of transplanted non-syngenic tumours (Visintainer, Volpicelli & Seligman, 1982). It may be that the ability of the animal to make a coping response, even if this does not remove the shock itself, has physiological consequences (Davis *et al.*, 1977). It has been suggested that fighting might also act as a coping response (Anisman & Sklar, 1984): mice who engage in fighting do not show any enhancement of tumour growth when their housing conditions are changed (Sklar & Anisman, 1980), and they also show increased resistance to a sarcoma virus (Amkraut & Solomon, 1972).

13. *Change in conditions* per se. It has been suggested that some of the observed effects of stressors may be a result of the *change* in conditions the animal experiences, and not the conditions themselves. For example, the effects of social isolation on tumour enhancement are greatest in mice who were previously reared under social conditions, and previously isolated mice exhibit marked tumour enhancement if subsequently placed in communal cages (Dechambre, 1981; Sklar & Anisman, 1980).

14. *Timing of stressor.* It seems that stressors can themselves have 'stress inoculation effects' under some circumstances. A number of studies suggest that the temporal relationship between the stressor and the cancer induction procedure is of critical importance in determining the effect of the stressor on the tumour. In general, if the stressor is presented prior to the microorganism or antigen the

effect is one of inhibition of tumour growth or incidence. If, on the other hand, the stressor occurs after the antigen there is increased mortality and enhanced growth. Palmblad (1981) has suggested that the stressor initially depresses host defence, after which a period of enhanced resistance follows. Amkraut & Solomon (1972) observed that four hour/day periods of unpredictable electric shocks given for three days prior to inoculation with a sarcoma virus produced a reduction in the size and incidence of tumours. Electric shock following inoculation, however, significantly increased tumour incidence and growth. Riley (1981) found that dexamethasone administered a week before lympho-sarcoma implantation resulted in inhibition of tumour growth. Administration of a chemical closely related to dexamethasone, at different stages after implantation, enhanced growth to a degree related to the time after transplantation. No effects were present after 21 days. Rotation stress four to six days after sarcoma virus inoculation significantly enhanced tumour growth, whereas mice rotated three days before inoculation showed tumour inhibition.

Reasons for Inconsistencies in the Animal Literature

In attempting to review the evidence on how environmental psychological factors affect the incidence and course of animal cancers, one is struck by the variability and inconsistency present in the evidence. The major question to be addressed is whether this lack of consistency reflects the fact that no (strong) relationship exists between such stressors and cancer, whether it reflects inadequate conceptualisation of the 'stressors' in relation to the cancers investigated (as implied by the findings on stressor predictability, control, and change *per se*), or whether it is a result of differences in methodological procedures, species, and tumour systems considered. Some of these aspects are discussed below:

Strain differences

There are marked differences between strains in cancer susceptibility for 'spontaneous' tumours, virally inoculated induced cancer, and tumour–host histocompatibility. Some strains are highly susceptible and others highly resistant to cancer. For example, mice strains C3H/A and C3H/Afb show almost 100% incidence of sponta-neous liver and mammary tumours (Sabine, Horton & Wicks, 1973). Strains CBA/Ht and WHT/Ht, on the other hand, show few spontaneous episodes (Hewitt, Blake & Walder, 1976). Careful study of different rat strains also reveals marked differences in incidence rates for many cancer sites (MacKenzie & Gardner, 1973). In studies involving tumour implantation, histocompatibility is strain dependent and tumour growth interacts with the effects of the stressor. For example, under non-stressful conditions, C3H/He mice exhibit minimal growth with regression of an implanted lymphosarcoma, while the more histocompatible C3H/Bi strain show a rapid sustained increase in tumour volume. When subjected to 45 revolutions per minute rotation stress for 10 minutes of each hour four to six days after implantation, however, the C3H/He strain develop tumours with almost identically shaped growth curves as the C3H/Bi strain (Riley, 1981). Strain differences can be relatively subtle, which makes it difficult to control all relevant variables. The C3H strains, for example, are unlike some other strains inasmuch as they do not show a significant reactivity/age decline to haemagglutinin challenge. Moreover, genetic–environmental interactions can be quite marked. For example, Sabine *et al.* (1973) found that the same C3H strains demonstrating 100% spontaneous tumours when reared in the United States showed an almost 0% rate when reared in Australia! Kakihana, Noble & Butte (1968) found that although two mouse strains showed similar corticosterone responses to a range of stressors, ethanol increased the response in one strain and decreased it in the other.

Species differences

There are differences between species in cancer incidence and sites affected. Purchase (1980), for example, in a large review, observed that 8% of the 250 chemicals he investigated were non-carcinogenic in mice only, compared to 38% in rats only. Furthermore, in the species-common carcinogenic substances, 36% produced tumours with no species-common site. Different species may show different patterns of reaction to other challenges. For example, Fox (1981) suggests that few cancers in humans are thought to be viral in origin, whereas a large number of spontaneous rodent cancers are viral. Mice show a significant propensity to develop viral mammary cancer. Rats, on the other hand, rarely develop mammary cancer spontaneously (Newberry, 1981). Thus the rat work has developed using chemically induced tumours, or transplanted tumours. DMBA-induced mammary carcinogenesis (a common substance in these cancer studies) occurs as a result of its hormonal action through the adreno-corticolytic system, which is why it is thought to be particularly stressor-sensitive. In mice, however, subjecting animals to daily *unpredictable* stress restraint regimes from 59 to 445 days resulted in 42% tumour incidence, compared to 7% for mice given the same amount of restraint which was *predictable*, and 13% for control mice (Newberry, 1981). Using the same restraint procedures with rats, on the other hand, Newberry *et al.* (1976) observed that restraint administered from 35 to 108 days inhibited DMBA feeding-induced tumours. In fact a whole array of stressors facilitate mammary cancer in mice, but have none or the opposite effect on induced rat cancers (Newberry, 1981).

Treatment differences

Tumour systems. For experimental and theoretical reasons it does not always make sense to wait for spontaneous neoplasms to develop. Whilst animals can be bred to show enhanced propensities to develop particular cancers, many treatments are adopted to examine the influence of stressor on cancer growth. This may involve the feeding or introduction of chemical carcinogens (e.g. DMBA), inoculation with' viruses (e.g. the Maloney sarcoma virus-induced tumours, or MSV), the transplantation of tumours to a host animal (e.g. 6C3HED lymphosarcoma), and so on. Whilst such procedures are perfectly valid, and allow an examination of stressor effects on different aspects of immune functioning and neoplastic development, there is a considerable need for careful orthogonal comparisons of the effects of a range of particular stressors on different tumour systems. The use of histocompatible tumour systems means that the observed effects of stress may be a result of the allograft rejection response.

Stressor regimes. We have already seen that different types of physical restraint used to stress mice may have quite different effects. Restraint unpredictability may be considered quite a subtle stressor. Other stressor differences have been investigated. One major dimension likely to be of considerable importance is that of acute–chronic stressors. Chronicity is a matter of degree, since 'acute' stressors usually involve the animal being subjected to the stressor a large number of times and often in repeated sessions. Neiburgs *et al.* (1979) used Sprague-Dawley rats in seven experiments to investigate the effects of different numbers and times of stressor administration on various indices including DMBA mammary tumorigenesis, blood lymphocytes, thymus and adrenals. Unfortunately the statistical analysis is rather crude, but a number of findings are relevant here. The effects of stressors on tumorigenesis were different for the different stressors used and the length of the stress period after DMBA administration. Exposure for five minutes every 96 hours on a 90-day regime of cold swim and handling enhanced tumour induction, whilst mild electric shock to the tail inhibited tumour induction but enhanced the rate of growth. A 150-day stress regime, however, produced more tumours, but all three stressors produced much smaller tumours compared to the controls. This inhibited tumour growth was also associated with more large lymphocytes and fewer small lymphocytes in the handling and cold swim conditions. Sklar & Anisman (1979) report an experiment exploring the effects of acute and chronic stressors using the viable syngenic P815 mastocytoma injected in DBA/2J male mice. The acute stressor consisted of 60 six-second, electric shocks in one session, 24 hours after transplantation. Chronic stressor conditions involved repeated daily sessions for either five or 10 days. Compared to non-shocked controls, the acutely stressed animals exhibited earlier tumour appearance, considerable enhancement of tumour growth and shorter survival times. These effects were, however, mitigated in the 10-day group, who exhibited inhibition of tumour growth. Sklar & Anisman (1981) also report that this inhibition is not simply a consequence of the stressor being applied later after transplantation, since a single session on day 5 results in tumour enhancement.

The experiments of Nieburgs *et al.* (1979) suggested that the type of stressor used may affect the chronicity outcome. Sklar & Anisman (1981) have suggested that stressors which are social rather than physical in nature are not affected by the chronicity of the exposure. They quote well-known studies by Andervont (1944), Henry, Stephens & Watson (1975) and Riley (1975), which involved (respectively) social isolation (vs. eight mice per cage), social change (of various types including same and mixed sex groups, large mixed colonies, removing litters after birth), and environmentally unprotected cages with frequent handling (vs. protected cages, little handling). In each case animals could be examined at different stages of a long period (e.g. 19 months in Henry *et al.*). Whilst the various stressors had significant effects on tumour incidence, no changes in the qualitative nature of the stressor/ neoplasia relationship occurred.

An alternative explanation of the failure to find chronicity effects in these studies is that they all involve spontaneous tumours. However, in experiment 4 of Newberry (1978) DMBA rats subjected to restraint stress for various lengths of time from day 30 until day 150 showed similar rates in increased tumour appearance once the restraint regime ceased, although the no-restraint controls and the continual-restraint group produced no such quadratic trends. This suggests that stressor chronicity did not affect the stressor-inhibition effect. It is difficult to say whether the different effects are tumour- or species-specific, especially since the terms 'acute' and 'chronic' have been defined relative to the stressor regimes adopted by different experimenters.

Housing conditions.   Riley (1981) has suggested that one reason for some of the contradictions in the literature are differences in the general housing conditions of the animals. He maintains that conventional rodent housing facilities "are not suitable for the maintenance of quiescent baseline values of the stress-associated hormonal and cellular elements that influence or control immunological and thus pathological processes" (p. 1101), and this makes it impossible to perform critical experiments with any confidence. His laboratory have developed 'low stress housing' which provides control of a number of variables which may be important in cancer research. Animals housed in these conditions also show baseline corticosterone levels 10–20 times lower than those housed under conventional conditions. The protective housing requires no air recirculation, soundproofing, elimination of noises, vibration and draughts, reduction of handling and cage-cleaning procedures, control of light, segregation of males and females and experimental from control animals etc.

Definitional problems

These differences do reveal the difficulties of using an imprecise or unclear concept of what is meant by stress. This imprecision is a consequence of the concept itself, and has led to different writers adopting different strategies to cope with the problem. Fox (e.g. 1978) uses the term 'psychological factors and/or stress'. Newberry (1981), on the other hand, side-steps the definitional problem with his consistent use of 'presumably stressful conditions'. Riley (1979) suggests that it might be helpful to employ a wider set of descriptive adjectives instead of the word 'stress' (or rather 'distress' in Selye's terms—see Chapter 1) and distinguishes between mild 'anxiety-stress' for stressors such as slow speed rotation; 'fear/rage stress' for physical restraint, electric shock, and social or territorial conflict; 'metabolic stress' for extremes of temperature, physical exhaustion or calorific intake. It seems that such distinctions beg the question if one considers the 'psychological' consequences of the stressors on the organisms, which clearly have somatic consequences.

Hormonal effects

If hormonal and immune systems are independent to the degree that stressors can have direct effects on immunological functioning without concomitant changes in hormonal balance, the interaction of hormonal factors needs careful examination. Riley (1981), for example, has observed that plasma corticosterone concentration increases linearly with rotational stress speed. Rotation stress (45 revolutions per minute) also enhances tumour growth after MSV inoculation, compared to controls. Mice with implanted slow-release corticosterone pellets, however, show more than twice the tumour volume growth 11 days after inoculation compared to the rotation stress animals. The fact that Riley also reports that the injection of a non-oncogenic virus (e.g. lactate dehydrogenase-elevating or LDH) also enhances tumour growth shows that assaults of different types on the organism may subtly affect neoplastic development, and suggests that the interactions of these different assaults require careful analysis.

HUMAN STUDIES

In the first part of this section the evidence that suggests environmental psychological stressors cause cancer will be reviewed. In the second part some of the research implicating personality factors as moderators of cancer susceptibility will be outlined. Whether or not psychological factors cause human cancer, they have been shown to discriminate cancer patients from controls. For example, Cramer *et al.* (1977) report that responses on a psychosocial questionnaire successfully discriminated between 40 cancer and 40 matched controls with more than 95% success rate. Factors such as perceptions of isolation, repression of aggression and of somatic symptoms, denial of fears, change in core family size and religious moralism were used in the discriminant function analysis.

Some Considerations

A number of points need to be borne in mind when considering the human work on stress and cancer. First, we have seen from the animal literature that acute stressors may have quite different effects on neoplasia compared to chronic stressors. In the human literature the distinction is difficult to make, as is the distinction between the contribution of stressors and personality or individual differences: the response to a stressor will depend partly upon personality differences. There is a sense in which the death of a loved one is an acute stressor. Such events do, however, usually have chronic consequences and this is, to some extent, dependent upon how the person reacts emotionally to events, as well as their social circumstances. They may change the social network of the surviving partner as well as having long-term effects on their psychological health. The role of social support in health is important (e.g. Cohen & McKay, 1984) and plays a major role in some models of stress (e.g. Payne & Fletcher, 1983). The relationship between depression and cancer has also received considerable attention (see below). It is very difficult to say that the loss of a significant person, rather than any resulting depression, is a contributory cause in the appearance of a tumour. This difficulty is, however, due to methodological and empirical problems, not to a lack of theoretical clarity.

Second, in human research it is very difficult to know what type of controls to employ. It would, of course, seem important to make sure that standard cancer risk factors are controlled (e.g. smoking history, age, social class), although this is often not done. A common technique is to compare people with a malignant cancer of a particular site to matched controls who have a non-malignant disorder of the same site. Sometimes this can be done without the subjects being aware of the diagnosis (e.g. breast carcinoma group vs. fibrocystic disease as in Biondi & Pancheri, 1985). However, such comparisons reduce the likelihood of finding any effects because patients with benign diseases may have higher stress levels than non-patients. Thus the otherwise well-designed study of 165 female breast biopsy patients by Muslin, Gyarfas & Pieper (1966), which failed to find any difference between malignant and benign groups in the loss of a significant close person or relative, leaves open the possibility that loss contributed to growths in both groups. The same could be true of similar studies which have failed to find effects between malignant and benign groups in terms of the amount of life changes that they have experienced.

Psychodynamic models of disease (e.g. Graham, 1972) also leave open the possibility that particular attitudes predispose a person to site-specific diseases without the corollary that they be disease-specific. To ensure that any observed difference between such groups is due to premorbid factors (and not a result of the knowledge that something major may be wrong, for example) prospective studies may seem necessary. However, even the use of such studies does not exclude two important possibilities. The supposed strength of prospective studies is that causal attribution can be made with greater certainty if measured psychological variables discriminate between cancer and case-control subjects. It should be borne in mind, however, that psychological stressors may have nonspecific disease effects (just as Selye's GAS posits nonspecificity) and that it is how the disease is manifested that is largely a matter of chance, even if the occurrence of *a* disease is under the control of psychological variables. Recent work, for example, shows that so-called 'coronary-prone personalities' may have generally enhanced risks for a number of diseases. Rime *et al.* (1989), for example, examined nearly 2000 adults and found that type A subjects were more likely to report not only CHD but also peptic ulcers, thyroid problems, asthma, and rheumatoid arthritis. Bahnson & Bahnson (1964) have suggested that "cancer is an alternative to psychosis", and that stressors may manifest themselves in different ways. Witzel (1970) reports that cancer patients, compared to patients with other diseases, were less likely to have experienced other illnesses, had less operations, or been out- or in-patients. Rassidakis (with Kelepouris, Goulis & Fox, 1971; with Kelepouris, Goulis & Karaiossefidis, 1972; with Erotokristov, Volidou & Collarou, 1973) shows that schizophrenic patients have a low cancer risk. One should also not forget that over time (and especially many years, as in the case of prospective studies) many variables change in a person's circumstances, lifestyle, self-perception, attitudes, and aspects of personality. Only some of these (or an aggregate, or interaction of any or some of them) are likely to have a bearing on disease. Prospective studies need to account for such dynamic changes. (Discussions of methodology and psychosocial oncology can be found in Cooper, 1988; Paykel & Rao, 1984 ; and Temoshok & Heller, 1984).

Third, if psychological stressors may *inhibit* cancer development, as they have been observed to do in the animal research, the impact of the psyche on cancer will necessarily be underestimated in the human work. This is particularly the case in prospective studies where the discriminatory analyses of cases versus controls will decrease the likelihood of detecting such factors.

Fourth, if the effects of stressors on cancer are as subtle as the animal literature would make it appear, human studies need to do more than take cognisance of a only a few broad psychological factors.

Fifth, as has already been touched upon, the attribution of causality in this field is difficult, principally for methodological reasons. There are two broad options in assessing the possible evidence. We can take a hard line from the outset by comparing alternative likely classes of causes (e.g. physical carcinomas vs. psychological causes) which are considered independent and mutually exclusive. Effectively, this is admitting that no evidence of the type we are likely to be able to collect relevant to psychological factors could produce proof of a causal link. Alternatively, we can use the term 'cause' in a relativistic manner. That is, we ask the question 'How well do the studies demonstrate a strong association within the pragmatic constraints under the control of the investigator?'. The former criterion is usually adopted on the grounds that it is more 'scientific' or 'objective'. In their review of stress and cancer, for example, Sklar & Anisman (1981) conclude their evaluation of the human research by saying "It is, of course, inappropriate to infer causation or modification of cancer development from these human studies…causal relations between these variables remain to be demonstrated" (p. 374). What could, in principle, count as such a demonstration? Is it not rather peculiar to hamstring such investigations from the outset: such a criterion need only be adopted when there are better ways of deciding on the potentially causal role of psychological factors in cancer *in practice*.

Unfortunately, the human literature, like the animal research, is full of positive findings on the one hand, and failures to replicate these findings on the other. There is, therefore, not simply the problem of using inappropriate criteria to assess the work, but variability in the results. This is clearly a serious problem when trying to draw patterns of interpretation from the research findings. This has led some writers to question whether there is any link between premorbid psychological variables and cancer onset. It also makes easy fodder for those wishing to espouse a purely 'physical' basis for cancer (for example, the idea that cancer may be a product of purely chance exposure to cosmic rays, natural radiation, etc.). Questioning whether psychological factors may cause cancer is not synonymous with having no evidence and having to accept this variability in data as a demonstration that there is no causal link. Fox (1978, 1982) is very critical of what evidence is available, but is careful to point out that there is nonetheless some evidence, and in any case the failure to produce very strong positive evidence "does not prove the null hypothesis. It is merely not inconsistent with it" (1982, p. 289). It is important to belabour this point for a number of reasons. We have already considered some of the pragmatic methodological difficulties which make finding positive evidence something of a long shot. We have also reviewed the literature which demonstrates that psychological factors can exert marked effects on endocrine and immune system function. For example, emotional stimuli have been shown to affect the reactivity of both B and T cells (Monjan & Collector, 1977) and antibody response (Edwards & Dean, 1977). In humans, Greene and his associates (1978) have shown a positive relationship between life event change and lymphocyte cytotoxicity. We have also discussed some of the extensive animal work which supports a role for direct effects of stress on tumour development. There is also considerable work on the relationship between neurochemistry and tumorigenesis (see e.g. Sklar & Anisman, 1981; Anisman & Sklar, 1984). Rao (1970), for example, reports a discriminant function analysis based on steroid abnormalities which was better than 90% accurate in categorising lung cancer and non-cancer patients.

A number of conclusions might be drawn from considering this body of evidence:

1. Those aspects of the immune system and the neuroendocrine system which have been shown to be modified by psychological factors/stressors may not play a significant role in neoplastic growth.
2. The research on animals, whilst more direct in implicating a role for stress in cancer, cannot be applied to humans.
3. Psychological factors may play an important role in the onset and growth of cancer, although there is not yet sufficient evidence to warrant strong conclusions about what role.

Whilst (1) is a possibility, the evidence so far presented would not make it reasonable unless further work on the immune and/or neuroendocrine system revealed such mechanisms. Point (2) has been seriously discussed by Fox (1978). There are good reasons to question the generalisability of the animal work to human beings, but there are also good reasons to believe there is sufficient commonality of mechanisms to make some aspects of the comparison reasonable. It would seem particularly perverse to take the stance that psychological factors can affect animal but not human cancer. It would seem reasonable to think the effects may be more marked in humans, but also rather more subtle.

PSYCHOLOGICAL STRESSORS IN CANCER

Life Events as Carcinogens

The work of Holmes & Rahe, which we have discussed in Chapter 2, was an attempt to quantify the life changes that occur, and to demonstrate that the degree of such change is related to the likelihood of physical illness. Some of the most heavily weighted life events in the SRRS refer to the death of a family member or other significant person. The experience of such actual or threatened significant loss has been attributed as a possible causal factor in the onset of cancer.

Paediatric cancer

A study by Greene & Miller (1958) on paediatric lymphocytic and myelogenous leukaemia showed that 31 of the 33 children had experienced at least one loss or separation within the previous two years, and many within the previous six months. Subsequent work by Greene & Swisher (1969), which implicated psychological stressors in the onset of leukaemia, was also able to rule out genetic predisposition as a major factor by using monozygotic twins who were discordant for the illness.

Jacobs & Charles (1980) studied the families of 25 children with various cancers and a comparison group of children with other diseases over a two-year period. The Holmes & Rahe Schedule of Recent Experiences was used to form the basis of a semi-structured interview with the children and at least one parent. In addition, an open-ended interview explored other relevant aspects of the children's domestic background. It was found significantly more of the cancer group were the result of unplanned pregnancies. More importantly, however, the mean score of Life Change Units (LCUs) of this group was more than double that of the control group, and they had also experienced more than twice the number of significant life events in the preceding year. This suggests that it was the cumulative effect of several life events, and not a single significant event, that distinguished the history of the two groups. It was noticeable, however, that 12 of the 43 individual life events produced significantly different frequencies of occurrence across the two groups, nine of them being more frequent in the cancer group. These included marital separation (32% vs. 12%), death of a close family member (20% vs. 4%), change in residence (72% vs. 24%), change in the number of arguments with spouse (20% vs. 4%), change in the health of some other family member (60% vs. 24%) and change in schools (56% vs. 32%). This study suggests, therefore, that psychologically important

factors may play a major role in the development of childhood cancer, although it
does suffer the weaknesses of being a retrospective study.

Adult cancer and the role of early child–parent relationships

There is evidence which supports the view that emotional factors in childhood
may affect propensity to develop cancer in adulthood. Bahnson (1981) suggests that
early family patterns may make people defensive, repressive and lacking in self-
communication, and subsequently affect their cancer risk. He reports two studies
of relevance in this context. The first (Bahnson, 1979) utilised the Roe Parent–Child
Relationship Questionnaire and showed that cancer patients, unlike various types
of control groups, saw their parents as having been cold, and uninvolved with them
as children. The second (Wryc, 1979) analysed the written responses of women
to topics including 'dialogues with my mother'. Apparently, careful analysis of the
texts revealed that breast cancer patients perceived their childhood relations with
their parents as stressed or lacking in aspects of the normal parental role, compared
to the responses of a matched group of women without breast cancer. An early study
by Bacon, Renneker & Cutler (1952), using psychoanalytic methodology, also
reported that breast cancer patients tended, amongst other things, to exhibit unresolved
conflict with their mothers which dated back to childhood.

The studies reported above were retrospective in nature. A major prospective
research project by Thomas and her associates (Duszynski, Shaffer & Thomas, 1981;
Shaffer, Duszynski & Thomas, 1982; Thomas,1976; Thomas & Duszynski, 1974;
Thomas & Greenstreet, 1973; Thomas, Duszynski & Shaffer, 1979), however, reinforces the view that *closeness to parents* is a critical factor discriminating between
people who subsequently develop cancer and others. A cohort of 1337 students who
graduated from Johns Hopkins Medical School between 1948 and 1964 were initially
screened physiologically and psychologically. To investigate family relationships
the Family Attitude Questionnaire was developed (Thomas *et al.*, 1979) which considered aspects of how the students perceived their parents' attitude to them, their
attitude to their parents, aspects of closeness to parents, and of relationships between
parents. The group have been monitored for many years. The investigators' aim was
to isolate any psychophysiological precursors of the onset of disease with particular
attention being paid to six classes of disorder (hypertension, coronary heart disease,
malignant cancer, suicide, mental illness and emotional disturbance). The finding
of relevance in this context was that students who subsequently developed cancers
(especially the major cancers, as opposed to squamous and basal cell carcinoma)
tended to perceive themselves as less close to their parents than those with none
of the disorders. In particular, father–son relationships demonstrated the strongest
link with cancer. Indeed the closeness to parents reported by the cancer patients
was the same as that shown by the individuals who later committed suicide or
suffered affective disorders, although cancer patients rated much lower on matri-
archal dominance.

Although the prospective nature of this study has resulted in small numbers of cancer patients, the questionnaires used have not been well validated, and the results are applicable only to males, the study is impressive. It does suggest that unresolved psychological problems related to child–parent interactions may have consequences for the appearance of particular disorders many years later. It is important to note that the inclusion of a number of disease categories, and the differential pattern of results for each one, suggest that the findings have specific relevance to cancer. Moreover, since the cancer groups did not produce higher scores than healthy controls on the scales that measured depression, anxiety, and anger (using the Habits of Nervous Tension Questionnaire—Thomas & McCabe, 1980), the study suggests that these are not part of the causal nexus in the etiology of the cancers. Later analysis of 913 men (Shaffer, Duszynski & Thomas, 1982) statistically controlling for various known cancer risk factors (smoking, drinking, radiation exposure) has substantiated the earlier view that the cancer–healthy group differences may have a psychosocial basis. In this study the nature of father–son relationships still discriminated cancer from control subjects after possible mediating and artifactual variables were statistically controlled. Closeness to parents is, of course, likely to be affected by many factors (e.g. family size, parental work, other relationships) and prospective studies of this type cannot possibly take into account such factors, except by the use of case–controls, which is a technique with inherent weaknesses despite its apparent attractiveness. It should also be noted that this Precursors study failed to find that the frequency of a number of traumatic life events during early childhood (including death of a parent or sibling, parental divorce, being the youngest child for less than two years) was related to illness in later life (Duszynski, Shaffer & Thomas, 1981), although the trend was in the predicted direction. Sampling only four events from early childhood does not, of course, provide a full picture of possibly significant life events.

Loss of a significant person during adulthood

The loss of a significant close person has been associated with cancer patients in many studies, although like most studies in this field they have been the subject of considerable criticism (e.g. Bieliauskas & Garron, 1982; Cooper, 1988). There does seem to be a discrepancy between clinical judgments of contributory factors and the perceived status of scientific evidence. LeShan (1977), who has studied more than 400 cancer patients, has reported that 72% of the patients had suffered the loss of a significant close relationship within the eight years preceding the illness. The comparable loss of control groups was 10%. In his early major review of psychological states as factors in the development of malignant disease, LeShan (1959) had concluded that the loss of a major relationship prior to the first noted symptom of neoplasia was the most consistently reported psychosocial factor. Greene (1966) reports on the psychosocial setting of 109 men and women with leukaemia and lymphoma. He presents well-structured clinical analyses which suggest strongly that loss, or threat of the loss, of a significant relationship through death or divorce may have contributed to the reticuloendothelial malignancy. For example, in a study of 32 women patients there were 105 such losses or separations which occurred during the four-year prodromal period, the median point being at 12 months. Greene suggests that such losses bankrupt the psychological resources of the person 'engendering shame and hopelessness', which may be relevant to the pathogenesis of the malignancies.

A number of scientifically controlled studies do not support these observations. Muslin, Gyarfas & Pieper (1966) considered losses of first-degree relatives and close friends in the first nine years of childhood and in the immediately preceding three years, in 165 women undergoing breast biopsy. Standard questionnaires were administered before the outcomes were known. After the diagnosis 37 patients found to have malignant growths were age/education matched with those with benign growths. No difference was found in the number or type of losses these two groups had experienced. Greer & Morris (1975) report a similar negative finding. Other studies utilising various measures of life event change and trauma (e.g. Holmes & Rahe's Schedule of Recent Experience, in which relationship loss is a major event) have failed to observe cancer–control differences (Biondi & Pancheri, 1985; Hagnell, 1966; Grissom, Weiner & Weiner, 1975; Graham *et al.*, 1971; Schonfield, 1975; Snell & Graham, 1971), although it should be pointed out once more that these studies have primarily concerned themselves with women who have breast growths where a benign group acts as a matched control for those with malignancies. Inadequate control comparisons may result in underestimation of the role of psychological factors in cancer onset. For example, in the study by Snell & Graham (1971) more than half of the control group had cancer of a site other than the breast. Moreover, those studies which research women prior to the results of breast biopsy are probably more likely to obtain emotionally distorted data for all women, because the patients doubtless realise that they may have malignant cancer. This may not be such an obvious possibility with other cancer sites (e.g. lung, stomach, colorectum).

There are a number of reasons to believe, in spite of this evidence, that the loss of a significant relationship may have effects on cancer onset. The first are the numerous methodological issues we have already raised which make type II errors more likely than is comfortable. Second, there is evidence from other studies which supports the contention that loss is implicated in cancer. In a review by Joseph & Syme (1982), for example, nine out of 10 studies were consistent with this view. Moss (1979) reports on a large number of individuals followed for nine years. Those suffering from divorce or marital separation had three times the risk of dying from cancer which was not attributable to smoking behaviour or cancer present before the loss. Kissen (1966) interviewed patients admitted for chest disorders prior to diagnoses, and determined cases from controls after 'blind' data collection. Lung cancer patients revealed a significantly greater number of cases of the death of a parent during childhood. In another study of lung cancer, Horne & Picard (1979) reported that the experience of a 'recent significant loss' (which included the loss of a job as well as significant persons) was the best of five subscales in predicting the actual diagnosis of the subsequent medical investigations (the others being childhood instability, job stability, marriage stability, lack of future plans). Prior to data collection all 110 subjects had an undiagnosed subacute or chronic lung lesion which was visible by roentgenographic examination. Forty-four patients were found to have malignant tumours. Interestingly, the psychological data derived from the patients were up to twice as good a predictor of final diagnosis as smoking history. A greater number of the malignant group were separated or divorced. This study also showed that job instability and lack of future plans were more marked in the malignant patients.

Other studies show that life events discriminate cancer patients from others. Smith & Sebastian (1976) used structured interviews to examine critical life incidents of 44 cancer patients and their matched controls with other physical disorders. The critical events examined were very wide-ranging and were rated for frequency, intensity and duration on a 15-point scale. The cancer group had experienced such events more frequently and with greater emotional intensity than the control patients. This study is useful in demonstrating one possible weakness of using the Holmes & Rahe scale to measure life events. The Schedule of Recent Experiences or Social Readjustment Rating Scale does not, by its very design, permit individual perceptions (of the patient or the clinician) of the impact of life events to be given additional weight. The score obtained on the scale is determined by reference to average perceptions of others. It may be, of course, that cancer patients react differently to life events compared to other patients. Indeed the work reviewed in the section on cancer and personality suggests this is a very important aspect of cancer etiology.

It may be that the SRE or SRRS is particularly unsuited to the job it has been put to so often in this area. The desire for objectivity of measurement has ignored the rich tapestry of human experience. We should not be surprised, therefore, that clinical report and some studies using such measuring instruments apparently contradict each other.

There are, nonetheless, some other studies which have shown cancer–control differences using the SRRS. For example, Lehrer (1980) obtained Life Change Unit scores from 40 colorectal cancer patients, 14 gastric cancer patients and 10 healthy controls. He found a significantly higher LCU score relating to the two years prior to the onset of first tumour symptoms in the stomach cancer patients (mean = 181), compared to either the colorectal patients (110) or the healthy controls (93). In addition, Lehrer observed a significant negative correlation between age and the amount of life change for those with gastric cancer (−0.68). No such trend was found in the other two groups. The data, therefore, support the view that life change, or the concomitant emotional stress it produces, may be a predisposing factor in gastric cancer, and that a smaller amount of life change is necessary to precipitate the onset of such cancer in older people.

These studies might also suggest that some cancer sites are more likely to be affected by psychological variables than others. This has to remain a moot point since there is simply not enough evidence to begin making such assertions, although Fox (1978) has suggested some reasons why we might expect this to be so. Breast cancer has been most extensively studied and has resulted in the greatest controversy. However, even if the evidence implicating loss or other life events in the etiology of this cancer is not sound, there is a considerable body of evidence suggesting that other psychological factors play a major role.

Hopelessness, depression and cancer

One reason why life events and cancer onset have produced conflicting results may be that some people are affected more than others by such events, or affected in different ways, only some of which are pathogenic. We will be considering personality variables in the next section. Of relevance here, however, is the role of felt hopelessness or depression in cancer. Engel (1968) and Schmale (1972) have proposed that a psychological state of hopelessness or helplessness may be a precursor to illness in general. This general idea has been put to the test in relation to cancer in excellent work by Schmale & Iker (1964, 1966a, 1966b, 1971). These studies are particularly good because all the subjects were women who had positive cervical smear tests (class III Papanicolaou cells, which is considered suspicious but not diagnostic of cancer) and were reporting for a cone biopsy. Thus all patients had the same pre-neoplastic condition at the time the psychological investigations were conducted. None of them exhibited any other abnormalities indicative of cervical cancer. The women were interviewed and given psychological tests prior to diagnosis. As well as investigating aspects of general health and sexual history, the interviews considered aspects of the patients' reactions to life events, their feelings of self-esteem and pleasure, coping ability, propensity to self-blame and feelings of doom and loss of gratification, in the six months prior to the first positive Pap test. Based on the results of the interview the patients were categorised in terms of felt hopelessness. From this classification the investigators then proceeded to predict which of these asymptomatic women would develop malignant cancer. In the 1966a study, for example, they were able to predict accurately with a success rate of over 75% (31 out of 40) from the interview data alone: eight out of 14 malignancies and 23 of 26 non-malignancies. The malignant group scored higher on hopelessness than the non-malignant group. The depression scale of the Minnesota Multiphasic Personality Inventory (MMPI) produced a difference approaching significance. Whilst Bieliauskas & Garron (1982) have criticised this study because of the use of non-standard interview procedures and an unclear definition of 'hopelessness', it does suggest that hopelessness may be a useful concept in this context, especially since recent work on coping processes and social supports has flourished. More recently, in a prospective study of 69 patients with early breast cancer, Greer, Morris & Pettingdale (1979) have shown that recurrence-free survival five years later was significantly worse in women who initially responded with feelings of stoic acceptance, helplessness or hopelessness, than in those who exhibited a 'fighting spirit' or denial of the cancer. Clearly, however, more research is needed on hopelessness and cancer.

Although there is evidence to suggest that hopelessness may be a precursor of some cancers, there does not appear to be much evidence that psychometrically quantified depression plays a significant role (Bieliauskas & Garron, 1982; Fox, 1982). In the study by Schmale & Iker (1971) the cancer patients did not score significantly higher on the depression scale of the MMPI. Other studies, several of which have been prospective in design, have reported similarly negative results using a range of measures of depression and a range of cancer sites (e.g. Gillum *et al.*, 1980; Greer & Morris, 1978; Koenig, Levin & Brennan, 1967; Plumb & Holland, 1977; Schonfield, 1977; Watson & Schuld, 1977. The reader is referred to Fox, 1982, for a discussion of the negative results). In fact, there are some examples of cancer patients obtaining lower scores on the depression scale of the MMPI (e.g. the prospective study by Dattore, Shontz & Coyne ,1980). Shekelle *et al.* (1981), on the other hand, found the opposite. They report the results of a prospective study of 2020 men in whom depression was measured 17 years earlier. They categorised depressives using the MMPI, and were able to control for age, smoking and drinking behaviour. They found that cancer deaths were more likely to occur in the men scoring high on the depression scale, at each time period examined after the initial screening. Of the 379 classified in the depression group 7.1% suffered death from cancer, compared to 3.4% for the remaining 1641 men. Depression seemed to have a smaller effect on other causes of death (16.4% vs. 13.2% respectively). As Bieliauskas & Garron (1982) have concluded, the evidence would suggest that "While certain cancer patients may be significantly depressed, it is clear that the widespread notion that cancer patients are generally depressed is not supported by the evidence" (p. 193). It should be also be noted that most of these studies deal with depression scores which are not in the pathological range.

In summary, the work implicating life changes, and reactions to such changes, in the pathogenesis of cancer is not clear-cut. There are may hints of influences which, added together, should convince one that psychological factors probably play a very significant role. One persisting message is that there is something of a disjunction between the clinically assessed factors and those derived from more standardised techniques. There are two interpretations of this contradiction. The first is that the standardised measures do not adequately tap the range or depth of experience or feelings that are relevant to cancer etiology. They are simply too crude. Alternatively, clinical judgment may be too coloured by non-objective criteria. My own view is that we should reject this latter interpretation for three principal reasons. First, the prospective nature of some of the interview-derived data (e.g. Schmale & Iker, 1971) makes this interpretation unlikely. Second, whatever the contribution of psychological factors in cancer onset their effect is likely to be dependent on subtle factors and the interplay between a number of such factors.

This may require the development of rather more sensitive measures than have hitherto been available. Third, personality might be expected to moderate whatever stressor–strain relationships exist. It is to this aspect that we now turn.

PERSONALITY FACTORS AS RESISTANCE WEAKENERS

Krantz & Glass (1984) distinguish between two categories of causal role for personality factors in disease. The first proposes that personality can produce pathology: that is personality plays a significant causal role in changing somatic functions which themselves are precursors of clinical symptoms. For example, the 'nuclear conflict theory' of Alexander (1950) suggests that unconscious conflicts may immediately or later activate emotional reactions which have somatic consequences. Other related theories (e.g. Graham, 1972) propose that specific attitudes which are discernible by clinical interview are related to the particular type of somatic disturbance or illness.

The second category proposes that personality plays no role in the initial appearance of the symptoms, but once present the illness itself becomes a stressor and the way the individual perceives the illness may affect the course of the disease and the outcome. This point of view is obviously important in discussions of how patients cope with their cancer and the effect this has on the course of the disease, although it is possible that a psychological reaction to a non-cancerous illness may itself have somatic consequences which are themselves related to neoplasia.

The majority of research on personality factors in cancer provides a mix of these two approaches. We will consider below the psychodynamic perspective which emphasises such factors as the lack of a loving childhood, the role of childhood trauma and the effects of denial, repression and object cathexes in the onset of cancer. In addition, we will consider evidence relating to personality factors in 'reactiveness' to life events (including illness) and the effects such reactions have on cancer etiology. Since the primary concern is with personality variables which may be precursors of cancer onset, little attention will be paid to factors influencing how patients cope with the knowledge they have cancer, and the subsequent effect this may have on tumour growth.

As with the animal research, there is considerable debate concerning the status of the findings. Fox (1978, 1982), in particular, has pointed to a number of difficulties in methodology, statistical analyses, interpretation of, and inconsistencies present in, this literature. Whilst the present author agrees that the results should be interpreted with considerable caution, and are certainly not of sufficient established status to have pragmatic implications, a number of significant patterns do emerge. It is all too easy to be critical of research in this area. The use of poor measures, the number of retrospective and quasi-prospective studies, the use of inappropriate control comparisons, the 'fishing' for psychologically relevant variables and attempts to make site-specific interpretations with small numbers of cases, the failure to report negative results, and so on, are largely problems necessarily inherent in the work for practical reasons. Indeed, the tendency to downplay the results of retrospective studies, and the special status given to prospective studies in virtually every review on psychological factors in cancer etiology, seems to ignore to an unhealthy degree the particular difficulties which beset the interpretation and implications of prospective studies: 'cause' is no less elusive here. Of particular importance is the point that only a few psychological variables have been investigated in prospective studies, and the nature of many prospective investigations makes it difficult to use some statistical techniques which require large sample sizes. Moreover, it does not follow that observing small or zero effects of the examined psychological variables entails that psychological variables do not have a major influence.

There have been some theoretical attempts to explain paradoxical results. People who score high on neuroticism scales, who might be expected to be more affected by stressors, do not seem to have an increased cancer risk: on the contrary there is evidence that they are protected to some degree (Eysenck, 1984). Eysenck has called this the 'inoculation effect' which is that "repeated stress will inoculate or desensitise the individual against future stress, so that this later stress does not have the same kind of effect on cancer growth, immune reaction" (p. 161). Such a view would predict differential effects of acute and chronic stressors, and we have seen that the animal literature supports this to some extent. Monjan & Collector (1977) have shown that acute noise stress (for 14 days) depresses B- and T-cell activity, but that chronic noise stress has the opposite effect. Sklar & Anisman (1981) also report that inescapable shock administered a few days before tumour transplantation eliminated the tumour-enhancing effects of post-transplantation acute shock. Stressors may, therefore, have bipolar effects depending upon previous exposure to stress and the way it is perceived.

Using a variety of methods, from judgments based on clinical impressions, Rorschach tests, draw-a-person tests, MMPI/EPI, with retrospective and long-term prospective studies, a whole host of personality factors or dispositions have been connected to the onset of cancer. Fox (1982), for example, lists evidence for 15 which can be described as personality traits or variables with a psychodynamic root.

The Cancer-prone Personality

Broadly speaking the work on personality predisposition and cancer can be classified as suggesting that three different characteristics of a person may increase susceptibility:

1. *Suppression of emotions*, especially anger, which may result in defensive reactions, as well as an 'internalised' perspective, to events that would normally result in a strong emotional reaction.
2. *Repression*, or failure to take an objective view of events and people including oneself. This repression essentially affects how such things as life events are perceived and coped with. This may also be related to the concept of rationality/anti-emotionality (Grossarth-Maticek *et al.*, 1982). Another dimension called

'harmonisation' represents suppression of emotions (quarrels, forthright behaviour, etc.) in order to keep a level of harmony amongst people who might otherwise be divided on an issue (Eysenck, 1988). Self-blaming may be one outcome of such repression, as may depression and feelings of hopelessness. Repression can also be viewed in straight psychodynamic terms, with its consequential effects on self-ego and sexuality.

Clearly items 1 and 2 are similar concepts. One distinction between them is that repression may be considered to occur more automatically, unconsciously, or without attentional mediation. The suppression of emotions requires more active cognitive effort to achieve.

3. *Reactive inconsistency or ambivalence*, which may lead to making ambiguous or irregular responses on different occasions. The lack of consistency is presumed to reflect some underlying weakness in the cognitive structures which guide our behaviour.

Cancer-proneness as schema–system inconsistency

All three aspects are closely associated, and may all be manifestations of an underlying failure to perceive matters with a clear 'worldly' view and to adopt a realistic set of cognitive schemata to assimilate and accommodate incoming information to structure future actions and reactions. If one were to postulate a distinction between schemata which organise incoming perceptions and information, and schemata which are responsible for organising the type and consistency of emotional reactions to these events, these aspects of personality can be seen as being the result of conflict between information schemata and emotion schemata. Adopting a 'realistic' or 'worldly' outlook on events and their consequences could be seen as adopting a balanced perspective based on both information schemata and emotion schemata.

The lack of, or suppression of, emotion could be viewed as showing too much reliance on information schemata, and would account for apparently inconsistent characteristics which have been associated with cancer such as impaired self-awareness and introspection (Abse *et al.*, 1972), self-blaming (Nemeth & Mezei, 1963; Biondi & Pancheri, 1985), and the many suggestions of emotional inhibition or poor emotional outlet (Booth, 1964; Kissen, 1963). The repression of emotions is, according to this view, a result of trying to take an overly rational view of evidence, or a 'reality' view. It would also predict that cancer patients would exhibit passive, rather than active, strategies to cope with stressful experiences (Grossarth-Maticek, Seigrist & Vetter, 1982), if the former is viewed as more 'information-schema-based' than the latter. The reactive inconsistency (Betz & Thomas, 1979) or ambivalence suggested in such things as human figure drawing (Harrower, Thomas & Altman, 1975) is also a result of this conflict between information and emotion schemata, where the actual (unconscious) behaviour is a consequence of vacillation between one and the other. Felt hopelessness (Schmale & Iker, 1971), depression (Shekelle *et al.*, 1981), lower neuroticism scores (Kissen, 1964; Berndt, Gunther & Rothe, 1980; which Eysenck, 1984, interprets as the absence of emotion, rather than its suppression) and extroversion (Coppen & Metcalfe, 1965; Kissen & Eysenck, 1962) may be more permanent consequences of this essential conflict but we might expect such effects to be less stable than their precursors (Fox, 1982) simply because they are not necessary consequences of the underlying difficulty. It may also exhibit itself in a number of other ways such as psychosexual disturbances and feelings of unresolved conflicts (Bacon, Renneker & Cutler, 1952; Reznikoff, 1955), lower perceptions of 'personal integration' (Grissom, Weiner & Weiner, 1975), and 'sub-stability' (Hagnell, 1966) and, of course, elevated scores on exhibited repression (Dattore, Shontz & Coyne, 1980).

Some Empirical Evidence

Suppression of feelings

There is a wealth of evidence that emotional inhibition, especially the internalisation of anger, is associated with increased cancer risk. Whilst this evidence is certainly of variable quality, the repeated demonstration of its relevance as a core concept in risk should be accepted. LeShan (1959) provides an excellent review of the early literature, although it is worth describing some of these studies, to give a flavour of the research. They report the work of Cobb (1952), who concluded from her study of 100 cancer patients and controls that the cancer patients invariably considered that emotional attachments should be avoided. This may have been the cause or the consequence of their negative reactions to their families and to their general difficulty in establishing adequate social relationships. The 'internalisation' effect is also demonstrated in Bacon, Rennecker & Cutler (1952). Some 88% of the psychiatric assessments of breast cancer patients showed a 'masochistic character structure', and 75% revealed no techniques for discharging or dealing appropriately with their anger. In later work Booth (1964), using the Rorschach test on 175 lung cancer patients and tubercular controls, found that the former were more emotionally repressed and, in particular, directed their felt anger inwards.

Of course, the early work shows a marked absence of control groups, objective measurement, statistical or other assessment of the role of traditional risk factors, and prospective studies. Other research has utilised more sophisticated psychometric tools and research designs.

In more recent work, Greer & Morris (1975) have carried out psychological investigations of 160 women admitted to hospital for breast biopsy. Interviews and a battery of psychological tests were completed before diagnosis was known. Patients were assessed for their degree of suppressed or expressed anger and other feelings. Compared to the 91 benign controls, the 69 patients who turned out to have malignancies were much more likely to have been rated as 'extreme suppressors' (e.g. had not openly shown anger more than twice in their life), and less likely to be rated as 'apparently normal' or 'extreme expressers' (i.e. those who did not conceal their feelings). To support these clinical judgments they found that their ratings were significantly correlated with the 'Acting Out Hostility' scores of Caine & Foulds (1967) personality questionnaire.

In his clinical examination of 161 lung cancer patients and 174 controls admitted to chest clinics, Kissen (1963) also observed that cancer patients exhibited an obvious difficulty with emotional discharge, tending to "conceal or bottle up their emotional problems" (p. 28). This difficulty seemed to be present from the early childhood reports he obtained, too, suggesting it was not a new phenomenon. The lung cancer patients reported many fewer episodes of release such as temper tantrums, truancy or delinquency, phobias, anxieties and bed-wetting. These differences could not be interpreted as cancer patients showing less aggression or lack of sociability since cancer and control patients had similar scores on these measures.

A prospective study by Hagnell (1966) of 2550 Swedes, begun in 1947, had produced 42 cancer cases (20 men, 22 women) by 1957. At the outset of the study the subjects completed a personality test which measured intellectual ability or 'capacity', suggestible or labile 'solidity', energetic forcefulness, certainty or 'validity' and emotionally controlled 'stability' or sense of coolness. For the first three of these scales, cancer rates showed no deviation from age-specific expected rates. However, for the dimension of 'stability' 20 of the women (as opposed to the 14.2 expected frequency) scored in the substability range. The observed/expected difference was also more marked for those women with evident as opposed to slight substability. These women, according to this scale, have a tendency to be more emotionally affected by incidents, to become dysthymic, and to inhibit any emotional expression, although they are warm, hearty, sociable and interested people. Thus, substability would appear to be a cancer risk, although the absence of any similar effect for men, and the fact that the breast was the most common cancer site for women (accounting for nine of the 22), suggests a site-specific effect. Fox (1978) has also statistically analysed the mediostability figures for the women and suggests that scoring within this range proffers a protective effect from cancer.

In a comparison of breast cancer patients and fibrocystic mastopathic controls, Biondi & Pancheri (1985) observed different patterns of response on their Reaction Scheme Test. Patients did not, at this time, know what diagnosis had been made, and the affected anatomical sites were the same for both groups. Of relevance here is that the cancer group obtained higher scores on 'self-blaming' and 'denial-suppression' scales suggesting their introjection of aggressiveness and assumption of guilt, and use of defence mechanisms to annul the impact of stressful events.

Kissen & Eysenck (1962) administered the Maudsley Personality Inventory to patients at chest units before diagnoses had been made. They found that the 116 lung cancer patients had significantly *lower* neuroticism scores than the control group.

This was true of subgroups with and without psychosomatic disorders. In addition, extroversion scores were higher for the lung cancer group with psychosomatic disorders. Higher extroversion scores have also been reported in cancer patients, compared to non-cancer and healthy controls, by Coppen & Metcalfe (1963). The low neuroticism scores of lung cancer patients have been observed in a number of studies by Kissen (1963, 1964, 1966, 1969). Interestingly, he also found that non-inhaling smokers who developed cancer produced very low neuroticism scores.

Greer & Morris (1975) did not substantiate either the neuroticism or extroversion differences in patients with breast cancer. Huggan (1968) and Fox (1978) have argued that the patients in Kissen's work may have been 'faking good' answers, or may have known that they had cancer. Nonetheless, the weight of evidence from other studies (e.g. Berndt, Gunther & Rothe, 1980; Biondi & Pancheri, 1985; see also Eysenck, 1980, 1981, 1984), and other positive aspects of Kissen's work (e.g. the use of controls with other lung diseases who also smoke—but see Fox, 1978, p. 103), make the link between cancer and neuroticism more certain. Indeed Kissen (1964) has calculated lung cancer mortality rates based on neuroticism scores. As an aside, both Fox (1978) and Eysenck (1983, 1984) have suggested that low neuroticism scores of cancer patients might demonstrate the *absence* of emotions rather than their *inhibition* or suppression. The earlier evidence presented in this section would cast doubt on this interpretation. That evidence supports the idea of some active inner channelling of feelings. In addition, there could also be unconscious aspects of repression (see below) which may make it appear as if the patient is emotionally neutral because they rely more on information schemata than emotion schemata.

Other studies have shown other personality measures to be associated with increased risk, although with less frequency than the ones discussed so far. However, even one of the most commonly used instruments to measure personality in such studies, the MMPI, has produced a bewildering set of inconsistencies. Fox (1982), in his review and discussion of these studies, has concluded that "one simply cannot take seriously the results of some of the cited papers. In view of the wide variety of tumours and stages, how can one conclude anything about the MMPI in general, or any single variable in particular" (p. 287).

Taken together, the research done does suggest that emotional suppression may play a significant role in the onset of cancer. There is other evidence which demonstrates that how a person responds or copes with cancer also affects the prognosis for survival. Derogatis, Abeloff & Melisaratos (1979) have shown that the survival time for patients with metastatic breast cancer is shorter for those unable to express hostility and anger outwardly, and Achterberg *et al.* (1977) have shown that denial has a similar consequence. Furthermore, patients with cancer who more readily adjust to the diagnosis (i.e. they base their response on information schemata rather than showing an emotional bias) are more likely to suffer relapses, as Rogentine *et al.* (1979) demonstrated in their prospective predictions of 33 melanoma patients.

Unconscious repression of action

In addition to the research of Greer & Morris (1975), suggesting that cancer patients show extreme suppression of emotions to anger as a consciously adopted strategy to situations (by 'bottling up' feelings), there is also evidence that unconsciously adopting a rational and anti-emotional approach to life situations carries a cancer risk. During informal observations of cancer patients, Grossarth-Maticek (in Grossarth-Maticek, Siegrist & Vetter, 1982) concluded that they showed an unusual propensity "towards passive responses, compliance and acceptance of overt and latent repressive cues" (p. 493) in their style of communication. This idea was empirically tested in a prospective study of a selected sample of 1353 people from the 15 000 population of a rural village in Yugoslavia. The study began in 1965, when full psychosocial data were collected, and there was continual medical monitoring until 1970 by a doctor who did not have access to this information. A rating system for interpersonal repression was developed which took into account whether the subject was a 'receiver' or 'emitter' of repression (i.e. passive or active), how long-lasting the repression was, whether the behaviour was implicit (e.g. withdrawal) or explicit (e.g. shouting), the degree of social support experienced in the repressive situation, and the degree of repression of the needs and emotions. The results clearly supported the idea that those who subsequently developed cancer ($n = 204$) were passive receivers of repression, whereas those who developed circulatory diseases ($n = 414$) were active emitters. For example, correlations between cancer incidence and the four different aspects of passive repression were all significant. Eysenck (1988) also reports data from this study, comparing high and low scorers on the rational–anti-emotionality scale. This is shown in Table 4.1.

Table 4.1. Comparison cancer risk for high and low scorers on the rational–anti-emotionality scale (adapted from Eysenck, 1988)

	Low scorers (0–9)		High scorers (10/11)	
	Observed cases	Expected cases	Observed cases	Expected cases
Lung cancer cases	0	26	38	12
Other cancer cases	8	84	120	44

Grossarth-Maticek has also presented strong evidence that the effect of physical risk factors in cancer can be significantly amplified by the degree of rational–anti-emotionality. For example, the regression coefficient between smoking and lung cancer was raised from 0.046 to 0.384 by adding in the rational–anti-emotionality scores (Grossarth-Maticek, 1980). Grossarth-Maticek, Bastiaans & Kanazir (1985) also show that the lung cancer risk from smoking cigarettes is only present for those who score highly on the rational–anti-emotional scale: for those individuals who smoked in excess of 21 cigarettes a day, none of those who scored less than 10 died of lung cancer, although 22% of those with scores of 10 or 11 did. In general, the relationship between physical and psychological risk factors is synergistic (i.e. both factors account for more of the variance in the outcome than either does separately).

Psychodynamically, one may expect repression to exhibit itself in other significant ways, such as sexual disturbance. There is evidence to support this view. In what they considered a preliminary study, Tarlau & Smalheiser (1951) found that Rorschach tests and interviews highlighted a number of similarities (and differences) between cervical and breast cancer patients which had been present before the appearance of physical symptoms. Both groups exhibited the same pattern of mother dominance and consequent rejection or repression of a feminine role, including negative attitudes towards sexuality. Interestingly, this psychosexual disturbance is also revealed in the work of Bacon *et al.* (1952), who found that 63% of the women had never experienced orgasm or liked intercourse, and all except one had received no sex education from their parents. Reznikoff (1955) also reports that women who showed difficulties identifying with the female role were more frequent among the group who turned out to have cancer rather than benign growths.

Reactive inconsistency and ambivalence

It seems necessary to consider this as a possible risk factor in cancer for a number of reasons. First, there is some evidence from the studies discussed above that some cancer patients exhibit extremes of behaviour in the opposite direction of the bulk of such patients. Greer & Morris (1975), for example, found that there were significantly more cancer patients than controls who exhibited 'extreme expression' of anger. Second, it may be that a balance between expression and suppression—a medium or balanced line—is protective. Fox (1978), for example, suggests that mediostability may reduce cancer risk. Third, some integration is required to explain inconsistent findings and some of the patterns of results obtained. For example, one needs to understand why higher extroversion, lower neuroticism, and inward channelling of emotional responses may each be a risk factor. The dimension 'stability' in Hagnell's work (1966), discussed earlier, also contains aspects which could be considered to demonstrate ambivalence.

There is some evidence of inconsistency and ambivalence in cancer patients. Harrower, Thomas & Altman (1975) report the results obtained from the draw-a-person test which was introduced into the Johns Hopkins Precursors study in 1951. In all, 870 medical students completed the test and by the time of the report 20 had developed malignancies. In this test the subject is asked to draw a male and female person. Harrower *et al.* classified the drawings into eight categories depending upon the attitude depicted: neutral (e.g. arms at the side, legs together), outgoing (e.g. arms outstretched, legs apart), self-related (e.g. arms crossed, slightly hunched look), ambivalent (e.g. one arm outstretched, the other at the side), profile or side view, incomplete, bizarre, and action pictures. The drawings of the cancer group were compared to healthy controls. Their most characteristic posture was one of ambivalence or dual orientation (15 out of 40 drawings) which appeared five times as often as in the control group (i.e. 37.5% vs. 7.5%). The cancer group also produced proportionately fewer incomplete, bizarre or action pictures (2.5% vs. 17.5%). Whilst this study has been criticised because of its inappropriate statistics (Fox, 1978) it does demonstrate that cancer sufferers had an unconscious propensity to ambivalent behavioural manifestations many years before the onset of the disease. The fact that none of the other disease groups studied showed a similar propensity adds weight to this conclusion.

Betz & Thomas (1979), using the typological criteria of Gesell & Ilg (1943), classified the data from 45 subjects in the Precursors study into three temperament types: the alpha types who were cautious, dependable, solid, and self-reliant; the beta types who were adaptable, articulate, cool and facile; and the gamma types who showed irregular or uneven responses, over- and underreactiveness and confusion. The data suggested that gamma types were more likely to exhibit early disease. When applied to a further 127 subjects, which included 20 cancer patients, morbidity was highest for the gamma classified subjects, with the pattern being particularly marked for the cancer patients.

The ambivalence characteristic, however, was not confirmed as a cancer risk in the Yugoslavian and Heidelberg studies by Grossarth-Maticek and co-workers (1982), although their 'ambivalent' dimension may be better described as 'reactive inconsistency' since Eysenck (1988) suggests that "in individuals of this type, we have an alternation of feelings of hopelessness/helplessness and of anger/arousal" (p. 64). The study showed that those classified as the ambivalent types had low cancer rates in the Yugoslavian and Heidelberg studies whether or not they were normals or part of a 'highly stressed' group. The question of whether ambivalence is a characteristic of any importance as a cancer risk variable cannot be answered with any certainty on the present evidence, although if it does play a role it would seem secondary to some of the other factors outlined previously.

Stress reactions and personality types

An alternative approach to investigating which personality traits may or may not be associated with cancer risk is to classify individuals in terms of how they react to stressors. To some extent this is inherent in much of the research on hopeless/helpless reactions. Grossarth-Maticek and co-workers have taken this approach one stage further by categorising people according to one of four types (see Eysenck, 1988; Grossarth-Maticek & Eysenck, 1990):

• *Type 1:* those who do not get close enough to an emotionally valued object (person, position, etc.) and suffer stress as a consequence.
• *Type 2:* those for whom the emotionally valued object is also the cause for their distress, although they continually strive for it (somewhat analogous to type A behaviour).
• *Type 3:* the person who responds inconsistently (see above).

- *Type 4:* those who avoid the stress reaction through realistic approach and avoidance behaviour/strategies.

The Heidelberg and Yugoslavian studies strongly supported the view that type 1 individuals have an excess cancer risk. For example, in the Yugoslavian study 46.2% of them died from cancer, compared to 8.3% of the type 2, and less than 5% of type 3 and type 4. In the Heidelberg study (which cannot be directly compared with the Yugoslavian study because the sample characteristics are different) 17.4% of type 1 individuals died of cancer, compared to 5.9% of type 2, and almost none of the type 3 and 4 groups. The fact that stressors may amplify the effects of having a 'risky' personality was also supported by the finding that in a 'stressed' group (which, incidentally, contained a much greater proportion of type 1s than the normal group) the percentage of type 1s who died of cancer was 38.4%, compared to 2.3% of type 2s. Smoking also behaved in a synergistic manner with personality types, such that being a smoking type 1 person was associated with considerably elevated lung cancer risk. Thus, it may be important in future research to ensure that stress reactions are considered in relation to the interaction of personality, life events, and physical risk factors: consideration of any in isolation will not meet with the same chance of success in predicting cancer outcomes.

The important role played by psychological factors in cancer is also shown by recent demonstrations that behavioural strategies can be applied to reduce cancer likelihood and to prolong the lives of cancer sufferers. Grossarth-Maticek & Eysenck (1991) and Eysenck & Grossarth-Maticek (1991) report that one technique (Creative Novation Behaviour Therapy) is very successful for both cancer and coronary heart disease. The technique requires individuals to develop new behaviours through self-observation and experience of the consequences of actions. Their results suggest that such therapy may dramatically reduce cancer incidence, increase survival times, reduce days spent in hospital, and act synergistically with chemotherapy.

CONCLUSION

Although far from conclusive, the research reviewed does support the view that psychological factors play an important role in the onset of cancer. The animal research is inconsistent, but the inconsistencies are probably primarily a consequence of experimental differences and interactions between stressor conditions. The human research does reveal suggestive evidence that both personality variables and life events may increase cancer susceptibility. Given the increasing evidence of links between the immune system, hormonal influences and tumorigenesis, the real questions to be answered relate to the relative weight played by psychological factors in the causes of cancer, and the way they are likely to interact with other environmental carcinogens.

Chapter 5

Stress and Coronary Heart Disease

This chapter considers whether psychological factors play a central role in the onset of heart disease. Much of the research concentrates on personality factors in heart disease, particularly the concept of type A coronary-prone behaviour and its physiological and psychological correlates. This work is considered in detail. The chapter also reviews the evidence that environmental psychological stressors play a causative role in heart disease. It concludes with a discussion of the psychological dimensions of hypertension and blood pressure—an important risk factor in the development of heart disease.

HEART DISEASE

The function of the heart is to supply the bodily tissue and organs with sufficient oxygenated blood to maintain normal metabolic functioning under a range of more or less demanding conditions. In the adult this requires it to pump between five and 15 litres of blood per minute whilst maintaining healthy and constant arterial, venous and intracardiac pressures.

Coronary heart disease (CHD) or ischaemic heart disease are generic terms for a number of cardiovascular disorders. Most of the research documented here concerns some form of *coronary atherosclerosis*. This is a chronic symptomless degeneration of the coronary arteries which supply the heart (or myocardium) with blood. The degeneration can be a result of the deposit of atherosclerotic plaque, formed from excess cholesterol and related lipids, which become attached to the arterial walls. This 'narrowing of the arteries' may eventually show itself in the form of some clinical symptoms. The person may periodically experience *angina pectoris*, or severe chest pains, when the heart is insufficiently nourished or placed under extra demands (e.g. physical exercise). Another clinical manifestation of atherosclerosis is *myocardial infarction*, or heart attack, which destroys heart tissue, sometimes fatally. There are also minor coronary events which are not manifested clinically but which result from oxygen insufficiency at the myocardium. These are sometimes referred to as *silent ischaemias*. Myocardial infarction can be precipitated by *coronary thromboses*, or clots, which may occlude the coronary arteries, although cardiac (and person) death can occur suddenly in the absence of thrombosis.

An essential of normal heart functioning is that there is prescribed rhythmic electrical activity of the cardiac tissue. This electrical activity is measured by the electrocardiogram (ECG) which represents particular wave-form deflections from the baseline, or isoelectric line. The deflections are designated by the letters P, Q, R, S, T and U, and have characteristic curve shapes in the normal ECG. Disturbances in cardiac conduction occur in the coronary diseased person and these show up on the ECG trace under certain conditions. The ECG is, therefore, a useful index of cardiac condition because it offers a diagnostic window before clinical symptoms occur. Disturbances of rhythm, the cardiac arrhythmias, may be present in the ECG for a number of reasons other than chronic disease.

There are many subclinical indices of the state of the cardiovascular system. These include abnormal ECG tracings (e.g. abnormalities of the QRS complex may show previous silent infarctions or left ventricular hypertrophy), heart wall motion abnormalities (which can be detected by radionuclide ventriculography and are indicative of silent ischaemia), the presence of corneal arcus, respiratory volume and oxygen uptake, left ventricular ejection fraction (which is a measure of myocardial flexibility as determined by the ratio of the volume of blood in the heart at the end of the ejection phase to the volume at the end of the filling phase), abnormal heart rate, high systolic and/or diastolic blood pressure, ventricular ejection time, and so on. Clearly, some of these measures are more direct than others. The distinction between subclinical signs and CHD risk factors is also a fuzzy one. The standard risk factors include high blood pressure, cardiac and endocrinological reactivity or lability, serum cholesterol, triglyceride and beta/alpha lipoprotein ratio, serum clotting times, serum clotting factors and fibrinogen concentrations; all of which have been implicated with varying degrees of support to manifest CHD. In addition, epidemiologists and clinicians would take account of smoking behaviour, obesity, age, sex, exercise, socioeconomic status, glucose intolerance and related conditions (e.g. diabetes mellitus), and aspects of endocrine functioning (e.g. high serum catecholamine levels serve to mobilise lipid stores from adipose tissue, enhance platelet aggregation and thrombosis, and increase blood pressure and flow turbulence).

Psychological Factors in Heart Disease

The report of a World Health Organisation Expert Committee on the prevention of CHD (1982) noted that

> Several behavioral patterns and psychological and social variables have been related to CHD risk.... With respect to 'stress', or 'response to stress', the lack of definition and quantitative measurement is severely limiting.... The Expert Committee noted the danger that public and professional misconceptions about 'stress', whereby it is assigned a primary role in the genesis of CHD, may divert attention from the demonstrated needs in prevention (p. 32).

It is not clear, however, whether it is a misconception to believe that medical science is close to understanding the causes of CHD. The standard physiological or medical risk factors for CHD are not good predictors of the degree or incidence of its clinical manifestation. For example, an Inter-Society Commission for Heart Disease Resources in 1970 showed that only 10% of men who exhibited two or more of these risk factors went on to develop CHD over the next 10 years. Over 40% of those who developed CHD within the 10-year period did not have two or more of the risk factors. Moreover, when reading the epidemiological literature relating to CHD, one is struck by the inconsistencies and failures to confirm many traditional risk factors.

The potential importance of psychosocial variables in CHD is suggested by the results of a prospective study by Lehr, Messinger & Rosenman (1973). The authors measured 12 biochemical and other biological risk factors, and 12 social variables (these were simply factual descriptions relating to the social background of the individuals such as parental country of birth, parent's occupation, subject's education, residence, etc.). Despite the fact that these variables do not encompass the rich tapestry of psychological factors and individual-based perceptions and life events, the social variables were important predictors of CHD. In a discriminant analysis comparing CHD cases with CHD-free controls, a 'parental religious difference factor' was the second-best discriminant, and 'father's occupation' and 'behaviour pattern' were more discriminating than eight of the biological risk factors. Of the biological risk factors, only age, systolic blood pressure, smoking and serum cholesterol levels contributed in the discriminant analysis, and these did not account for much of the predictable variance.

An excellent experimental study by Rozanski *et al.* (1988) can be used to demonstrate the potential causal role of psychological variables or mental stress in CHD. Their research, which utilized CHD patients, showed that some mental stressors can induce elevations in arterial pressure and abnormalities of heart wall motions comparable to that induced by exercise in CHD patients. Moreover, the mental-stressor-induced minor ischaemias occurred at lower heart rates than that produced by exercise. Four mental stress tasks were compared with the effects of exercise (simulated public speaking on a personal subject, doing arithmetic, reading aloud, and the Stroop colour–word task). Nearly 60% of the patients had heart wall motion abnormalities (assessed by radionuclide ventriculography) whilst doing the mental tasks, with 36% showing a fall in left ventricular ejection fraction of at least 5 percentage points (an indication of the heart failing to respond flexibly). The vast majority of the ischaemic changes were 'silent' or symptomless. The public speaking task also produced ischaemic changes as large as exercise, even though it was not rated more tension-producing, anxiety-provoking, or arousing–challenging than the arithmetic or Stroop tasks by the patients. This study provides a powerful demonstration that mental stress can have silent and significant effects on the cardiovascular system which may be functional in clinical manifestations.

It is also interesting to note that a recent review of stress-management approaches to the prevention of CHD shows that such approaches (e.g. relaxation, management training techniques, problem-solving, anger control, assertiveness training) can reduce serum cholesterol, high blood pressure and coronary-prone behaviours (Bennett & Carroll, 1990). If psychological techniques can play a significant role in reducing CHD risks it may also be that they play a role in the genesis of the disease.

PERSONALITY AND HEART DISEASE

In his Lumleian lectures on angina pectoris in 1910, the cardiologist Sir William Osler observed that "It is not the delicate, neurotic person who is prone to angina, but the robust, the vigorous in mind and body, the keen and ambitious man, the indicator of whose engine is always at full speed ahead". The view that personality factors play a significant role in the development of heart disease has received considerable recent scientific support, notably from the influential work of Friedman & Rosenman, and their co-workers.

In their original 1959 study, Friedman & Rosenman considered the possible influence of behavioural patterns on clinical CHD and subclinical indices (corneal arcus, serum cholesterol levels, blood clotting time). Three groups of male subjects were selected as exhibiting different behavioural types:

1. Eighty-three men were designated as group A because they exhibited intense sustained drive towards poorly defined goals, competitiveness and desire for advancement and achievement, with extraordinary mental and physical alertness. During a subsequent interview session these men also showed excessively rapid bodily movements, muscular tenseness with teeth and hand clenching, explosive conversation, and impatience.
2. A control of 83 men were designated as group B if they exhibited the converse of overt behaviour pattern A.
3. Group C, consisting of 46 men, were similar in behaviour pattern to group B but, in addition, were chronically anxious or insecure.

Friedman & Rosenman found that the A-group subjects had much higher average levels of serum cholesterol than the other groups (253 mg/100 ml vs. 215 mg and 220 mg), and were more likely to have clinical coronary disease (28% vs. 4% and 4%), arcus senilis (38% vs. 11%, no measure for group C), and a positive parental history of heart disease (36% vs. 27% and 15%). However, whether these differences were due to their specified behaviour patterns or a result of higher levels of smoking behaviour (67% vs. 56% and 61%), smokers using more cigarettes per day (23 vs. 12 and 15), group A's getting less sleep at night (7.3 hours vs. 7.8 and 8.0), or working more hours per week (51 vs. 45 for group B), is impossible to say. Dietary fat intake showed no significant group differences.

The study was very poor in a number of important respects. For example, the selection of subjects for each group was done by laymen without any psychometric aid. Furthermore, those in group A came from a whole range of occupations, those in B primarily from accountancy, and group C men were unemployed, blind and nearly half institutionalised. The study is, of course, retrospective in nature and this makes it difficult to conclude that the personality differences were causes or consequences of heart disease and its precursors. Other existing differences between the groups (e.g. the greater incidence of smoking and positive parental histories of the group A subjects) may also have been responsible for the pathological differences without there being any separate contribution from personality dispositions and behaviour patterns. For these reasons, amongst others, Friedman & Rosenman undertook a major longitudinal predictive study of CHD which started with initially healthy subjects with groups controlled for the presence of any of the traditional risk factors. This has become known as the Western Collaborative Group Study (WCGS).

The Western Collaborative Group Study

This prospective study was initiated in 1960 and Rosenman *et al.* (1964) outline the basis and methodology of the research. Some 3524 men aged 39–59 years, who believed they were free of CHD or other serious illness, were given an in-depth initial examination to assess their personal history, serum lipids and lipoprotein fractions, blood coagulability, the current state of their cardiovascular system, and their overt behaviour pattern. The behaviour patterns were assessed by tape-recorded interview and a polygraph test (Friedman & Rosenman, 1959) which classified them as exhibiting fully developed type A behaviour (A-1), less developed type A (A-2), fully developed type B behaviour (B-4), or less developed (B-3).

From these initial examinations 113 men were excluded from the prospective phase of the study because they showed signs of manifest CHD. Interestingly, these men were more likely to be sales and publicity personnel, have a higher level of job responsibility, a history of high blood pressure, be smokers, have higher cholesterol levels and beta/alpha lipoprotein ratios, and were more than twice as likely to exhibit the type A coronary-prone behaviour pattern.

In all, some 3182 men who were free of manifest CHD were re-examined annually by electrocardiograph for the presence of abnormalities indicative of the development of CHD. Rosenman *et al.* (1966) present striking evidence showing that *of those free of manifest CHD* at the outset of the follow-up study there were no clinically relevant differences between the type A and B on almost all the traditional CHD risk factors (exercise, smoking, serum lipid values, blood coagulation, blood pressure, socioeconomic status).

After a mean follow-up time of 2.5 years 70 of the 3182 men had suffered the advent of CHD (Rosenman *et al.*, 1966). Fifty-two had had myocardial infarctions, and 18 exhibited the classic symptoms of angina pectoris. Nine of the men had fatal infarctions. Eight of them had been classified as type A on initial examination in 1960/1961. An examination of the initial 1960 profiles of these 70 new cases of CHD with the average of the 3182 men showed that the CHD men were less likely to have never smoked (10% vs. 22.7%), more likely to never take exercise (21.4% vs. 13.9%) and earned more; they had a greater prevalence of parental CHD (31.4% vs. 16.3%), diastolic blood pressure greater than 95 mmHg (27.1% vs. 9.4%), higher mean serum cholesterol (249 vs. 224.9 mg/100 ml), beta/alpha lipoprotein ratios (2.46 vs. 2.03), and triglycerides (159.6 vs. 147.7 mg/100 ml). There were no significant differences in calorie, alcohol, cholesterol and fat intake, or in mean height and weight, schooling, job-related physical activity, and prevalence or amount of current cigarette smoking.

Of particular importance here, however, was the finding that 77.1% of the new CHD cases had been originally classified as exhibiting type A or coronary-prone behaviour, compared to 49.8% of the entire sample. Classifying subjects into high or low risk categories on the basis of the 1960 examinations showed that type A men were 3.4 times more likely to have become a new CHD case than type B men (13.6/1000 vs. 4.0/1000 incidence rates). The young (39–49-year-olds) type A men were 6.48 times more likely to have developed CHD within the 2.5-year period than the type B men. Type A/B behaviour pattern was a better predictor of relative CHD risk than other prognostically significant indices such as high/low beta/alpha lipoprotein ratios (>2.36, <2.37), serum cholesterol levels (>270, <271 mg/100 ml), or the presence or absence of parental CHD. Moreover, whilst the type A diastolic hypertensive was more than three times more likely to have developed CHD than the type A normotensive, the type B men showed virtually no such excess hypertensive risk with even hypertensive type B men showing less CHD risk than normotensive type A men.

A 4.5-year follow-up of the men was published by Rosenman *et al.* in 1970, and the empirical data collection continued through an 8.5-year and a 22-year follow-up. At the 8.5-year stage (Rosenman *et al.*, 1975) the death rate per 1000 person-years was 2.10 for CHD events and 3.78 from non-CHD causes. CHD rates for type A men were 2.92 and for type B men only 1.32. Type A men also showed a higher death rate from non-CHD causes than type B men (4.38 vs. 3.21). In all, some 257 men (of the 3154 followed to the end) developed CHD after being free of any signs of it in 1960/61. Of the 135 men who developed symptomatic myocardial infarction (accompanied by definite ECG and serum enzyme changes or postmortem pathology) 93 had originally been classified as type A personalities, which represents an excess risk 2.2 times greater than those classified as type B. Of the 71 men with "unrecognised myocardial infarction" (ECG indicated during annual resurvey, but not clinically present), 48 were type A—an excess risk of 1.71 compared to type B. Finally, 37 of the 51 men with classical angina pectoris without infarction were type A—an excess risk of 2.45. Overall, type A men were 2.24 times more likely to have become CHD cases, compared to type B men. In order to dismiss the claim that these differences in prospective CHD rates with personality type were a result of the association of personality type with specific risk factors, or a combination of them, the authors stratified the CHD risk of A and B types by eight classes of risk factor (parental history of CHD, smoking habits, current cigarette usage, systolic blood pressure, diastolic blood pressure, serum cholesterol, fasting serum triglycerides and serum beta/alpha lipoprotein ratio). Even after adjusting for all these risk factors, each of which differentiated type A from type B by equivalent magnitudes, the remaining relative risk for type A over type B men was 1.87 for those aged 39–49 years (reduced from 2.21) and 1.98 from those aged 50–59 years (from 2.31). Thus the predictive relationship between behaviour pattern and CHD incidence could not be explained by these risk factors.

In order to provide a more direct estimation of predictive strength, and to provide some indication of the relative importance of different risk factors in the CHD cases, Rosenman *et al.* (1976) report the results of multiple logistic risk analysis of the Western Collaborative Group Study on the 8.5-year data. Only three of the 17 'risk' factors produced statistically significant Standardised Relative Risk scores (this is the relative risk [odds ratio] for a change in the risk factor by an amount equal to its standard deviation) for both age groups. These were type A/B behaviour pattern, serum cholesterol and smoking behaviour. The 39–49-year-olds also showed significant risk from age, the presence or absence of corneal arcus and systolic blood pressure. The type A/B behaviour pattern was shown to have the greatest predictive strength for CHD presence of all the factors for the 50–59-year-olds and was the second-best predictor (behind cholesterol levels) for the younger men. The relative risk for type A compared to type B was 2.16 for 50–59-year-olds and 1.87 for the 39–49-year-olds.

A recent 22-year follow-up of the WCGS men has cast some doubt on the long-term predictiveness of the type A concept. Raglan & Brand (1988a) report the results of a cohort in 1982–1983 when some 214 of the men had died of CHD. Univariate analyses showed that systolic blood pressure, serum cholesterol level, cigarettes smoked and age were all predictive of CHD mortality to at least the $p<0.001$ level. Type A/B personality produced a corresponding value of $p=0.08$ when the whole sample was considered, and much higher non-significant p-values when each age category was considered separately. Multivariate proportional hazards analysis produced a relative risk hazard of 0.98 for type A/B, although the numbers were significantly in excess of 1.0 for the other risk factors (indicating that type A men had almost the same CHD mortality risk as type B men). Splitting the follow-up period into different quarters even resulted in the type A personality producing a significant negative risk in one of the time intervals.

These results should not be ignored. There are, however, a number of reasons for holding the view that type A is truly a risk factor for CHD, despite these findings. First, it should be recalled that the WCGS assessed personality many years previously. It may be that personality measured some 20 years previously is not representative of behaviour in later years. Although the structured interview is relatively robust, even after only one to two years apart the classification agreement on type is only about 80% (Jenkins, Rosenman & Friedman, 1968). If test–retest unreliability is added to personality change over the time period, this could result in deflated estimates of type A risk. Second, it may be the case that type A behaviour has a synergistic relationship with other risk factors, and that over time these other risk factors are diminished. For example, younger men may have to cope with more life and work changes/demands than older men, and the effects of this may interact with personality type. Thus, although the Raglan & Brand (1988a) study confirms that type A personality is associated with increased CHD mortality risk after 8½ years, one may not expect the risk to be present at all life stages. Third, there may be other changes which go hand in hand with being a type A person that offer some protection from type A risk, as the person gets older. For example, it has been suggested that type A subjects achieve higher occupational status because they devote more of their discretionary time to work (Byrne & Reinhart, 1989), and that company performance and growth is better in companies with a greater proportion of type A individuals (Boyd, 1984). It has also been shown that type A subjects report more life events than type B and that this difference is primarily due to type A individuals self-initiating the events (Jarvikoski & Harkapaa, 1988). The extra work load involved in success may result in excess CHD risk during the time of occupational advancement (see the section later on work load and CHD). Once successful, however, the benefits of high status may confer a health advantage (Fletcher, 1988a).

Type A behaviour has, however, been associated with benefits as well as costs. Many of the aspects of the concept are positive attributes for organisational productivity, individual motivation and self-gratification (Ivancevich & Matteson, 1988), and have been related to profitability and sales performance (Boyd, 1984). Moreover, it may be that the prognosis after a heart attack is better for type A individuals. Raglan & Brand (1988b) studied the survival rates of 257 males who suffered coronary events. These men were from the 8.5-year stage of the WCGS. Of the 231 who survived for at least 24 hours the mortality risk was only 19.1/1000 person-years for the type A, compared to 31.7/1000 for the type B. The association was also stronger for those with symptomatic myocardial infarction, rather than silent infarction or angina pectoris.

Friedman & Rosenman have published many tens of papers, and several books, on coronary-prone behaviour. The idea that there is a reliably measurable behaviour pattern which is predictive of CHD has, however, received a number of challenges (as well as considerable support). Before considering some of this work, however, one important point should be noted. Whilst "it is impressive that a relatively straightforward behavioral classification of people permits the subsequent prediction of coronary heart disease independently of other recognised risk factors" (Syme & Seeman, 1983, p. 63) Friedman & Rosenman have brought attention to only one dimension (albeit possibly a major one) of the psychological universe of potential relevance to heart disease. That psychologically rooted factor has been shown by their work to be at least as important as traditional risk factors. There remains the possibility that other psychological factors (perceived or not, aspects of personality or the environment) are similarly important in either the genesis of CHD or in promoting its behavioural (e.g. cigarette smoking) and physiological precursors (e.g. cholesterol). For example, research has outlined ways in which stress-related hormones can contribute towards elevated levels of serum lipids, and their deposit on arterial walls. One major reason for the importance of the Western Collaborative Group Study was precisely that it allowed for the relative assessment of the behavioural risk factor and the traditional ones. There must be very limited value in prospective studies of risk factors in heart disease which do not include the measurement of psychologically relevant variables too (e.g. Shaper *et al.*, 1985).

The Measurement of Type A Behaviour

The measurement of the type A behaviour pattern is not without its difficulties. Some researchers have even suggested the construct should be abandoned (Ray, 1991). Price (1982) has argued that a major problem with the research has been the lack of clarity about precisely what the type A behaviour pattern is. In her review of over 100 studies she lists the frequency with which certain characteristics have been cited as underlying the type A person. Some 31 characteristics were cited. Nine of these were mentioned in more than one-fifth of the studies (in rank order: competitiveness, time urgency, aggressiveness, drive, achievement striving, preoccupied or subject to deadlines, ambition or the desire for advancement, accelerated pace, impatience). Price argues that we still do not have a theoretical rationale as to how these different components relate to each other, or how they are acquired and maintained. She attributes this partly to the generally atheoretical nature of epidemiological research. She proposes a *cognitive social learning model* which outlines how the different components of the type A pattern may fit together (see Figure 5.1).

   The prognostic value of the type A/B personality in CHD relies not only on the adequacy of its conceptual basis but also on the soundness of the measurement procedures used to identify the behavioural patterns. There are a number of assessments of the measurement techniques which have been used (e.g. Matthews, 1982; Matthews, Jamison & Cottington, 1985; O'Looney, 1984). There are four principal scales for use with adult populations and two for children. The *Hunter–Wolf A–B Rating Scale* shows some relationship to the intensity or pace with which children perform tasks (Wolf *et al.*, 1982) and to children's systolic blood pressure (Hunter *et al.*, 1982) but it has not shown any relationships to other risk factors or the later development of CHD. The *Matthews Youth Test for Health* (Matthews & Angulo, 1980) is designed to be filled in by an adult who rates the children on 17 scales. Previous research has shown predicted behavioural concomitants of type A scores (e.g. Matthews & Siegel, 1983) as well as expected cardiovascular response to challenge (Lundberg, 1983). The work with children is, however, in its infancy.

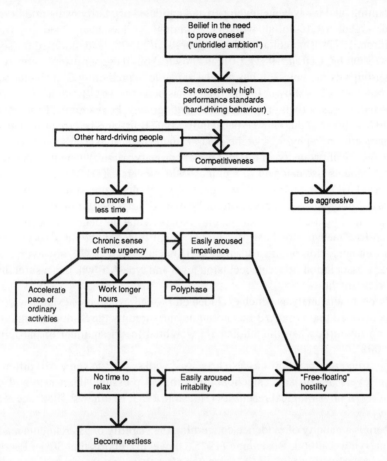

Figure 5.1 Price's (1982) overview of how the type A components fit together (reproduced by permission)

The adult measures have been used in many studies:

The structured interview (SI)

This developed from the clinical observations of Friedman & Rosenman (Rosenman, 1978) which has developed into an interview-based continuous scoring system of 39 indicators summed to provide a total score (Friedman *et al.*, 1982). The individual can be classified into one of five categories, A1, A2, X, B3, B4, where X represents equal amounts of A and B behaviours. The interview method (which may involve videotaping and subsequent scoring) can be time-consuming, and it has been developed and validated primarily using middle-class, middle-aged, white-collar workers. Although it has been used on women (Waldron, 1977), blue-collar workers (Kittel *et al.*, 1978), and modified for adolescents (Siegel & Leitch, 1981), little is known about its general applicability with such groups. Nonetheless, it has proved valuable in predicting CHD incidence, as the above work has shown. In addition, it has been shown to predict the degree of coronary atherosclerosis as measured by angiography. For example, Blumenthal *et al.* (1978) observed that of 85 type A and 57 type B patients referred for diagnostic coronary arteriography, 93% of the group with the highest TOTCI scores (a measure of the degree of occlusion of the four major coronary arteries) were type A patients. Type A patients also made up 70% of those with moderate TOTCI scores. Covarying standard CHD risk factors of sex, age, smoking, blood pressure and cholesterol levels did not remove the association. Williams *et al* (1980) report an analogous finding on 424 patients. In addition, they observed that the degree of occlusion was related to a measure of hostility: higher hostility scores being associated with increased occlusion on the arteriogram (Dimsdale *et al.*, 1979, however, did not find any association between occlusion level and type A/B when measured by the interview method).

A recent meta-analysis which excluded cross-sectional studies (Matthews, 1988) has confirmed that type A/B behaviour as measured by the SI does predict CHD risk, particularly when the studies are weighted for the number of participants ($p=0.008$).

The structured interview has also been used with success to show A/B differences in the levels of cortisol, catecholamines, blood pressure, heart rate and other measures of physiological reactivity (Houston, 1983; Matthews, 1982; see section below).

There is a paucity of evidence concerning the stability of assessments made by the interview method. Rosenman (1978), however, reports that 80% of subjects were similarly classified up to 20 months after their first interview.

The Jenkins Activity Survey (JAS)

This scale (Jenkins, Rosenman & Friedman, 1967; Jenkins, Zyzanski & Rosenman, 1971, 1979; Jenkins, 1978) was developed in close association with Friedman & Rosenman and the Western Collaborative Group Survey. It is a self-report multiple-choice questionnaire measure, is easily administered and can be automatically scored. More than 45 000 subjects have completed the questionnaire. There are different editions of the instrument. The questionnaire provides a measure of type A behaviour, but with the use of different weighting scales it also provides scores on three subscales of behavioural pattern which were derived from factor analysis of an early version. These measure job involvement, speed and impatience, and hard driving and competitiveness. Using the Western Group Survey data, Jenkins, Zyzanski & Rosenman (1978) have shown that different types of CHD subject show different responses on the questions: those with symptomatic myocardial infarction were more hard-driving and competitive and took fewer vacations when younger; those who developed unrecognised infarctions found job deadlines more stimulating and reported changes in appetite when under stress; those with angina pectoris (without infarction) became particularly irritated by interruptions to their schedules. The Jenkins Activity Survey has successfully predicted CHD in initially healthy subjects (Jenkins, Rosenman & Zyzanski, 1974; Jenkins *et al.*, 1978), and predicted the risk of new myocardial infarction in those with manifest CHD (Jenkins, Zyzanski & Rosenman, 1976). It also correlates with the degree of atherosclerosis revealed by arteriogram (Zyzanski *et al.*, 1976; but see Dimsdale *et al.*, 1978). However, it showed no ability to discriminate survivors from non-survivors when administered within two weeks of an acute infarction to 516 patients (Case *et al.*, 1985). In the same study type A score was not related to total mortality, cardiac mortality, time to death of non-survivors, left ventricular ejection fraction or duration of stay in the coronary unit. One reason for this lack of effect is that the Jenkins Activity Survey is only about 20% better than chance, when compared to the structured interview, at correctly classifying the behavioural patterns (Kittell *et al.*, 1978). Thus, compared to established physiological measures, it is a relatively insensitive measure with quite high error variance. The measure also has a rather low test–retest coefficient. Jenkins, Zyzanski & Rosenman (1971), for example, report a coefficient of 0.66 after one year based on a large sample ($n=2800$).

The JAS has not been found to be predictive of CHD risk in meta-analyses which exclude cross-sectional studies. Matthews (1988) reports that only three out of 11 tests in studies using the JAS type A/B classification are significant at the $p<0.05$ level, and the combined z-score taking account of the number of participants in each study has a p-value of only 0.464. Friedman & Booth-Kewley (1988) have even asked "What is the JAS measuring, and why should anyone care? In other words, research involving the JAS should provide a detailed conceptual justification for why it is of interest in that study.... There is little reason now to conduct studies of health that only use the JAS" (p. 383).

The Framingham Type A Scale

This scale is derived from 10 items of a 300-item questionnaire designed to investigate the role of a range of psychological variables in CHD in the Framingham Heart Study (Haynes *et al.*,1978a). Unlike the previous instruments, however, it was specifically developed for use with women (working women and housewives) as well as men, and has been shown to predict myocardial infarction and angina pectoris in these groups in an eight-year prospective investigation (Haynes, Feinleib & Kannel, 1980). Multivariate analysis, which includes the standard coronary risk factors and a number of psychological ones derived from the Framingham study, has also shown it to have independent predictive power of CHD for some blue- and all white-collar 45–64-year-old men and for working women of the same age range.

When considering specific CHD disorders the eight-year incidence of angina pectoris was higher in the 55–64-year-old type A women (11.8%) than in type B (3.5%), and the 65–74-year age group (5.9% vs. 0%). Myocardial infarction showed enhanced risk of type A behaviour for 45–54-year-old men (8.4% vs. 3.9%) and the 55–64-year-olds (9.1% vs. 4.4%). The 65–74-year-old men, however, showed lower type A risk (5.9% vs. 20%). This reversal was principally due to retired blue-collar workers. Multiple logistic regression of the data of the females aged 45–64 also showed that type A behaviour was an independent risk factor both when considering total CHD and angina pectoris cases (Hayes *et al.*, 1980). For both men and women there was also a clear synergistic relationship between type A/B and the other CHD risk factors (cholesterol level, blood pressure, cigarette smoking) (Haynes & Feinleib, 1982).

However, when compared to the methods used in the Western Collaborative Group Survey, the relative risks for both myocardial infarction and angina pectoris of type A behaviour are consistently lower. This suggests that the Framingham scale is not as sensitive, although the occupational differences between the subject cohorts may have contributed to this discrepancy. Indeed, the Framingham scale agrees with the structured interview classifications in only about 60% of cases (i.e. 10% better than chance) (Hayes *et al.*, 1980), and the distinction between type A and type B is statistically rather than conceptually based: the top 50% of scorers are designated as type A and the bottom 50% as B. Undoubtedly, the small number of items used to measure the behavioural type also contributes to the scale's insensitivity. Each of these factors may explain why the Framingham type A/B distinction has failed to show significant relationships with cardiovascular reactivity to psychological challenge (Dembrowski *et al.*, 1979a).

The Bortner Rating Scale

This scale requires subjects to place a vertical line between two extreme phrases or words, separated by a 1.5-inch horizontal line, which indicates how they perceive themselves. There are 14 rating scales (although the best seven are sometimes used) and the measured sum of distances from the type B end provide the score (Bortner, 1969). It shows 75% agreement with the structured interview (Rustin *et al.*, 1976) and correlates around 0.7 with the Jenkins Activity Survey (Johnston & Shaper, 1983). The scale has been used with success in a prospective study of heart disease by the French–Belgian Collaborative Group (1982). In this study 2811 CHD-free men aged 40–60 were followed for over six years. Bortner type A scores were higher in those men who suffered Rose-questionnaire-assessed angina or myocardial infarction or sudden death (although they only reached the 5% level of significance when total CHD was considered). Moreover, this score had predictive capacity independent of age, cholesterol, systolic blood pressure and smoking behaviour. Recent research, however, suggests the scale may be made up of two dimensions (speed and competitiveness) which, overall, have unacceptably low reliability (Edwards, Baglioni & Cooper, 1990).

PSYCHOPHYSIOLOGY OF TYPE A RISK

What, then, accounts for the apparently increased risk that type A persons exhibit of developing CHD? One suggestion is that type A individuals have enhanced sympathetic nervous system arousal responses to stressful situations. In an early biochemical study Friedman *et al.* (1960) observed that type A individuals have higher catecholamine levels than type B subjects during the working day. The same study showed that the catecholamine levels of the two behavioural groups were similar at night, which suggests that the daytime differences were a reflection of different patterns of reaction to daily events. Byers *et al.* (1962) also found that type A individuals exhibit higher levels of noradrenaline and its metabolic end-state 3-methoxy-4-hydroxymandelic acid during tense working days, even though evening levels are similar to type B subjects. Whilst it should be noted that other studies, using individuals with less well-established behavioural patterns, have failed to confirm these results (e.g. DeBacker *et al.*, 1979), there is considerable supporting evidence that type A people show greater cardiovascular changes, with concomitant changes in central nervous system and neuroendocrinal functioning, when placed under challenging or stressful conditions. That is, type A people show greater *reactivity and lability* to environmental situations than type B people. Reactivity refers to the change which may be observed in the resting or baseline levels of physiological indices when the subject is presented with psychological or physical stressors. The fact that type A individuals may show larger autonomic nervous system responses to particular stressors does not show they have excess CHD risk, although there is evidence from a 23-year prospective study that diastolic blood pressure change to the cold pressor test (limb immersion into cold water) is a strong predictor of future CHD (Keys *et al.*, 1971).

The range of stressors used in reactivity studies includes cognitive tests of varying difficulty (e.g. mental arithmetic, medical quiz, history tests), speeded reaction time tests and video games, dealing with threatening interpersonal situations (e.g. verbally hostile challenges, interview, competition), aversive stimuli (e.g. shock avoidance), and tasks which place the subject under physical demands (e.g. isometric hand-grip, cold pressor test).

Psychophysiological reactivity has been suggested as one of the major precursors of CHD independent of its relationship to type A behaviour (see Krantz & Manuck, 1984, 1985; Krantz & Raisen, 1988, for reviews and Light, 1985; Obrist, 1981, for examples). Although little is known about how acute changes become translated into chronic morphology, it is established that there are marked individual differences in reactivity (Engel & Bickford, 1961). Whilst there is evidence from twin studies suggesting a genetic component to physiological reactivity (Rose, Miller & Grim, 1982), there is also a considerable body of research showing that cardiovascular functioning can be operantly conditioned in humans as well as primates (e.g. Engel, 1977) which provides one mechanism for learnt dysfunctional responses. Ernst (1979), for example, has shown that dogs can be trained to control their coronary blood flow. It may be that persistent reactive responses to environmental stressors gradually result in morphological changes relevant to CHD. Necropsy of monkeys exposed to a mild stressor (gloves used for their catching) revealed that those with large heart rate changes had developed greater coronary and aortic atherosclerosis than those with low reactivity (Manuck, Kaplan & Clarkson, 1983). It should also be noted that in this study the atherosclerotic changes were present even though the mean reactivity differences between the monkey groups were not particularly large (61% vs. 88% above resting levels). In humans Dembroski, MacDougall & Lushene (1979) have reported that patients who have suffered myocardial infarctions exhibit greater increases in systolic blood pressure than case-controlled non-infarct subjects when given a history quiz (although no differences were observed for a challenging interview situation). No group differences were found for heart rate changes, but this may have been a result of most patients being on beta-blocking medications (Krantz & Manuck, 1984).

Behavioural Pattern and Physiological Reactivity

The evidence linking reactivity to type A/B behavioural patterns appears relatively convincing at first sight (reviews are provided by Glass, 1985; Houston, 1983; and Krantz & Manuck, 1984). Krantz & Manuck (1984) report that 70% of all studies, which include a variety of subject populations, have found greater reactivity during stressful situations among type A people on at least one of the measured cardiovascular or endocrine indices used. For example, Dembroski *et al.* (1978) required subjects to perform three different tasks (speeded reaction time task, an electronic game, a time-limited anagram test). In all tasks type A subjects showed greater systolic blood pressure and heart rate responses compared to type B. MacDougall, Dembroski & Krantz (1981) have also reported greater systolic pressure changes in type A than type B women under quiz and interview conditions.

David Glass, from the City University of New York, has completed a considerable amount of research on reactivity and behavioural patterns. In one study (Glass *et al.*, 1980) the reactivity of type A and B men was observed when they played games with and without competition and a harassing (confederate) opponent. Arterial systolic and diastolic blood pressure and heart rate were monitored every two minutes over a baseline period and during nine different games. The levels of plasma catecholamines (adrenalin and noradrenalin) were determined from blood samples taken during baseline and after each set of three games. The subjects were all screened and free of the major CHD risk factors. As is usual, no differences were observed in the baseline measures of the type A and type B men, and all five dependent measures showed increases as a result of game playing. For type B subjects there were no differential increases in any of the measures as a result of playing with a hostile or harassing opponent. Type A men also showed no greater reactivity, compared to type B, when playing under the normal competitive conditions. However, type A subjects playing with a harassing opponent showed significantly greater reactivity compared to the other three groups: their mean systolic blood pressure changes exceeded the other groups by more than 13 mmHg, heart rate by more than 8 bpm, and adrenalin levels by nearly 100 pg/ml. Noradrenalin levels produced a similar trend. There is some evidence that such task-induced reactivity is relatively stable over time within individuals (Glass & Contrada, 1983; Manuck, Corse & Winkelman, 1979; Obrist, 1981).

Stimulus and Response Characteristics

It should be noted that different types of stressor have differential effects on various reactivity measures which are likely to show significant patterns of interaction with type A/B behaviour. Noradrenalin secretion is more marked in response to the physical stress of exercise than the psychological stress of public speaking (Dimsdale & Moss, 1980) and to the cold pressor test and venipuncture than mental arithmetic (Ward *et al.*, 1983), whilst the opposite is true for adrenalin. Such findings, together with only moderate correlations between reactivity scores across different tasks (Krantz & Manuck, 1984, 1985), suggest the need for more research on task/ dependent measure interactions, although the field is a difficult one in which to do meaningful research (Dimsdale, 1985; Obrist, 1985c) not least because of the inherent variability of reactive complex mechanisms. More research is necessary to establish precisely which task characteristics cause which physiological changes in which individuals under what circumstances.

It may be that psychological task characteristics affect aspects of the cardiovascular system in different ways in different people. Dembroski & MacDougall (1983), for example, distinguish three categories of systolic blood pressure reactive individuals. When presented with psychological challenge most individuals show blood pressure increases which are primarily a result of increased cardiac output and not a change in peripheral resistance. Some, however, show increases in cardiac output and stroke volume together with a decrease in resistance. The third group exhibit increased peripheral resistance together with decreases in cardiac output and stroke volume.

Greater refinement of the type A/B distinction is necessary to isolate what aspects of type A behaviour carry CHD-related risk. Perhaps then we will have a better understanding of why "Most Type A's will not develop CHD and some Type B's will" (Dembroski *et al.*, 1983, p. 66). Some 45–76% of the population demonstrate type A behaviour (Rosenman *et al.*, 1964; Howard, Cunningham & Rechnitzer, 1976) yet the incidence of CHD among type A subjects is relatively low (e.g. 13.2/1000 men at risk in Rosenman *et al.*, 1975), especially when considered in terms of type B incidence (5.9/1000 per year). Thus, despite the relative success of the behavioural dichotomy in predicting CHD rates, a considerable amount of the predictable variance remains unaccounted for. In the factor analysis of structured interview data from 186 men from the Western Collaborative Group Study, of the five factors derived only those of *competitive drive* and *impatience* were predictive of later CHD

(Matthews *et al.*, 1977). These factors have also been shown to be predictive of physiological reactivity to challenge (Dembroski *et al.*, 1978; 1979a).

Self-involvement and Control

There is some suggestion (Glass, 1977, 1983; Matthews & Glass, 1984) that type A individuals attempt to exert more *control* over their environment, and that active efforts to do so are reflected in physiological reactivity as well as behaviour. In contrast to type B subjects, type A subjects exposed to noise showed worse performance on a subsequent reaction time task if they could control the termination of the noise bursts by pressing levers. When the noise could not be controlled, however, type A subjects showed enhanced performance. The results suggest that type A subjects attempt to impose some control over uncontrollable events, thus enhancing short-term attention. In the long term, however, such attempts must result in failure and poor coping/learned helplessness (Seligman, 1975). The work of Frankenhauser, Lundberg & Forsman (1980a,b) suggests that type A subjects placed in uncontrollable situations ('effort with distress') show enhanced secretion of sympathetic adrenal–medullary adrenalin *and* adrenal cortisol. When under controllable demands, however, enhanced adrenalin secretion is accompanied by a suppression of cortisol ('effort without distress'). Type B subjects, however, are not affected by demand controllability and thus exhibit less adrenal–cortical reactivity. We have seen in previous chapters that control and predictability are important dimensions of task stressfulness and that some models of stress incorporate discretion as an independent predictor of strain. The evidence concerning control reactivity and behavioural pattern is, however, ambiguous (Dembroski *et al.*, 1983), although Rosenman & Chesney (1980) propose that type A individuals are particularly affected by stressors where the locus of control is uncertain.

This emphasis on control by type A subjects is also related to another aspect of behaviour which differentiates type A from type B subjects. The work of Scherwitz, Berton & Leventhal (1978) suggests that type A individuals may be more 'self-centred' than type B individuals. The investigators observed that type A subjects who used more references to themselves in the structured interview situation also displayed the highest systolic blood pressures.

SELF-AWARENESS OF TYPE A CHARACTERISTICS

One important question, which has considerable relevance to the reduction of any type A coronary risk, is whether such individuals have conscious insight regarding their behaviour. An additional question is whether or not the reactions which type A subjects demonstrate are mediated by conscious mechanisms. With respect to the first issue there is evidence which suggests that type A subjects show a greater disjunction between knowledge and behaviour than type B subjects. For example, when performing a treadmill task Carver, Coleman & Glass (1976) found that type

A subjects did more physical work than type B subjects, although they did not admit to being as fatigued. Pittner & Houston (1980), using a digit repetition task, found that type A subjects, compared to type B subjects, exhibited greater heart rate under all conditions, and greater systolic and diastolic blood pressure changes after being told that they needed to respond more quickly (the 'threat to self-esteem' condition). Type A subjects, however, reported significantly less subjective distress relative to their level of psychophysiological arousal than did type B subjects, and more evidence of using the cognitive coping strategies of denial and suppression. This tendency to use denial by type A subjects led Pittner & Houston (1980) to conclude that they "are more likely to *consciously* try to cope with the situation—that is, consciously try to suppress thinking about the aversive aspects of the situation...it may lead them to endure stress longer and/or to endure higher levels of stress than Type B individuals" (p. 156). This denial of negative aspects of experience may be one reason why type A subjects delay seeking medical help for the early symptoms of CHD, even though patients with angina pectoris show a propensity to complain about somatic symptoms (Bakker & Levenson, 1967; Haynes *et al.*, 1978b).

Type A Behaviour During Surgery under Anaesthesia

Cognitive or conscious strategies, however, cannot entirely account for type A/B differences since some evidence demonstrates physiological reactivity when the subjects are not conscious. Two studies of patients anaesthetised for coronary bypass surgery report greater increases in intraoperative systolic blood pressure for type A compared to type B patients (Kahn *et al.*, 1980; Krantz *et al.*, 1982). The latter study, an extension of the former, assessed the contribution of interview and Jenkins-questionnaire-measured type A/B personality to three blood pressure measures: peak operative increase compared to admission, peak operative increase compared to first operative pressures, preoperative increase from admission to first operative. Whilst type A behaviour was not related to systolic blood pressure changes which occurred prior to surgery (the third measure), the systolic changes during surgery (the first and second measures) showed marked behavioural influences. Intraoperative changes for type A1 subjects exceeded those of type B subjects by more than 30 mmHg, whilst peak operative measure compared to admission was over 45 mmHg greater for type A1 subjects. In addition, 12 of the 27 patients who underwent surgery had complications recorded during the surgical and postoperative course which involved sympathetic nervous system activity (mainly arrhythmias—pericarditis alone being excluded). All 12 were type A men (either A1 or A2). It is interesting to note that the Jenkins questionnaire was not found to be a discriminating instrument with respect to the blood pressure effects.

These findings led Krantz & Durel (1983) to propose that there may be an underlying psychobiological basis for interview-defined type A behaviour and that full conscious mediation and appraisal is not a necessary prerequisite for such behaviour as has previously been assumed. They suggest that "the impatience, hostility, and speech patterns exhibited by Type A individuals may, in part, *reflect* an underlying sympathetic nervous system responsivity". They suggest that such a view is divergent from the idea that type A behaviours *produce* elevated sympathetic responses. They provided a further test of this view by showing that a pharmacological manipulation which reduces sympathetic responsivity (the beta-adrenergic blocking drug propranolol) decreased the actual intensity of type A behaviours during interview. Coronary patients given propranolol showed less evidence of speech which was loud/explosive, rapid/accelerated and evidenced rapid response latency and potential-for-hostility, compared to non-treated patients, although the content of interviews and Jenkins-questionnaire-type A assessments were similar for both groups. No other medications (diuretics, nitrates, CNS-active drugs) showed such effects (Krantz *et al.*, 1982).

Inconsistencies

Despite the considerable body of evidence supporting the various aspects of coronary-prone behaviour, the research work shows a number of inconsistencies (see Evans, 1990). For example, Keith, Lown & Stare (1965) and Ahnve *et al.* (1979) did not find significantly more type A individuals in their CHD patients, compared to non-CHD controls. Two studies by Dimsdale and his colleagues (1978, 1979) failed to find any relationship between arteriogram-determined coronary atherosclerosis and behaviour pattern. In physiological reactivity work, Manuck, Corse & Winkelman (1979) failed to replicate type A/B differences in response to task conditions used in earlier studies. Moreover, whilst there is a large measure of agreement, despite these broad failures to replicate, about the tasks that do or do not produce reactivity, it should be noted that there are many inconsistencies between studies when one considers specific reactivity measures (e.g. systolic and diastolic blood pressure, heart rate). This is further confounded by inconsistent sex differences (see Houston, 1983).

For these and other reasons some of the inconsistencies can probably be attributed to measurement, methodological and subject population differences, rather than to the theoretical bareness of the type A/B distinction. Any measure of behaviour based on crude atheoretically derived and developed metrics which classifies entire populations into (essentially) two categories is certain to produce occasionally inconsistent findings with high variance scores. This is especially so when the categories are derived in several different ways. In an empirical investigation Myrtek & Greenlee (1984), for example, found that the correlation between the Structured Interview and the Jenkins Activity Survey was only 0.23. In their analysis of previous studies the average correlation was a little higher (0.34) but even this higher figure indicates only 11% of the variance as being common to both measures. Restricted range and large variance are poor bedfellows of consistency.

Different subpopulations (e.g. patients, white- or blue-collar workers, specific occupational groups, students) may also show different patterns of results. Haynes,

Feinleib & Kannel (1980), for example, report that retired blue-collar 65–74-year-olds show a reversal of the usual pattern between type A/B behaviour and CHD incidence.

Krantz & Manuck (1985), in a discussion of the reactivity literature, suggest that some inconsistencies may be due to: (a) inadequate adaptation and baseline measures, (b) the lack of reliable and standardised test procedures applicable to a wide range of subject groups, (c) failure to control task duration and timing of the measures in relation to the task, (d) the recording of too few physiological indices with the concomitant omission to consider individual response variations, and (e) a failure to pay adequate attention to subject characteristics such as age, race, sex and the subjects' task appraisals and capabilities.

It has to remain something of an article of faith that the type A/B distinction has pragmatic and/or theoretical use. The numbers of studies which report evidence in support of a psychophysiological basis of the distinction are outweighed by the non-replications. Myrtek & Greenlee (1984) provide an analysis of some 45 investigations on type A and type B men which were pertinent to the view espoused by Williams *et al.* (1978) that type A men have enhanced sympathetic nervous system activity. This hypothesis entails that type A individuals, compared to type B, should exhibit higher blood pressure and heart rate values, lower pulse volume amplitude, shorter pulse transit times, more skin conductance responses with shorter latencies and higher levels, and higher uric catecholamine levels. For these 10 physiological measures, and considering resting, strain and change scores, these 45 studies produced 49 main effect differences between type A and B individuals (at 5% or better level) out of 367 possible effects (i.e. 13%). This is not greatly in excess of chance levels. If one considers only the change scores (baseline–challenge differences) 27 of 132 are significant (this excludes the catecholamine measures) which represents only a 20% 'hit rate'. Even for specific indices where we might expect a better picture we do not find much solace. For systolic blood pressure changes to task challenge, 16 of 38 main effects are statistically significant (42%), and for adrenalin and noradrenalin only four of 28 tests were significant, and one of those was in the wrong direction!

Myrtek & Greenlee (1984) also report an experiment in which they obtained data from 58 subjects on three occasions over a one-year period in an attempt to evaluate the existence of physiological differences of type A/B individuals. Since the experiment is unique in the scope and depth with which it considered the psychophysiology of the type A/B dichotomy, it will be described in some detail. All subjects were classified separately by both the structured interview and the Jenkins questionnaire. Some 27 physiological dimensions were measured under a variety of experimental conditions including rest, mental arithmetic during acoustic distraction, reaction time, preparation and presentation of a speech, cold pressor, bicycle ergometric exercise and a 1000 metre run. Monetary incentives were given to enhance competitiveness. The measures taken included blood pressure, heart rate, different measures of impedance cardiography (stroke volume, cardiac output, ventricular ejection time), pulse volume amplitude, pulse transit time, pulse wave velocity, various measures of electrodermal activity measured by skin conductance, eyeblink activity, various respiratory variables and catecholamine excretion. In addition, 11 dimensions of emotional state were measured (at rest and during experimental phases) which were relevant to the behavioural dichotomy (tense, angry, insecure, cramped, ill-humoured, active, nervous, helpless, indifferent, competitive, annoying).

The results were very clear-cut and provide no support whatsoever for the assertion that there are psychophysiological differences between type A and type B individuals. For example, of the 834 possible physiological main effects of behavioural type only 29 (i.e. 3%) were significant at the 5% level when subjects were classified by the structured interview, and only 62 (i.e. 7%) when using the Jenkins Activity Survey. Thus, overall only 5% of the effects were significant at the 5% level! In addition, not only did the different behaviour pattern classifications show different patterns for the significant results, but some important physiological measures produced significances in the opposite direction to those predicted. For example, there were no main effects for type A subjects showing higher systolic blood pressures (at rest, during strain, or change scores measured by arithmetic difference or as autonomic lability scores) although there were 14 effects of *lower* systolic pressures in the type A samples. Not one of the self-ratings of subjective state was significant.

Whilst this study is not beyond criticism it is comprehensive. The fact that it utilised fit young students should also not be held against it since, as the authors point out, some 60% of all the studies in the literature have also used student subject populations. The study does raise a number of significant issues which question the whole basis of the type A/B distinction. The behavioural patterns may well be useful (if unreliable) predictors of future CHD pathology. There is, however, considerable reason to be unhappy with the evidence that there are identifiable physiological differences between these subgroups. There is even less justification for the proposal that such acute physiological indicators are the precursors or risk factors in the onset of later chronic pathological changes. Perhaps the best we can do is to conclude rather cryptically that "the hypothesised physiological differences between Type A and B persons remain, for the time being, missing" (Myrtek & Greenlee, 1984, p. 464).

OTHER PSYCHOLOGICAL FACTORS IMPLICATED IN CHD

A large number of retrospective studies, and a small number of major prospective studies, have investigated the role of dispositional and personality characteristics other than type A/B behaviour in the onset of CHD. The principal factors which have been implicated in 'normal' population samples essentially free of clinical psychiatric disorders are *anxiety, depression* and *neuroticism*, although a whole range of other dimensions have been studied to a lesser extent (e.g. Jenkins, 1976a,b; 1982; Siegel, 1985). The psychometric properties of the measuring instruments vary considerably from simple questions presumed to have high face validity (e.g. as in major studies by Medalie *et al.*, 1973; and Paffenbarger *et al.*, 1966), through those with considerable study-specific piloting (e.g. Haynes *et al.*, 1978a), to those which have utilised established personality profiles with extensive reliability and validity data such as the Eysenck Personality Inventory (e.g. French–Belgian Collaborative Group, 1982) and the Minnesota Multiphasic Personality Inventory (MMPI) (e.g. Ostfeld *et al.*, 1964).

Psychological Traits and Self-reported Symptomatology

One major problem in assessing the link between personality factors and CHD is that some manifestations of CHD are difficult to diagnose unambiguously independently of the subjective reports of the patient. This is particularly problematic when considering any causal link between psychological traits with a clinical root and angina pectoris. Angina is often diagnosed in studies by simply questioning the subject (e.g.with the clinical interview instrument used by Medalie *et al.*, 1973, or the Rose questionnaire) about the type and presence of chest pain (plus radiating left arm pain) and the effects of physical exertion on symptomatology. Moreover, angina patients do not form a homogeneous group since they are often classified into different categories (e.g. nocturnal, exercise-provoked, postprandial, emotionally provoked sufferers with or without infarction history). If the heart condition is not diagnosed independently of the self-report (e.g. by confirmatory horizontal depression of the ST segment of the ECG under stress or evidence of stenosis) it may be that it is the psychological state of the subject which causes him to present with the symptoms irrespective of the presence of angina. Elias *et al.* (1982), for example, found that patients with angina pectoris but no stenosis scored higher on Spielberger's State–Trait Anxiety Scale and the Zung Self-rating Depression Scale than those angina patients with stenosis. This led the investigators to suggest that "neuroticism may bring the patient to the cardiologist for examination and diagnosis but does not predict ischaemic heart disease or myocardial infarction" (p. 49). Earlier reviews of the scientific literature (e.g. Mai, 1968; Jenkins, 1976a) conclude that there is little support for a connection between personality factors and myocardial infarction, although there is some evidence that angina pectoris is related to such factors as anxiety, depression and neuroticism. The 'relationship' could not be seen as being a causal one, however.

The results of a number of major prospective heart disease studies support this view to some extent. In the French–Belgian Collaborative Group Study (1982), a prospective design which began with over 3000 factory workers and civil servants, and lasted from just under four and a half years in Paris to over eight years in Marseilles, neuroticism (measured by the Eysenck Personality Inventory) was found to be the best discriminator between CHD and healthy groups. However, when only those men with 'silent' CHD (i.e. only ECG manifestations, no symptoms) were considered, neuroticism was no longer predictive. In the Israeli Ischaemic Heart Disease Project some 8528 CHD-free men aged 40 years or over, of an initial population sample of 10 059, were followed for five years with three periodic comprehensive examinations. This study, discussed in greater detail below, observed that a number of psychological factors (anxiety, problems and conflicts in various areas of life) were predictive of later angina pectoris assessed by questionnaire (Medalie *et al.*, 1973a; Medalie & Goldbourt, 1976) but were not predictive of myocardial infarction endpoints (Medalie *et al.*, 1973b; Goldbourt, Medalie & Neufeld, 1975). Thus, we are left with the uncertainty as to whether there is a causal link between such psychological variables and CHD, or whether individuals of a certain predisposition are more sensitive to somatic occurrences.

Unfortunately, it is not uncommon for angina patients to have clear ECG stress tests and for some groups of healthy subjects to show positive records. One must remain particularly wary of reports which do not provide objective evidence of heart disease (be it confirmatory ECGs or death from infarction!). A further complication, however, is that some groups of subjects with a higher risk of CHD have been shown to exhibit a greater propensity to deny symptoms and unpleasant experiences (see the section on 'Self-awareness of type A characteristics'). It is unclear whether these apparent inconsistencies can be attributed to different types of CHD and their specific related psychological factors, or to difficulties of diagnoses.

The Western Electric Company Study

An early prospective study of the relationship of personality factors to CHD is reported by Ostfeld *et al.* (1964). In this study 1885 men of a Chicago company, aged between 40 and 57 and free of CHD at the outset, were followed for five annual examinations. Each person completed both the MMPI and the Cattell 16PF near the beginning of the study. Fifty men developed angina pectoris and 38 were diagnosed as having myocardial infarctions (with or without angina) by ECGs. The MMPI data revealed some significant differences between the angina group (*n*=48) on the one hand, and the infarction (*n*=37) and disease-free control (*n*=1771) groups on the other. The angina subjects showed higher scores on both the *hypochondriasis and hysteria* scales, suggesting that they are more likely to perceive somatic symptoms. Indeed, a multiple discriminant analysis revealed that hypochondriasis was the variable which most discriminated the angina from the no-CHD group. Lebovits *et al.* (1967) also report that living angina sufferers scored higher than infarction survivors on psychopathic deviance, paranoia, psychasthenia and schizophrenia. They also show that the difference in hypochondriasis scores was still present on MMPI retesting in year 5, which suggests that the concern about health and the presence of physical symptoms or objective evidence of ill-health is not the cause of these elevated scores.

Both angina and infarction groups revealed higher scores on the 16PF scales *self-sufficiency* and *suspiciousness* compared to the controls, but there were notable differences between the CHD subgroups on the *emotional stability* scale: angina subjects demonstrating greater emotional lability.

A re-examination of the MMPI of this study by Lebovits, Lichter & Moses (1975) provided additional support for the view that different CHD groups have different personality profiles, and that these are different in structure to healthy individuals. Each group was split into high and low scorers on a validity scale and the analysis considered the relationship between the MMPI profiles and physical coronary risk factors. The healthy individuals were distinct from the CHD groups inasmuch as they showed different profiles, independence of the physical and personality factors, and no difference in the validity scale. The factor loadings also differentiated an angina group from a combined infarction and sudden death group, but these groups showed considerable overlap of the physical and personality variables which also varied with the validity scale score.

Lebovits *et al.* (1967) report more analyses of the Western Electric Company study relating to changes in MMPI scores from the first to the fifth year, and the profiles of CHD survivors compared to those who died. Non-survivors of infarction scored more highly on some scales than survivors (hysteria, psychopathic deviance, psychasthenia), although the living angina group exhibited similarly elevated scores on these scales as well as higher scores on hypochondriasis, schizophrenia and paranoia. In addition, although there were no differences between survivors and non-survivors on the depression scale, non-survivors more frequently had elevated scores on this scale, as they did on others. It may be that a subset of CHD patients are psychiatrically labile and become profoundly disturbed by their heart attacks. Wolf (1969), for example, found that 10 patients who had recently suffered an infarction were particularly depressed when assessed, and all 10 died within the four-year study (two committed suicide and the others had fatal heart attacks).

The analysis of MMPI changes, however, suggests that some of the personality differences revealed may have been a consequence of perceived changes in health rather than the cause of such changes. First, both the angina and infarction survivors had increased scores on the *neurotic triad (hypochondriasis, depression and hysteria)* in their fifth year compared to their first. Second, although the angina survivors did not differ from the healthy controls on this triad at the beginning of the study (a finding supported by a study of Maggini *et al.*, 1976/77, but which employed a control group who were on the average nearly 20 years younger), they did so at the end. A small study by Bruhn, Chandler & Wolf (1969) shows a similar effect for both *anxiety* and *depression* scales. A more recent study of 204 middle-aged (mean= 53 years) men who were potential patients for coronary bypass surgery also demonstrates the need for multivariate analysis (Jenkins *et al.*, 1983). In this investigation angina was univariately correlated with the depression subscale of the Profile of Mood States, but was not a significant predictor in the multivariate analysis which controlled for physical risk factors and any overlap between the personality scales.

The Framingham Heart Study

The Framingham Heart Study is a major examination of the development of CHD in a population of more than 5000 men and women in Framingham, Massachusetts. Since 1949 the individuals, initially free of CHD, were monitored biannually for signs of CHD. From 1965 to 1967, when the participants were aged between 45 and 77 years, a 300-item questionnaire/interview was successfully administered to 1822 members of the study with the aim of investigating the possible contribution of psychological factors in CHD (Haynes *et al.*, 1978, outline the methodological and questionnaire details). The biannual examinations included extensive physical examinations, serum cholesterol determination, and ECG measurement. Those free of CHD were followed for an eight-year period for various clinical manifestations of CHD (Haynes, Feinleib & Kannel, 1980). Some 10-year incidence data have also been reported (Haynes & Feinleib, 1982).

Various CHD categories were used in subsequent analyses:

- *Myocardial infarction* was defined by unequivocal ECG changes (e.g. S-T segment elevation) and/or diagnostic elevations of serum enzymes indicative of muscle necrosis.
- *Coronary insufficiency* referred to those with a history of ischaemic chest pain accompanied by transient S-T segments and T-wave abnormalities (without Q-wave changes).
- *Angina pectoris* primarily included those with classic emotional or exercise substernal discomfort of less than 15 minutes' duration which was relieved by rest or nitroglycerine. It should be noted that this category included all those with these symptoms irrespective of the co-occurrence of other clinical manifestations of CHD above.
- *Sudden CHD death* was death within one hour of the first symptoms of CHD in apparently well individuals.

Although the study did not incorporate previously established psychometric tests, 20 different scales were specifically developed to ascertain the potential contribution of psychological dimensions in CHD development. One of these scales—the Framingham type A measure—has already been discussed. Each scale was subjected to prior item and factor analysis to remove those items with poor intercorrelations. Although some of these scales apparently dealt with external or environmental situations, rather than person-based properties, the person's subjective evaluation of the situation was what was measured.

The scales of relevance here measured: the personality traits of *emotional lability* or reactivity, *ambitiousness*, '*easygoingness*'; two scales concerning worry about ageing and personal matters; interpersonal perceptions about the supportiveness of boss and spouse; and seven scales which measured the behavioural responses of individuals to stressors including tension, daily felt strain, anxiety, and anger scales which differentiated suppressed anger ('anger-in'), externalised expression ('anger-out') and coping by talking ('anger-discuss').

At the outset of the study none of these 15 variables correlated with any of the four CHD risk factors (systolic and diastolic blood pressure, serum cholesterol, smoking behaviour) with a coefficient of greater than 0.14 for either men or women.

Some correlations were significant at the 5% level or better (for men six of the 60, for women 10 of the 60) the most notable being: ageing worries with systolic and diastolic pressure (men only); anger-in, anger-discuss, anxiety symptoms, and tension with diastolic pressure (women); anxiety symptoms with diastolic and systolic pressures (women); cholesterol with anger-out (women); cigarette smoking with easygoingness and anger-in (men) and ambitiousness and marital dissatisfaction (women) (Haynes *et al.*, 1978). Thus, it can be seen that as well as any effects being very small, there is a virtually total lack of consistency for any given psychological factor. This situation is made even worse when subsamples are considered (e.g. white- and blue-collar workers).

The usefulness of the same psychological factors in predicting the eight-year incidence of CHD was no better. For men the univariate analyses produced lower anger-out scores (and work overload scores) for 55–64-year-olds, and higher anxiety symptoms for 65+-year-old CHD cases. None of the variables were significant for 45–54-year-olds. In multiple logistic regression, which controlled for identified risk factors, the only significant psychological predictor which remained was anger-out—and this only for white-collar men. In the female sample, only the 55–64-year-olds produced any significant univariate effects: CHD cases had more anxiety symptoms, higher tension scores, higher anger-in scores, and lower anger-out and anger-discuss scores, compared to non-cases. In the multivariate model only the anger-discuss variable remained a significant predictor for women aged 45–64 (although it did this for the categories of total CHD and angina pectoris when all women in this age group were considered—but this was relevant only to working women, not housewives, as shown by separate analyses). Tension scores and easygoingness scores taken during the 1965–67 period were also independent predictors of total CHD in the housewives group. This maze of different types of analyses, using different variables, different age range configurations in different analyses, and different diagnostic CHD categories, itself illustrates that the data have had to be 'trawled' to quite a sophisticated level to catch any significance. Such analyses are rather *post hoc* and, as such, of dubious status.

It should be noted that although some of the statistical analyses are significant, the general level of predictability is not much better than chance (which would allow for 5% of the analyses to be significant). Of the psychological variables the only one with any consistent pattern is the type A scale. The appearance of other correlations here and there is largely meaningless without *a priori* reason to predict that pattern (as opposed to any other). Consider, too, that when specific CHD manifestations are considered separately, the predictability is reduced even further. Whilst one reason for this is the small number of cases in each category, the reason for the lack of reported specific analyses for each diagnostic category of CHD is presumably because they produced no significant pattern of results. Thus, the large Framingham study suggests that these psychological variables are not very useful in predicting CHD incidence (and that the traditional risk factors do not account for much of the predictable variance either). It must be remembered, however, that the majority of the scales used have only the smallest degree of external validity.

Other studies provide further support for the assertion that personality and related psychological variables are not useful consistent predictors of CHD. In a 30-year prospective study of 281 initially healthy men, for example, Gillum *et al.* (1980) did not find any relationships between MMPI scores and CHD. Elias *et al.* (1982) report a negative correlation between the number of diseased arteries and the hypochondriasis and hysteria scales. The MMPI Depression Scales and the Zung Self-Rating Depression Scale produced quite different patterns of results. Indeed, one major reviewer has concluded that "The prospective studies on personality and CVD (cardiovascular disease) as a group provide little encouragement for future research endeavours of this sort. None of these studies supported the importance of personality (as measured) as an etiological factor" (Siegel 1985). Siegel also lists a number of methodological reasons why this has been so. First, there has been generally inadequate assessment of the different types of CHD, particularly angina pectoris. Second, the assessment of personality variables has been too haphazard and relied on too many different measures with variable reliability and validity. Third, the sample populations, and the control groups used (sometimes other hospital patients, sometimes not), are often not representative of the general population. Fourth, only truly prospective studies can demonstrate that personality variables are not the consequence of heart condition changes. Finally, there has been insufficient use of multivariate analyses to demonstrate the independent contribution of psychological factors, rather than their dependence on other risk variables. It seems that the closer to the 'ideal' design the study is, however, the less likely it is to show any meaningful contribution of personality in the etiology of CHD, particularly myocardial infarction.

Meta-analysis of Psychological Predictors of CHD

The importance of type A behaviour and some other personality variables as a cause of CHD has been examined by a systematic meta-analysis of 87 published studies by Booth-Kewley & Friedman (1987). Meta-analysis is a statistical technique which allows a quantitative review of previous research, and is one way of determining whether obvious inconsistencies in the literature nonetheless hide statistically meaningful trends. It provides an estimation of the combined size of effects previously reported, as well as an analysis of variables which can be assessed only by collating a number of different studies. Booth-Kewley & Friedman (1987) included all significant objective studies of personality characteristics (particularly type A behaviour) and CHD which were published or reviewed between 1945 and 1985.

The analysis demonstrated a number of important factors. First, type A behaviour was reliably related to CHD. The combined correlation between all type A measures and all CHD outcomes was 0.136, which is rather modest. Second, with small sample sizes the correlation was extremely variable, suggesting that sampling error is a major factor with such studies. It is well known that ordinary least-squares regression coefficients are very dependent on the frequency of the outcome state being measured. Second, the link between type A and CHD was much weaker in prospective ($r=0.045$, $p=0.00009$) than cross-sectional studies ($r=0.175$, $p<0.0000001$), suggesting that prevalence rates are particularly prone to over-estimating cause–effect relationships if they exist. Third, the Structured Interview was a much better predictor of CHD than the JAS, probably because the JAS includes a scale relating to the degree of job involvement which is, if anything, negatively related to CHD outcomes. Fourth, measures of anger/hostility and competitiveness/hard-driving behaviour may be better predictors of CHD than other related type A characteristics. Fifth, other psychological characteristics are probably at least as predictive of CHD as the type A concept. Anxiety and depression were found to be particularly important characteristics despite the inconsistencies discussed in the preceding pages. For example, although we have seen that depression has not been found to be consistently related to CHD, in the meta-analysis it was a better predictor of all CHD disease outcomes ($r=0.205$, $p<0.0000001$) than any type A measure or single subscale. This was true when the analysis was restricted to prospective studies ($r=0.168$, $p=0.00008$) which rules out the possibility that CHD is itself the cause of the depression. The authors concluded:

> Overall, the picture of the coronary-prone personality emerging from this review does not appear to be that of a workaholic, hurried, impatient individual, which is probably the image most frequently associated with coronary proneness. Rather, the true picture seems to be one of a person with one or more negative emotions: perhaps someone who is depressed, aggressively competitive, easily frustrated, anxious, angry, or some combination (p. 358).

A subsequent meta-analysis by Matthews (1988), which included four new prospective studies, excluded cross-sectional studies, only included one report for each separate study sample, and weighted the analysis according to the number of participants in each study, has confirmed and extended the results of Booth-Kewley & Friedman (1987) in some important respects. Although Matthews reports that across all measures and all studies type A behaviour was not predictive of CHD ($p=0.26$), or in studies confined to high CHD-risk populations ($p=0.55$), there was a clear association for those studies utilising the Structured Interview to assess behaviour type ($p=0.008$), and for those using general populations (as opposed to high CHD-risk ones) ($p=0.001$). Moreover, the 'negative emotions' of anxiety and hostility were also associated with increased CHD risk ($p=0.005$ and 0.01, respectively), although depression was not ($p=0.39$). This latter finding does reinforce the somewhat fragile status of the role of depression in CHD, and suggests it may be dependent upon the person being aware of the presence of disease symptoms or a CHD diagnosis.

Individual Temperament and Premature Heart Disease

As part of Johns Hopkins Precursors study, discussed in the previous chapter, Betz & Thomas (1979) examined the hypothesis that individual temperament had predictive potency in CHD. Temperament refers to the individual's nature of affect as manifest in the mode of action and reaction and in behavioural style. It is conceived as a property originating from within the individual and with life-long effects on behaviour. Based on the work of Gesell & Ilg (1943), Betz & Thomas classified some students of the medical school into one of three temperament types:

- *Alpha types*, who were characterised as being slow and solid.
- *Beta types*, who were spontaneous, rapid and facile.
- *Gamma types*, with irregular and uneven behaviour showing mixed or confused responses.

Up to 30 years later the records of these physicians were examined for premature disease and death. In a small first study 49% of those who developed a disorder had been classified as gamma types, and 33% as beta. A second study examined whether these proportions were different from normal healthy controls. Sixty-three individuals who had developed a disorder were matched with 64 healthy controls. As in the first study, the individuals were primarily designated as exhibiting the gamma temperament (47%). Of this gamma group, however, 62% were individuals who had developed disease prematurely, suggesting that this type of temperament has disease risks. Of particular interest here, however, is that 11 of the 14 (79%) myocardial infarction sufferers had been designated as gamma types. This percentage was much larger than for the hypertension sufferers (12 out of 26, or 46%) or the major cancer group (12 out of 20, or 60%), supporting the view that gamma temperament may have specific heart disease risks.

Picture Drawings as Predictors

In the same Precursors study, Harrower, Thomas & Altman (1975) examined whether the human-figure drawings of 204 former medical students were predictors of CHD when examined 13–23 years later. This study, discussed in greater detail in the previous chapter, classified the drawings of disease groups and matched controls into various categories depending upon the attitude depicted in the stance of the figures which were drawn. The 15 individuals who had suffered a myocardial infarction, or were being treated for clinical hypertension (the data of these two groups were collapsed because they showed a similar pattern of results), were more likely than either their healthy control group or any of the other illness groups (malignant cancer, suicide, mental illness, emotional disturbance) to have drawn 'Category 2' figures. These were figures drawn with 'Arms extending outward, thought of as outgoing, inviting, or an input-demanding attitude' (Harrower *et al.*, 1975, p. 193) which are reflective of people who invite excessive input and demand on themselves. Of the eight possible categories 45% of pictures drawn by the CHD group were figures displaying this characteristic—this was twice as likely as for any other disease condition or their control group. Harrower *et al.* suggest that "a person's attitude toward the outside world, as mirrored in his human figure drawings, is an important factor in determining his specific vulnerabilities" (p. 198). What can be made of such findings is unclear.

ENVIRONMENTAL STRESSORS AND CHD

Life Change, CHD Survival and Sudden Cardiac Events

In the life events research discussed below, the methods used have primarily been based on those outlined in Chapter 2. They are generally open to the same range of methodological criticisms.

A range of studies have implicated psychological stressors as important factors in heart disease. One category of studies, those which assess the contribution of such stressors in sudden coronary death, suggest that acute factors may affect the likelihood of diseased or susceptible individuals surviving infarction, or affect the likelihood of fatal ventricular fibrillation without the evolution of acute myocardial infarction. (It should be remembered that in 25% of the victims of sudden coronary death no previous symptoms had been presented [Kuller, 1966], and 24% have only one or none of the major coronary vessels with 75%+ luminal stenosis [Perper, Kuller & Cooper, 1975]).

Myers & Dewar (1975) investigated the prior circumstances of 100 men who had died suddenly from ventricular fibrillation as far as could be determined by the coroner's necropsies. Acute psychological stress in the 30 minutes preceding the coronary event had occurred in 23% of cases, and 40% had experienced such stress within the past 24 hours (e.g. notification of divorce, being harassed by dogs, being involved in a non-traumatic car accident). Lown, Verrier & Rabinowitz (1977) have shown that an emotionally taxing interview can induce arrhythmogenesis in myocardial infarction patients who do not show abnormal rhythm at rest. Such rhythmic dysfunctions may be due to enhanced sensitivity to catecholamines under aversive situations (Verrier, Calvert & Lown, 1975; Verrier, DeSilva & Lown, 1983).

In an attempt to provide an understanding of why potentially damaging 'spontaneous' episodes of transient myocardial ischaemia occur (i.e. ST-segment depression and sometimes chest pain in the absence of an obvious provocation such as physical exercise) it has been hypothesised that such events are triggered off by changes in mental activity. Deanfield *et al.* (1984) subjected 16 CHD patients (41–74 years) and 13 non-CHD controls (28–50 years) to a bicycle exercise test and a simple mental arithmetic task, and measured myocardial perfusion with positron tomography. 'Silent' ischaemia (i.e. abnormal perfusion without chest pain or ST-segmentation) occurred frequently in the CHD patients when given mental arithmetic, but never under exercise. More importantly, however, was that the control subjects showed increases in the myocardial uptake of the isotope to arithmetic, whereas the CHD patients showed absolute regional decreases. A study of coronary heart disease patients by Rozanski *et al.* (1988), outlined at the beginning of this chapter, has extended this study by showing that a range of mental tasks can cause silent ischaemias, and that public speaking in particular may induce cardiac dysfunction. These studies suggest that everyday mental stress may effect important cardiac changes which, in the long run, can have major life consequences.

Although Myers & Dewar (1975) found no distinguishing effects of chronic stressors, Rissanen, Romo & Siltanen (1978) found that chronic stressors had been present in 25% of sudden-death CHD cases, as revealed by interviews with relatives. In addition 19% had suffered some acute stressor just before death. Acute myocardial infarction was also less likely among those with acute rather than chronic stress. It is true, of course, that people do try to give external causes for negative outcomes such as heart attacks. This 'effort after meaning' makes the need for longitudinal studies rather clear.

Chronic psychological stressors have also been implicated in the likelihood of an individual surviving a life-threatening coronary event. Rahe *et al.* (1974) compared the recent life events of a group of abrupt coronary death individuals with a group who had survived a myocardial infarction. Interviews with relatives showed that those who died had experienced more life changes in the immediately preceding six months compared to the survivors, although both groups had high change scores, compared to the same time period in the preceding year. Those who had died showed particular change in problems at home and work, as well as interpersonal difficulties with friends and family. In a more objective, quasi-prospective study, using case record charts of known CHD sufferers who had frequently attended an outpatients clinic, Theorell & Rahe (1975) compared those patients who had died after a second attack with others who had survived for more than six years. Clinicians ignorant of the CHD endpoint scored the record for life events in six-month blocks. It was found that whilst the survivors showed a relatively consistent score in each time epoch, the patients who died had a cluster of events in the seven to 12 months before death.

Life Events and CHD

In addition to the research showing that psychological stressors may have effects on the likelihood of an individual having or surviving a coronary event, there is also a body of evidence which suggests that such stressors may contribute towards the likelihood of a person developing CHD in the first instance. Rahe & Paasikivi (1971) obtained retrospective information concerning life changes (using the Schedule of Recent Experiences) from myocardial infarction survivors who had experienced their initial episodes one to four years previously. The life change information covered a four-year period in an attempt to exclude contamination of the effects of recent diagnosis. The patients showed a gradual increase in life change scores in the year-quarters preceding the infarction from about 25 LCUs to 55 LCUs per year-quarter. The reported life change scores reverted to baseline levels post-infarction.

Theorell & Rahe (1971, 1972) compared myocardial infarction sufferers with matched controls from the same social circles. Infarction patients generally exhibited higher life change scores in their preceding three years. There was also some evidence that recent life events contributed to patients experiencing their first infarction event: the patients with a history of CHD had consistently high scores in each of the time epochs studied, whereas those with their first infarction exhibited particularly high scores in the six months before the infarction. In an interesting attempt to exclude the argument that it is genetic susceptibility that influences the life event–CHD relationship, Ulf (1975) used the twins of myocardial infarction sufferers as controls. In such 'death-discordant' twins it was found that the infarction twins had higher life change scores, based on the preceding four years, than the non-suffering twins, although this was true for monozygotic—not dizygotic—twins. A study of chest pain patients by Byrne (1980; Byrne & White, 1980) attempted to exclude data contamination due to knowledge of diagnosed condition by collecting the life events information before diagnoses were made. Those patients whose pains were later attributed to infarctions did not previously report more events than those with negative ECGs but they did exhibit greater emotional distress to the events they experienced.

It is difficult to draw firm conclusions from the life events–CHD literature, partly because of the paucity of truly prospective studies to complement the retrospective ones, and partly because of inherent weaknesses and uncertainties about the general methodology. The studies which have utilised the Schedule of Recent Experiences are also inconsistent about which preceding time epoch, if any, is associated with peak change scores among the CHD groups (see Connolly, 1976). Nonetheless, it seems that those studies which have weighted the subjective impact of life events find CHD/no-CHD differences, whereas those that simply use event-counts have been less discriminatory (Wells, 1985). This is probably because cruder measures (even if more justifiable for theoretical and interpretive reasons) will necessarily be less discriminatory, especially if they are attempting to measure subtle influences. Connolly (1976), in a study of 91 myocardial infarction patients and 91 individually matched controls, utilised the rigorous interview method of Brown's Bedford College instrument to identify and examine life events in the previous three- and 12-week periods. Significantly more infarction patients than controls reported experiencing at least one life 'event' in the previous 12 weeks—the difference being particularly marked in the immediately preceding three weeks. The principal events which distinguished the two group comparisons were also rated as outside the control of the person, which diminishes the likelihood that the infarction patients were causal agents in the events because of their condition. Interestingly, when the infarction group were split according to whether they had experienced angina for at least some weeks ('anginal-onset') or with no premonitory angina longer than one week before the infarction ('point-onset'), only the point-onset patients were significantly more likely than their control group to have experienced at least one event in the 12-week period, although the trend was in the same direction for the anginal-onset patients.

Wells (1985) suggests that new research in this area should: (a) use specially formulated lists of events which eliminate events that might be confounded by pre-morbid states, (b) explore a range of dimensions of events (e.g. threat, emotional distress) rather than concentrate on readjustment, and (c) take account of social contexts, life-cycle stage and personality differences.

A number of studies have investigated the relationship between psychological life stressors and CHD using techniques which have been designed specifically for the study (e.g. Friedman *et al.*, 1971, Ochm, Reeder & Dirken, 1973). One of the better-known prospective studies is the *Israeli Ischaemic Heart Disease Project* (e.g. Medalie *et al.*, 1973a; Medalie & Goldbourt, 1976; Golbourt, Medalie & Neufeld, 1975) . This involved a random sampling of 10 059 male civil service employees aged 40 or over in 1963, who were examined extensively on a range of biochemical, CHD-related clinical, genetic, sociodemographic, behavioural, psychosocial and sociological variables. They were re-examined five years later. Of the original sample 8528 who were free of verified myocardial infarction, definite or suspected angina pectoris were included in analyses to investigate the possible role of psychological stressors on any subsequent manifestation of CHD within the five-year period. Some 300 new cases of angina (with or without infarction) developed. There were 29 questions which investigated psychological variables in relation to problems and conflicts in the areas of family, finances, work, co-workers and superiors. Medalie *et al.* (1973) report that, because so many of these questions were significantly related to the incidence of angina pectoris, the answers were combined to form a 'severity score' for each area and a 'combined severity score' for them all.

Each psychological area was related to the five-year incidence of angina. For example, if one calculates the relative risk ratio of the age-adjusted incidence rates of those with the highest severity score compared to those with the least, every area carries excess angina risk: family problems = 2.8; co-worker problems = 2.5; superior problems = 1.8; financial problems = 1.6; work problems = 1.6. The combined severity score of all areas showed the same positive relationship to angina incidence. Of course, this may suggest that those who are susceptible to angina pectoris are more likely to have problems in any of these areas, not that the relationship is causal even though the study was prospective. Medalie (1985) has presented evidence which supports the view that the relationships were not simply a result of having a 'soft' tool for the diagnosis of angina: the different categorisations based on their chest pain/angina questionnaire were predictive of the future development of myocardial infarction.

SOCIAL FACTORS IN CHD

Cassel (1976) proposed that the social environment in which a person lives can have marked effects on resistance to disease. In particular he argued that meaningful, and therefore relatively long-term, *social contacts* provide individuals with a network for receiving feedback about the effects of their intentions or behaviours. Without adequate social contacts the individual has a marked degree of uncertainty, as well as a poor network of support systems. For example, a study by Bruhn *et al.* (1966) suggests that reinforced social ties can be protective. The strongly patriarchal catholic Italian–Americans of Roseto in Pennsylvania, who have very cohesive social structures with clearly defined social roles, were shown to have less than half the myocardial infarction death rate of those in the ethnic and religiously mixed town of Bangor. The towns, of similar size, are about one mile apart, and the difference in death rates was not considered dietary in origin since the Roseto residents had a high-fat diet (41%) and were considerably more obese (Stout *et al.*, 1964). Although it seems that the impact of social support is greater on mental health measures than physical health indices (Ganster & Victor, 1988) this may be partly due to definitional difficulties and the relative lack of prospective investigations with physical health outcome measures.

Behaviours which interfere with the network of social contacts, or which prevent the establishment of an adequate network in some way, seem to be associated with higher levels of morbidity and mortality. Social networks and social supports should be differentiated. Berkman (1985), for example, makes the distinction that "If 'networks' is defined as the web of social relationships that surround an individual and as the characteristics of such linkages, 'social support' is defined as the emotional, instrumental, or financial aid that is obtained from one's social network" (p. 52). Cohen & Wills (1985) distinguish between two types of 'social support' which correspond to Berkman's distinction. On the one hand there is the 'support as a main effect' which is beneficial because "large social networks provide persons with regular positive experiences and a set of stable, socially rewarded roles...positive affect, and a sense of predictability and stability in one's life situation, and a recognition of self-worth" (p. 311). On the other hand, there is 'support as a stress buffer' in which "the perception that others can and will provide necessary resources may redefine the potential for harm...and/or bolster one's perceived ability to cope with imposed demands" (p. 312). This type of social support includes esteem supports, informational support, social companionship and instrumental support. Cohen & Wills (1985) provide a review of the research demonstrating support for both conceptualisations.

Social Networks and Social Ties

The relationship between social and community ties and disease has been extensively studied in a now 18-year prospective study of 6928 men and women residing in

Alameda County, California (Berkman & Syme, 1979; Berkman & Breslow, 1983; Kaplan, 1985). This is part of the work of the *Human Population Laboratory*, established in 1959 as a unit of California's Department of Health Service. As well as a range of other information, identified individuals were questioned about various aspects of their social networks (marriage, friends and extended family, religious or church contacts, other formal and informal group affiliations). The Social Network Index measured the number of social ties and weighted their relative importance to the individual.

Berkman & Syme (1979) present the mortality data based on a nine-year follow-up of 4725 30–69-year-olds from the first wave of the study (1965–74). The scores on the Social Network Index were classified according to how extensive the social networks of the individuals were from I (least connections) to IV (most connections). The results show that people who lacked social and community ties were more likely to have died than those with more extensive networks. The age-adjusted relative risks (I compared to IV) was 2.3 for men and 2.8 for women. Each age-band, for both men and women, showed a poor social network risk. Moreover, the social network/mortality risk was independent of a number of risk variables including self-reported physical health in 1965, socioeconomic status, smoking and alcohol consumption, obesity and physical activity. This pattern of results was also present for specific causes of death including ischaemic heart disease, cerebrovascular and circulatory disease, and cancer (Berkman & Breslow, 1983). Kaplan (1985) presents an analysis of 2352 respondents who were aged 50 years or over in 1965. Of those who died of ischaemic heart disease the relative risk of social isolation (least connected divided by most connected) was 3.4 for men and 2.7 for women. In addition, the relative CHD risk associated with social isolation was only reduced by some 4.8% when adjusted for life satisfaction, 3.9% when adjusted for depression, and 5.4% for perceived health. The relationship of each of these variables to CHD mortality, however, is reduced by a markedly greater amount by adjusting for the Social Network Index score (19.5%, 10.7% and 9%, respectively). In fact no variable had a significant effect on the relationship between social network and ischaemic heart disease mortality. As Kaplan writes:

> Social network participation also involves day-to-day activities which provide one with ongoing feedback regarding the structure, meaning and value of one's social relationships. The data...surely point to the importance of maintenance of these day-to-day social connections. Furthermore, the fact that measures of depression and helplessness do not account at all for the association between social isolation and increased risk suggests that there is something important about the absence of ongoing social feedback which is important far beyond any affective dysfunction (p. 263).

Other prospective studies broadly support the view that social integration is related to CHD mortality (e.g. House, Robbins & Metzner, 1982).

Marriage

There is considerable indirect evidence that such social processes as marriage provide a protective structure, with consequent reductions in morbidity and mortality. For example, married people have lower mortality and morbidity than single individuals (Bloom, Asher & White, 1978; Ernster *et al.*, 1979; Ortmeyer, 1974). When the network of the marriage breaks down many measures of morbidity are elevated (see a review of the effects of marital disruption by Bloom *et al.*, 1978). Moreover, when a spouse dies and that network is destroyed there is some evidence that the surviving person shows an increased risk of dying from CHD. Parkes, Benjamin & Fitzgerald (1969) followed 4486 widowers for nine years after the death of their wives. There was a 40% elevation in death rates in the six months following bereavement. Compared to the mortality rates of married men of the same age the bereaved men showed an excess risk of 1.7 times of dying from 'coronary thrombosis and other arteriosclerotic and degenerative heart disease', and 1.6 for 'other heart and circulatory diseases'. In fact these coronary diseases accounted for two-thirds of the total excess mortality risk from bereavement.

Mobility

There is some evidence that geographic, socioeconomic and job mobility each carry a CHD risk, although the evidence is not unequivocal (Syme & Seeman, 1983). Syme, Hyman & Enterline (1964) report that men who had made two or more significant moves in geographic location were twice as likely to develop CHD when compared to men with only one or no such moves. It may be that the disruption of social networks caused by the moving partly contributes to the excess CHD risk, although other factors (e.g. personality, whether the mobility is enforced or chosen) may also play a role. A person's social network is, in a sense, their microculture. Cultural changes on a more macro-scale have also been associated with the premature development of CHD. One particularly well-known study in this area was done by Marmot & Syme (1976). This was a cross-sectional study of 3809 Japanese migrants, aged 30–74 years, in San Francisco. The traditional Japanese society is very socially structured with less emphasis on the individual, more social interaction, group cohesion, social stability and clearly defined role structures. At the time of the study the Japanese had the lowest mortality rates from CHD of any industrialised country and the USA had one of the highest rates. Japanese–Americans showed intermediate rates. These differences in mortality could not be accounted for by the major coronary risk factors. Thus, Marmot & Syme suggested that social and cultural factors may play an important role. Their study included scales to measure acculturation (culture of upbringing, cultural assimilation, and social assimilation) as well as a range of biochemical and other CHD risk factors, ECG diagnostic, and sociodemographic variables. The prevalence of CHD was found to be up to 9.5 times greater for those who were most acculturated to the Western culture, compared to those who retained their Japanese culture, with an average excess risk of between 3 and 5. The Japanese–Americans with the more 'traditional' cultures showed smaller prevalence rates for angina pectoris and myocardial infarction as measured by the London School of Hygiene Cardiovascular Questionnaire, as well as fewer major ECG abnormalities. This difference in CHD rates was present when the data were controlled for the traditional CHD risk factors of diet, smoking behaviour, blood pressure, serum cholesterol, triglycerides and glucose levels, and relative weight. Thus, the evidence points to the importance of psychosocial factors in the development of CHD (see also Cohen *et al.*, 1979, who consider acculturation and type A behaviour in Japanese–Americans). Marmot (1983) has further argued that the higher rates of CHD in the lower income groups in the United Kingdom may also be partly associated with a low degree of social support, similar to that of the Japanese Americans in non-traditional cultures.

It should be mentioned that a recent study examining the impact of social networks on CHD of Japanese–Americans in Hawaii, casts doubt on the view that such structures can be considered to have a causal role in CHD (Reed *et al.*, 1983). After an initial examination before 1968, 4653 men returned a psychosocial questionnaire sent to them in 1971. Some 264 cases of CHD had been identified, and by 1978 a total of 218 more men had developed CHD. An examination of the 264 prevalence cases showed that two scales measuring social networks (a general one and one which considered only intimate contacts) independently predicted total CHD (but not myocardial infarction) when standard risk factors were included. When the 218 incidence cases were analysed, however, the social network factor was not an independent risk for any of the CHD dependent variables. This may indicate that the experience of the disease itself affects the nature of social networks.

Early studies by Syme and his colleagues (Syme, Hyman & Enderline, 1964; Syme, Borhani & Buechley, 1965) suggest that changing jobs, with the consequent effects this has on disrupting established or learnt social networks, may also carry an enhanced CHD risk. Men who had changed jobs three or more times showed up to four times the incidence of CHD, compared to those with less than one or two changes. Remaining in one occupational category for more than 30 years also appeared to have a protective effect. In the Framingham Study outlined earlier in this chapter, the 'number of promotions in the past 10 years' was found to be a significant independent predictor of the eight-year incidence of total CHD and myocardial infarction in men aged 45–64 (although in subsequent analyses the relationship was primarily due to blue-collar workers) (Haynes, Feinleib & Kannel, 1980).

Socioeconomic mobility has also been associated with CHD risk. Shekelle, Ostfeld & Paul (1969), in their prospective study of the Western Electric Company employees, also discussed earlier, found no independent relationship between socioeconomic class and CHD, but report significant relationships between CHD incidence and a number of status discordance variables. Men of a lower or higher social class than their parents, or who showed marked differences in their ranked positions on different social variables (e.g. education, income, residence, occupation), were found to have a markedly higher CHD incidence. Whilst this paper has been critically evaluated by Horan & Gray (1974), who inferred that it did not demonstrate any link between status incongruity and CHD, Shekelle (1976) presents a reanalysis and reaffirmation of the original position. The role of socioeconomic variables in heart disease is difficult to study, not least because there are numerous indices reflecting different theoretical stances (Morgenstern, 1985). The role of such variables, and their interaction with others we have outlined, is likely to be an important one: to quote Syme (1985): "to view social context as merely a background variable is to miss an important and possibly meaningful element regarding the psychosocial variables we study" (p. 39).

COGNITIVE ORIENTATION AND CHD

The relationship between personality, affective behaviour and actual behaviour in work settings remains largely unknown. One attempt to circumvent the problems this entails has been to pay more attention to the relationship between different types of belief and how these might guide behaviour. Kreitler & Kreitler (1976, 1982) have developed a theory of how cognitive orientation is related to behaviour. The theory has been successfully applied to the prediction of more than 50 behaviours such as punctuality, achievement, impulsivity and pain thresholds. It has recently been applied to the investigation of psychological factors involved in CHD (Drechsler, Bruner & Kreitler, 1987).

Broadly, the theory says that behaviourally relevant situations are assessed in terms of a constellation of beliefs to provide the appropriate behaviour. There are four types of beliefs which are necessary for an act to be selected. For example, for the act of 'working hard' these might be:

- *Norm beliefs*, which may be ethically, culturally, or socially desirable behaviours such as 'people should work hard for their money'.
- *General beliefs*, which reflect the person's view of people in general in situations such as 'most people do not work hard for their money'.
- *Beliefs about self*, such as 'I always work hard for my money'.
- *Goal beliefs* about future desired states, such as 'I wish I didn't care so much about the equity between my effort and my salary'.

The theory supposes that if the majority of the beliefs concerning an act are consistent with the act the *cognitive orientation* will cluster and support a *behavioural intent* such as 'working hard'. The major point here is that all four beliefs need to be considered before an action or behaviour is illicited.

Drechsler *et al.* (1987) tested the theory in relation to 'coronary-involved behaviours' such as 'time at work', 'disagreeing', 'being in control' and 'demands on oneself'. A questionnaire assessing endorsement of the four categories of belief was given to 44 men under the age of 60 who had experienced a myocardial infarction within the previous year, 28 healthy men, and 20 CHD-free men suffering orthopaedic disorders.

The results supported the cognitive orientation theory in three major ways. First the CHD group scored more highly on the beliefs concerning the coronary-involved behaviours than either of the two control groups. In other words the CHD group were generally more concerned about eight of the 12 behaviours assessed (being punctual, disagreeing with others, demanding a lot from oneself, not wasting time at work, caring a lot about order and cleanliness, being accurate at work, keeping promises, being in control). The CHD group had stronger norm beliefs and beliefs about self, but not general or goal beliefs. Second, the degree of inconsistency across the different kinds of belief (an indicator of potential physiological and psychological conflict) was greater for the CHD group than the control groups for half of the behaviours. Finally, the CHD group showed a much closer association between their beliefs about the coronary-involved behaviours and CHD risk factors such as systolic blood pressure, diastolic blood pressure, cholesterol levels, and high-density lipoprotein cholesterol. The control groups showed only a chance number of correlations between the beliefs and the risk factors, whereas the CHD group showed 3.8 times more.

The study shows, therefore, the potential contribution of beliefs to CHD. It also makes a contribution inasmuch as it does not rely on *exhibited* behaviours, but also accounts for their underlying psychological concomitants. Even if coronary-prone behaviour is not present the conflict between central belief systems may itself exert an influence on the cardiovascular system: "The findings suggest that CHD-proneness may consist in cognitive–motivational conflicts of beliefs in regard to certain behaviours rather than in the actual enactment of these behaviours" (p. 587). It also suggests that treatment could be usefully aimed at modifying beliefs instead of at changing aspects of the CHD-susceptible person which may be as much a part of that person as their genes.

PSYCHOLOGICAL FACTORS AND HYPERTENSION

Hypertension may be directly or indirectly responsible for up to 20% of all deaths through the effects it has on the heart and the coronary, renal and cerebral vessels. Blood pressure is a major clinical indicator of a whole array of dysfunctions. In addition, both systolic and diastolic blood pressures have been shown to have predictive value in virtually all the major heart studies discussed in the preceding sections. The CHD risks of such factors as elevated cholesterol, smoking, diabetes, and left ventricular hypertrophy are also greater when accompanied with higher pressure (Kannel & Sorlie, 1975; Insull, 1973). It has been used as a dependent variable in a large number of experimental psychological studies with animal and human subjects, as well in the large epidemiological investigations of risk factors in CHD.

In the majority of individuals, especially those over 35 years or so, chronically raised resting blood pressure cannot be attributed to any clear 'secondary' cause (e.g. various renal, endocrine, coronary and cerebrovascular diseases). In such cases the condition is labelled 'essential hypertension'. Essential hypertensives account for about 80% of all cases of hypertension (Bech & Hilden, 1975). Because essential hypertension has no obvious identifiable physical cause—although the condition does have a familial component—there has been considerable interest in the possible contribution of psychological factors in the development of the disorder. This interest in psychological factors has undoubtedly been boosted by studies showing that the blood pressure of hypertensives can be significantly reduced by psychologically based interventions (e.g. Agras & Jacob, 1979; Charlesworth, Williams & Baer, 1984; Goldstein, Shapiro & Thanopavaran, 1984; Peters, Benson & Peters, 1977; Seer, 1979; Shapiro, 1983), that some pharmacological interventions may not work to lower blood pressures when they might be expected to (e.g. Cappuccio *et al.*, 1985), and that traditional antihypertensive drugs (the thiazide diuretic bendrofluazide, the beta-blocker propranolol) have only minor benefits on stroke mortality, none on the influence of coronary events, but cause a large proportion of patients to suffer chronic side-effects (Medical Research Council Working Party, 1985). The impact of the stresses of Western living on blood pressure has also been suggested as a reason why men and women living in industrialised countries develop higher blood pressure with age (independent of weight change), whereas non-industrialised societies do not show such an age/pressure function (Waldron *et al.*, 1982).

Arterial blood pressure is determined by the interaction of cardiac output and peripheral vascular resistance. The hypertensive has raised blood pressure due to abnormal output and/or resistance. Of those with marginally raised pressures ('borderline hypertensives') about 30% show elevations in cardiac output with no increase in peripheral resistance (Julius, 1982; Julius & Esler, 1975), whereas those with established hypertension may have normal cardiac output, but increased peripheral resistance (Folkow, 1982). Increased cardiac output is often associated with increased sympathetic drive on the myocardium, and this has led to the proposal that adrenergic-mediated myocardial hyperreactivity may be a precursor in the development of established hypertension (Obrist, 1981, 1985a). Little is known about the transition from labile or borderline hypertension, although repeated acute elevations probably result in increased resistance in the arterioles due to hypertrophy of the vascular smooth muscle and autoregulatory arteriole constriction triggered by repeated excessive elevations in cardiac output beyond metabolic requirements, both of which lead to reduced venous return and lowering of cardiac output (although this view is controversial). Thus, much of the experimental psychological research has been aimed at understanding what factors affect such lability, and the mechanisms of their action.

'Definite' hypertension is often distinguished from 'borderline' and 'labile' hypertension. Although there are no agreed standards, definite hypertension may be considered as blood pressure in excess of 160/95 mmHg, and borderline hypertension above 140/90 mmHg (but less than 160/95 mmHg). Labile hypertension usually refers to a condition in individuals whose levels are not chronically raised, but who show a propensity to exhibit high levels under certain circumstances. Borderline and labile hypertensives are more likely to develop definite hypertension (Julius, 1977, 1981) and this is one reason why research has focused on them.

It is important to investigate the 'causes' of hypertension, not least because large surveys suggest that hypertension is a very common condition. In the USA more than 18% of adults aged 12–74 years have definite hypertension, either a systolic pressure of 160 mmHg or more, or a diastolic pressure of 95 mmHg (Health and Nutrition Examination Survey, 1977). A further 12% or more have borderline hypertension. In the UK large screening surveys of middle-aged men have revealed that around 40% have casual diastolic pressures 90 mmHg or above (Royal College of Physicians and The British Cardiac Society, 1976) In a recent survey of the blood pressures in a national birth cohort at the age of 36, over 17% of men and 9% of women had diastolic pressures over 90 mmHg (Wadsworth *et al.*, 1985) (in this survey the nurses recorded diastolic pressure by sphygmomanometer at the phase V, disappearance of Korotkoff sounds, endpoints. Use of the phase IV—muffling of sounds—point would increase the percentages. Moreover, the recorded pressures were those taken on a second reading). A recent Munich Blood Pressure Survey of 2216 people aged 30–69 years found that 23% of men and 19% of women were hypertensive, and that 39% had blood pressures exceeding 140/90 mmHg (1st and 5th phase Korotkoff; Hartel, Keil & Cairns, 1985).

One difficulty with hypertension, however, is that it is generally asymptomatic and only a small proportion of cases are caught by the usual medical practitioners' nets and the number receiving treatment is low. For example, in the national birth cohort study 88% of men found to have hypertensive blood pressure readings were previously unrecognised, and there were as many men being treated for hypertension whose readings were lower than 140/90 mmHg as there were men with hypertensive readings. In the USA Framingham study Kannel (1975) reports that as many as 50% of hypertensives are recognised, and around 50% of them are treated (of which some 50% are treated adequately). In Munich, a city with one of the highest physician densities in the world, 38% of men and 16% of women with definite hypertension were unaware of their condition prior to the investigation. In addition, 22% of men and 42% of women were both aware of their condition and had it under drug control (Hartel, Keil & Cairns, 1985). Even in risk categories (e.g. middle-aged men) it has been found that as many as 63% of patient records have no blood pressure record relating to the previous five years even in good practices (Oliver, 1984). Thus, audits of hypertension in general practice are to be recommended (Taffinder & Taffinder, 1984).

Traditionally, diastolic pressures have been considered most predictive of subsequent coronary and cerebrovascular events, and medical textbooks often concentrate on diastolic pressure in diagnosis and treatment recommendations. It is becoming clear, however, that systolic blood pressure is also a major predictor of ischaemic heart disease (e.g. Shaper *et al.*, 1985), if not a better one than diastolic pressure (Lichtenstein, Shipley & Rose, 1985; Lehr, Messinger & Rosenman, 1973).

Investigations of the possible contribution of psychological factors in hypertension have to bear in mind three important points:

1. Essential hypertension is not a single disease entity. Blood pressure control is complex, and the many physiological factors involved in its regulation are themselves affected differentially by a whole array of variables. Both Folkow's (1982) multifactorial model and Page's (1977) mosaic model of the etiology of essential hypertension recognise that the interrelatedness of the many dynamic regulatory mechanisms means that hypertension is likely to have different causes for different individuals, and that the nature of the individual and the way they are affected by stressors will affect how the mechanisms are affected. As Obrist (1985b) has noted "A fundamental problem in our efforts to relate some behavioral dimension to hypertension is that we tend to treat the BP (blood pressure) as a selfcontained entity, and at times even as a static event" (p. 657). At the simplest level, for example, diastolic and systolic pressures, although both used to diagnose hypertension, are influenced in quite different ways by different psychologically relevant task demands in different individuals. For example, the systolic pressure is increased most in tasks where beta-adrenergic influences are maximum (e.g. subject-controlled shock avoidance), although the diastolic pressure changes are very small. However, when beta-adrenergic influences are less (e.g. shock avoidance with no control, the cold pressor test) and in individuals who evidence small beta-adrenergic influences, the diastolic pressures increase more (Obrist, 1981, 1985a). As Obrist (1985b) has said, this also implies that the concept of a 'hypertensive personality' should be considered with great caution.
2. The definition of hypertension is arbitrary. It should be noted that both systolic and diastolic blood pressures in the general population conform to normal unimodal distributions, with only slight negative skewing. There is no distributional discontinuity to support a clinical segregation of normotensives from hypertensives. In addition, CHD risk increases continuously over the entire range of measured systolic blood pressure, with no sign of a threshold value (Anderson, 1978). (In the case of diastolic pressure re-examination of this Framingham data suggests that the curve flattens at the lower range of 70–80 mmHg [Anderson, 1978]). Thus, 'hypertension' is a matter of arbitrary degree and any contributory psychological factors should be considered in the same way. It does not make sense to say that certain causal factors are either necessary or sufficient.
3. Blood pressure is extremely variable or labile. For example, simply taking a second measure of blood pressure produces a marked decrement in levels. A second screening of those in the Hypertension Detection and Follow-up

Programme reduced the prevalence of 'mild' hypertension (diastolic pressures 90–104 mmHg) from 20.5% to 7.2% (Hypertension Detection and Follow-up Co-operative Group, 1979; Labarthe, 1985). Even individuals who would normally be described as normotensive show very marked variations in blood pressure: many individuals would exhibit blood pressures into the hypertensive range from time to time (Bevan, Honour & Stott, 1967; Littler *et al.*, 1975). Using 24-hour monitoring techniques, Richardson *et al.* (1964) report a normotensive with a 40 mmHg+ systolic and 35 mmHg+ diastolic variation in blood pressure, and a patient with essential hypertension whose corresponding variations were 120+ and 60+. All the healthy subjects showed occasional hypertensive values. Whilst many changes are made in response to metabolic requirements (blood pressure is low during sleep, and high during anaerobic exercise) Obrist (1985b,c) reports that young normotensives simply resting quietly in a lounge chair show changes in blood pressure (+ or −2 standard deviations) averaging 22 mmHg for systolic and 16 mmHg for diastolic blood pressure. Exposing the subjects to minor laboratory stressors increased the variability to 50 mmHg systolic, 35 mmHg diastolic, and put some subjects within the hypertensive range.

With such a range in blood pressure values two particular problems are posed. First, it becomes more difficult to establish that psychological factors are of causal importance in the development of hypertension, even if consistent elevations in response to them are observed. Second, the very lability of blood pressure makes it difficult to study and interpret the effects of psychological interventions, because the measurement error is high and the determination of the influence of subtle psychological factors likely to be masked. One can make the situation a little easier by taking account of factors such as metabolic requirements (e.g. by measuring O_2 uptake) or adrenergic reactivity, but such considerations are principally confined to limited laboratory experimental investigations. Much of the research implicating psychological variables to hypertension has been non-laboratory-based, correlational or epidemiological.

In addition, the lability problem does make it difficult to determine the clinical meaning of 'casual' blood pressure measures. There is evidence that casual pressures either overestimate or are not correlated with general levels (Obrist, 1985c). This certainly makes one feel uneasy when it is realised that antihypertensive drug treatment, which is often accompanied by adverse side-effects, is sometimes initiated on the basis of one casual reading in a potentially stressful doctor's consulting room. Parkin (1979) reports that 33% of patients had only one blood pressure recorded before treatment, and Taffinder & Taffinder (1984) report that only 18% of those given drugs for hypertension had had three or more measures taken. Since some measure of average cardiovascular load is more likely to be of pathogenic importance the use of casual measures of blood pressure is of dubious clinical as well as theoretical importance.

THE HYPERTENSIVE 'PERSONALITY'

Despite the multifaceted nature of blood pressure control, some researchers have suggested that it does make sense to talk of a hypertensive personality. Amongst the earliest of these was Alexander (1939) who, in a tentative hypothesis, characterised the hypertensive as exhibiting chronic *hostile and angry* impulses which were inhibited or repressed. Such an unconscious conflict results in an essential tension, chronic elevations of blood pressure, and anxiety. When these inner conflicts are allowed an external outlet—for example, when the individual can act aggressively and show hostility to the object of the feeling—there is evidence that acute elevations of blood pressure are more quickly normalised than when no such outlet is allowed (Hokanson, 1961). The repeated acute elevations in blood pressure probably result in a change in the sensitivity of the baroreceptors and increased peripheral resistance. There have been many studies suggesting that some groups of hypertensive individuals show greater suppressed hostility than normotensives (e.g. Gentry *et al.*, 1982; Kidson, 1973; Haynes *et al.*, 1978b; Kaplan, 1961; Sullivan *et al.*, 1981a,b).

The repressed-hostility view of the hypertensive, however, has not found general empirical support. As many commentators have pointed out (e.g. Krantz & Glass, 1984; Steptoe, 1981; Matthews, 1985) the literature contains many examples of contradictory findings. Even the studies mentioned above in support of the hypothesis have not produced unequivocal support for the position. In the Framingham study, for example, both 'anger-in' and 'tension' scales only showed significant correlation with diastolic blood pressure for women. None of the correlations with systolic pressures were significant, nor were any of those for men (Haynes *et al.*, 1978b). Other studies report significant results for systolic, but not diastolic, or for men but not women, etc. There are a number of reasons for these inconsistent results.

Loading the Dice

The first is that many of the studies have not adequately controlled the selection of subjects (e.g. for the hypertensive and normotensive groups) to ensure that there is no referral bias, or that the results are not contaminated with the subjects' expectancies or present mood. When this is done there is, at best, only minor support for the suppressed-hostility view. For example, Steptoe, Melville & Ross (1982) found no differences between essential hypertensives and matched controls in terms of trait anxiety (measured by the Spielberger, Gorsuch & Lusherne, 1970, STAI) or total hostility, intropunitive hostility or extropunitive hostility (measured by Caine, Foulds & Hope, 1967, HDHQ). In fact, the normotensives showed significantly higher state-anxiety than the hypertensives. This study is particularly good because, although the final number of subjects was quite small (based on an initial screening of 870 people), the categorisation of individuals into the blood pressure groups was based on very rigorously obtained multiple measures in different settings, which also eliminated the considerable problem of referral bias (of both groups) present in many studies. Another positive aspect of the study is that individuals were not aware of their diagnostic status until after all procedures were completed. It is also useful because it enabled an estimation of the within-subject correlation between self-monitored blood pressure and anger-hostility and tension when controlled for expectancies or reporting biases (by using a mood control scale). Thus, unlike previous studies (e.g. Pennenbaker *et al.*, 1982; Whitehead *et al.*, 1977), it provides a way of separating spurious associations from genuine effects. Self-monitored systolic and diastolic blood pressure was significantly correlated with each mood scale for both normotensives and hypertensives (in 11 out of 12 cases). However, when controlled for reporting bias, only the association of systolic blood pressure with the tension scale in the hypertensive group was significant. Thus, the study provides only limited support for the view that any factors relevant to the suppressed-hostility hypothesis are related to blood pressure when care is taken to measure blood pressure accurately and to take account of reporting biases.

A second reason for the lack of consistency in the literature is the use of a plethora of different measures of hostility and anger. As Krantz & Glass (1984) have pointed out:

> Investigations of personality and hypertension have defined 'suppressed hostility' in many ways (e.g., the tone or style of reporting anger; a lack of expressed anger on self-report scales; higher levels of observer-rated hostility; subjects' not admitting hostility; etc.). Some studies have measured suppressed hostility in a few specific situations... , where other studies have examined habitual patterns expressed in a variety of situations... . Relatively few studies have examined such variables as frequency and amplitude of expressed anger (p. 61).

With so many different measures, and the omission of important contextual and content aspects of hostility, it is not surprising that the literature is not uniform in its findings.

Matthews, Jamison & Cottington (1985) provide a good review of many of the scales used to assess anger and hostility in this field.

Cause or Effect?

The third aspect of the research which requires particular attention is to ensure that any 'personality' differences between hypertensives and normotensives are not a consequence of the *knowledge* of being classed as hypertensive. A number of studies suggest that at least some observed differences are a consequence, and not a contributing cause, of such classification. In the Munich Blood Pressure Survey (Hartel, Keil & Cairns, 1985) it is apparent that the patients' knowledge of their hypertensive condition led some of them to view other aspects of their health in a negative light. For example, for those under 50 years old the hypertensives who were unaware of their condition were as likely as the normotensives to report suffering other chronic diseases, although both these groups were less likely to report such diseases than any of the aware hypertension groups. Monk (1980) also observed that hypertensives who knew of their condition were more likely to produce lower scores on the General Well-being Questionnaire than those who had not been informed.

It is also possible that hypertension may itself be responsible for other changes in personal perceptions. In a study by Baer *et al.* (1979) the hypertensive group scored more highly on anxiety and hostility measures than normotensives. However, the hypochodriasis scale of the MMPI also discriminated the groups (whether the hypertensives had been detected at screening or referred), suggesting they were more sensitive to somatic functioning. Robinson (1962) found that hypertensive subjects scored as highly on the Neuroticism Scale of the Maudsley Personality Inventory as outpatients of a psychiatric clinic, although both the former groups were significantly more neurotic than normal community controls. In addition, unaware hypertensives (from the community control group) produced lower neuroticism scores than the aware hypertensives, and there was no significant correlation between neuroticism scores and blood pressure for the community sample. These three findings led Robinson to conclude that neuroticism played no causal role in hypertension, although being hypertensive may itself lead to significant changes in perceptions and behaviour. This conclusion is also supported by a study of the personality profiles of a group of outpatient hypertensives and non-patient controls by Kidson (1973). Hypertensives scored higher than normotensives on a number of scales including neuroticism, anxiety, depression, tenseness, anger and sensitivity (using the Cornell Medical Index, the 16PF and the EPI). However, when the non-patient controls were split into higher and lower blood pressure groups, none of the psychological variables referred to discriminated between them. If these variables did play a causal role in blood pressure elevation one might have expected to have found such differences. One is left with the conclusion that the hypertensive/non-patient differences were a result, and not a contributing cause, of the hypertension itself.

Hypertensive Types

The evaluation of the concept of the 'hypertensive personality' is complicated by the finding that different types of hypertensives produce different psychological profiles. Matthews (1985) has suggested that the conflicting results present in the literature may be due to the relative frequency with which these types are represented in the different studies. Esler and his colleagues, for example, have distinguished between borderline hypertensives in terms of their control of renin release by the kidneys. Some hypertensives have lower levels of plasma renin activity, which has been associated with lower levels of sympathetic nervous system activity. Others have elevated levels of renin which may be partly maintained by high catecholamine activity. In such patients, and not with normal-renin hypertensives, adrenergic blockers produce a significant reduction in peripheral vascular resistance, and beta-adrenergic-only blockage produces a greater reduction in cardiac output and heart rate in high-renin hypertensives than with normotensives or essential hypertensives with normal renin levels (Esler *et al.*, 1977). Of particular interest here, however, is that the Esler *et al.* (1977) study included the measurement of a number of psychological variables (using the IPAT Anxiety Scale Questionnaire, the 16PF, Buss–Durkee Personality Inventory, and the Harburg 'Anger-in/Anger-out' scale). Only the high-renin hypertensives exhibited elevated suppressed hostility and unexpressed anger scores. This group were also found to be more submissive than normotensives or hypertensives with normal renin levels. This study suggests, therefore, that borderline hypertensives with different underlying physiologies may also show quite different psychological attributes. Whether the psychic determines the physiology, or vice-versa, is unclear.

A study by Harburg *et al.* (1964) reinforces the need to adequately distinguish the parameters which define the borderline hypertensive groups. In this research, done on young college males, the personality profiles of those with sustained or reproducible systolic hypertension (in excess of 140 mmHg on nine consecutive occasions at college home and in the doctor's practice, including three readings following a 20-minute supine rest) were different in significant respects from those whose casual blood pressure was found to be elevated on two single measurements taken one month apart. Both the 'sustained' and the 'casual' hypertensive groups exhibited correlations between blood pressure and and the 'sensitive' scale of Cattell's 16PF. However, there were a number of differences between the groups. Adopting a significance criterion of 5% or better, the 'casual' group also showed significant correlations with 'submissiveness', 'warm-sociability', 'suspicion', 'neuroticism' and 'introversion'. The 'sustained' group, on the other hand, produced significant correlations with blood pressure only for 'anxiety'.

Active Control and Passive Acceptance

There is some indication that individuals who are more likely to perceive that they can effect active control in a situation are more at risk than those who are more passive and accepting. Obrist and his colleagues (e.g. Obrist, 1981; Obrist *et al.*, 1978; Light, 1985, Light & Obrist, 1983) have found that laboratory challenges which require active coping (e.g. a shock avoidance reaction time task where the individual perceives they can control the shock by their reaction time performance, or a reaction time task where they are in competition with another) produce greater blood pressure changes than challenges which have to be passively accepted, or which demand impossible levels of performance to succeed. There are marked individual differences in cardiovascular reactivity to such tasks. These differences are probably a reflection of differences in alpha- and beta-adrenergic responses to active coping tasks. Only individuals who demonstrate high reactivity to active coping tasks also show a marked reduction in sodium and water excretion under the competitive conditions (Light, 1985), suggesting that such psychological factors may affect these renal mechanisms which are involved in the longer-term regulation of blood pressure (Guyton, 1980). Little is known, however, about the relationship of this individual cardiovascular and renal lability to the individual's perceived need for active control. This would seem a fruitful area for future research on individual differences in hypertension.

Dominant and Subordinate Behaviour

Henry (e.g. 1976, 1982; Henry & Stephens, 1977) also suggested that how an individual copes with events determines the pattern of physiological response and, therefore, their susceptibility to, and severity of, essential hypertension. He proposed that the effects of a stressor could be dealt with in one of two ways:

1. Dominant challenged control leads to aggression or hostility. The stimuli activate the amygdala and the sympathetic adrenal medullary system, allowing the individual to maintain an alert readiness to cope with new stressors and to maintain the apparent value of this response. This 'defence reaction' results in elevated sympathetic activity with increased initial cardiac output, blood pressure, peripheral vascular resistance, fatty acids, glycogenolysis, and catecholamine activity.
2. Subordinate loss of control leads to depression, failure to act and behaviourally react. The stimuli activate the hippocampus–septum region and the pituitary–adrenal cortical system, producing conservation–withdrawal and inducing further uncertainty and lack of positive behavioural response. This 'submissive' response is associated with enhanced adrenocorticotrophin (ACTH) levels, vagal activity, blood pressure, gluconeogenesis, and pepsin levels, and decreased reticuloendothelial activity.

Henry (1976) equated activation of the second axis with learned helplessness, and suggested that it was more likely to occur as the individual loses resources for active coping. Additionally, one may consider that such a pattern of response reflects an individual's personality, however determined. This would imply that depression was not a necessary component of the pattern of response to challenge, although it may be present in a subset of individuals.

Henry's distinction is useful because it illustrates that the effects of stressors may lead to increased blood pressure in one of at least two ways, depending upon which component of the neuroendocrine system is pre-eminent. It also adds to the view that there is a need to consider the different psychological and endocrinal patterns of hypertensives, since these are not likely to be equivalent. It is, of course, not clear why some individuals exhibit greater responses of either system than other individuals (except by appealing to genetics and early experience). This is the central question of interest here. Part of the answer may revolve around understanding more

162 *Work, Stress, Disease and Life Expectancy*

about the stressors, support systems, and social structures within which the individual operates. What is needed is research which considers the individual differences in hypertension allied to their hypothesised neuroendocrinal mechanisms. Thus, future research needs to measure both physiological and personality profiles, and not simply attempt to correlate personality factors with measured blood pressure. After all, blood pressure control depends on many underlying mechanisms and its elevation is not likely to be a result of stressors influencing only one possible path. Understanding the multifaceted nature of the underlying pathophysiology of borderline hypertension only provides half the answers to why an individual is susceptible to, or becomes, hypertensive. We need to marry that understanding with the other half (which is likely to involve the interrelationship of many psychological variables too): the individual. The many apparent inconsistencies in the literature may well then disappear. Instead of being put down to the vagaries of imprecise measurement error, we might find that they have more to do with the many physiological and psychological differences between them.

Chapter 6
Transmitting Occupational Stress

This chapter documents some of the indirect health consequences of stress. People may be carriers of stress and infect others with its consequences. This chapter explicitly examines evidence that occupational stress may affect the life expectancy of the job incumbent and that these specific work stressors may be transmitted through psychological mechanisms to the worker's spouse. That work may spill over into the home may not seem surprising. The evidence presented here, however, attempts to demonstrate that occupational stress does play an important role in the life expectancy of both the worker and his/her spouse. Even more startling is the possibility that a person's cause of death may be related to the job *their spouse is engaged in.* If the evidence supported such a theory of the transmission of specific disease risks a number of important factors could be established. First, it would make a strong case indeed for the central thesis of this book that psychological factors play a causal role in the major diseases. Second, it would show that occupational stressors form one major category of possible causes of disease. This may also require some re-evaluation of the role of psychological factors in affecting matters concerned with everyday lifestyle such as smoking, drinking, exercise behaviours, etc., and would imply that occupational stress was all-pervading in its effects. Third, and as a consequence of the other two points, it would suggest that psychological effects should not be expected to be confined only to those directly exposed to the stressors. If psychological mechanisms were operating, occupational stress (and its disease consequences) should be revealed in those to whom these stressors may be communicated. Fourth, it would add weight to a view expressed throughout this book that occupational stress is not primarily consciously apparent in either its nature or effect.

These are strong claims. They need to be evaluated closely because the consequences of confirmation should be major both from a practical and theoretical stance. Before considering the more contentious evidence, however, the first half of the chapter provides an outline of some research which may act as a backcloth structure on which to paint the more abstract subject-matter. Two types of literature will be reviewed:

1. Evidence which shows that work may spill over into the home.
2. Evidence suggesting that the mental and physical ill-health of marital partners

is linked, and that there is concordance in the disease-specific mortality rates of marital partners.

The debate will primarily centre on the effect of occupational stress on male job incumbents and how this may affect the health of their wives. This should not be taken as implying that only this pattern of influence is possible. Risks may be two-way and affect others in other relationships to the job incumbent. If there is support for the central thesis of the chapter it would suggest that other indirect risks exist.

WORK SPILLOVER AND HEALTH

It will come as no surprise to anyone that aspects of a person's job affect factors outside the job environment. There are two rival hypotheses about how work affects non-work perceptions and behaviour: '*spillover*' and '*compensation*'. The spillover hypothesis proposes that job experiences are carried over into the domestic environment, thus determining the similarity in perceptions in both spheres. The compensation hypothesis, on the other hand, suggests that deficiencies in need-fulfilment in one sphere will be compensated for by activities and perceptions in the other. Staines (1980), in a review of the competing hypotheses, found general support for the spillover view in most areas considered (behaviour and subjective reactions). The major exception was that those who did physical work were less likely to be involved in physical leisure activity.

There have been many investigations of the relationship between work and non-work. In their well-known survey study of shift workers, for example, Mott *et al.* (1965) found that nightshift workers reported more marital problems than other shiftworkers whilst afternoon workers were more likely to exhibit difficulties with the parent role. Staines & Peck (1984), in an analysis of data from the *1977 Quality of Employment Survey*, show how working at weekends and working variable-day weeks results in less time involved in such family roles as child care and housework. Such non-standard work schedules were also associated with greater conflict between work and family life. Working certain shifts (afternoon and night) also resulted in considerably greater work/family conflict despite the fact that shift workers spent more time on family roles. Winnett & Neale (1981) also report marked effects of flexible work schedules on family time allocation. Research also suggests that the age of children, and whether or not the household is one in which both partners are in paid employment, will affect how work schedules impact on family life (Hood & Golden, 1984).

Young & Willmott (1973) report an in-depth examination of work and leisure in families in the London region. In one case study, Mr Fison, a deputy production manager, commuted from Reading to London. The interview showed that he was clearly troubled by the one-upmanship in his work environment. His wife was subjected to his dissatisfactions with work: "It's not so much that he's unpleasant to us. But he will come home and talk the whole problem out—he will talk for two hours on the trot" (p. 159).

The study revealed other ways in which work affected home and family matters. For example, 37% of men in full-time work found their work interfered with their family in significant ways. In addition, the higher the occupational class the greater the interference: 53% of professional and managerial men reported interference, as opposed to only 25% of semiskilled and unskilled workers. Work spillover was reflected in what men did at home (e.g. their leisure activities) and how they occupied their minds. One manager, for example, said: "I think about work continually when I'm at home. If you are digging a flower bed for a couple of hours you can have a marvellous think about some deep problems of organisation" (p. 166). Another said: "My concern for work interferes with my home. It would be nice if I could switch myself off and cheerfully help my wife with the washing up instead of doing it all with a long face" (p. 167).

Although Young & Willmott found that different occupational groups spent different numbers of hours at work Clark, Nye & Gecas (1978) report almost no relationship between the number of hours a husband worked and his wife's marital satisfaction.

The study by Young & Willmott (1973) did not consider how this type of work spillover affected the well-being of the job incumbents and their spouses. The work orientation of men, defined by their degree of type A behaviour, has, however, been shown to affect the well-being of wives. Burke, Weir & DuWors (1979) found that lower level of well-being and satisfaction among the wives of administrators in corrective institutions was associated with the type A behaviour of their husbands. Other investigations have shown that occupational stress has significant spillover into the home environment. Jackson & Maslach (1982) studied 142 police couples and the way they interacted at home. Strain was assessed by the Maslach Burnout Inventory, which measures feelings of emotional exhaustion, personal accomplishment and depersonalisation. The quality of family life of both marital partners was linked to the degree of job stress reported by the males. By far the most frequently used method for coping with work stress was talking over the problems with the wife, although the police officers were more likely than their wives to cope by smoking, having a drink, getting away from people and finding activities to take their mind off their problems. The study showed that the husbands who were under stress at work were more likely to show anger, to have unsatisfactory marriages, to be uninvolved with family matters and to spend time away from the family. In fact, 27% of the variance in the quality of family life was accounted for by the husband's strain score. There is a considerable literature suggesting that marital disruption can be a considerable stressor associated with increased incidence of psychiatric illness, motor vehicle accidents, cancer and other physical illnesses, suicide, and disease mortality in general (Bloom, Asher & White, 1978; Ernster *et al.*, 1979).

The effects of work stress affect the well-being of both marital partners. Burke, Weir & DuWors (1980) report the results of a field study of senior male administrators and their spouses. Eighty-five husband–wife pairs were questioned independently on a wide range of issues. The men were questioned about

18 occupational demands, and their wives about the degree to which they worried about life concerns (family sickness, friendships, etc.), perceived type A behaviour of husbands, stressful life events (à la Holmes & Rahe), negative affective states, impact of husband's job on family and home, life and marital satisfaction, psychosomatic symptoms, social support and coping behaviours. In general the study supported the view that the greater the occupational demands on husbands the lower the level of satisfaction and well-being of wives. Only 22 of the 159 significant correlations showed non-detrimental effects. Stepwise multiple regressions of the occupational demands with the various measures of wives' well-being resulted in a number of independent correlates with effects being most marked in those areas closest to the husband–wife relationship such as marital satisfaction and job impact on home and family. Several occupational demands were consistently associated with lower well-being in wives: quality pressures, communication at work stress and stress from rate of change. Other factors including number of work hours, job complexity, role ambiguity, quantitative overload, pay inequality, responsibility for things and boundary spanning had significant but less marked detrimental effects. Of particular interest is that five of the occupational stressors were significantly related to the number of wives' psychosomatic symptoms, with the stress of responding to change being an independent contributor in the regression. There were also some effects of husband's job demands on spouse health behaviour. For example, wives were more likely to smoke if their husbands experienced greater role ambiguity. Role ambiguity and the stress of change were also independent correlates of the number of cigarettes smoked. Wives' drinking behaviour was also associated with higher levels of rate of change stress. Husbands' job complexity was also an independent predictor of the time since a wife had taken a non-routine physical examination.

Other factors such as job mobility or job relocation (Cooper, 1979; Lewis & Knapp, 1989; Seidenberg, 1975), and the extent of job-related travel (Culbert & Renshaw, 1972; Renshaw, 1976; Sloan & Cooper, 1986) have also been shown to have stress effects on both marital partners and their children.

The interaction of work and family roles also appears to result in strain effects when they are considered together. For example, Bhagat *et al.* (1985) found that employee well-being was better predicted by taking account of the combined effects of both work and personal roles. Personal and family stressors appeared to spill over into the workplace too: personal life stress was significantly correlated with work dissatisfaction, lack of organisational commitment, job strain and job alienation. Such findings are important because they imply that families may act as stressors as well as sources of social support. Many studies have demonstrated that social support has a buffering effect to offset the impact of job stress, although there is a good degree of inconsistency in the studies which makes it difficult to assess if social support operates as a main effect or by interaction in different role domains (see Cohen & Wills, 1985; Dooley, Rook & Catalano, 1987; Kessler & McLeod, 1985; Payne & Jones, 1987). In the physical health sphere, Winnubst, Marcelissen &

Kleber (1982), for example, show that supervisor support has a strong buffering effect against employee blood pressure (both systolic and diastolic). La Rocco, House & French (1980), in a review and reanalysis of data from Caplan *et al.*'s (1975) sample, show support for the buffering hypothesis for mental and physical health measures (although no buffering for job-related factors). Considering families as a potential source of both stressors and supports by taking account of the whole life stress pattern may resolve the inconsistencies to some extent. The configural model of stress discussed in Chapter 2 considered such aspects.

Cooke & Rousseau (1984) tested two contradictory models on a sample of 200 teachers to examine the interaction of work and family roles. Social support theory predicts that family roles should serve to reduce strain, whereas role theory allows that family roles may exacerbate the effects of work stressors because it can cause inter-role conflict. This would be particularly marked for those workers who work excessive hours (8.2% of those in employment), overtime (10.5%), or work schedules that interfere with family life (26.7%; results from Quinn & Staines, 1979). Physical strain was measured by a 13-item list of physical symptoms used in the 1977 Quality of Employment Survey (Quinn & Staines, 1979), which included conditions such as 'trouble breathing or shortness of breath', 'pains in my back or spine', 'feeling my heart racing or pounding', 'spells of dizziness', 'becoming very tired in a short time'. As predicted by role theory, work strain was found to be related to work overload and inter-role conflict. Family roles interacted with work roles: the family roles–physical strain relationship was mediated by inter-role conflict. Although generally supportive of the role theory view there was some evidence that the presence of a spouse and children was related to physical well-being, as would be expected according to social support theory.

Frone & Rice (1987) investigated the effects of role involvement on work–family role conflict. Previous studies had been rather ambiguous about the effects of high work involvement on work–family conflict, partly as a consequence of methodological and measurement differences and partly due to the failure to consider the degree of family involvement. Using a questionnaire survey of 141 non-teaching professionals employed by a university, Frone & Rice found that the job involvement/job–spouse conflict relationship was affected by the degree of spouse involvement reported: for those low in spouse involvement there was no association between job involvement and job–spouse conflict, whereas those high in spouse involvement showed a marked positive relationship. Interestingly, job involvement was positively associated with the degree of job–parent role conflict irrespective of the degree of involvement in parental affairs.

A number of studies have demonstrated that women may be particularly prone to the role conflicts between work and home, perhaps because they have traditionally assumed a greater domestic responsibility. Employed women, at least those with children, experience considerable guilt and conflict as well as lack of sympathy from employers (Kamerman, 1980). It does not appear to be work overload, but role conflict or multiple-role stress, that married employed women are susceptible to. Mannheim & Schiffrin (1984), for example, measured the degree to which 419 professional women with children showed cognitive investment in their work role compared to other roles. Ninety per cent of the women experienced no work overload although they were highly work-centred. Neither the husband's attitude to wife's work, nor the way in which the family roles were divided, was related to the degree to which the women were work-centred. Fifty-three per cent said their jobs interfered with the family, and 26% reported their role demands were contrary to their personal values. Perhaps unsurprisingly Mannheim & Schiffrin also found that the women still performed the traditionally female jobs in the home despite their demanding jobs. Sekaran (1985) did an exploratory study of the causes of mental ill-health in 166 dual-career families. For wives, both multiple role stress and the number of children were predictive of mental ill-health.

The literature suggests that married women in paid employment are more likely to suffer strain if they have children, although the literature is not unequivocal (Haw, 1982; Lewis & Cooper, 1983). Davidson & Cooper (1980a), for example, report that married female executives with children showed higher levels of strain than either single or divorced executives. Crouter (1984), in an analysis of the effects of spillover from home to work, has shown that such spillover is highest for working women with young children at home. Haynes & Feinleib (1980) compared a sample of 350 housewives with 387 women working outside the home and 580 working men. All were free of CHD at the outset of the study and were followed for eight years. The working women experienced more daily stress, marital satisfaction and ageing worries, and were less likely to show overt anger than either the housewives or the men. They were also more likely to have moved jobs and received fewer promotions than men. Although the incidence of CHD was not overall significantly greater in the women working outside the home compared to the housewives (7.8% vs. 5.4%), women in clerical jobs showed excess rates (10.6%). Of particular interest, however, is that the CHD rates of working women increased with the number of children they had: for women with no children the rate was 6.5%, for those with one or two children 8.3%, and for those with three or more 11%. Haynes & Feinleib concluded that "These findings suggest that dual roles of employment and raising a family may produce excessive demands on working women" (p. 139). It might at first sight be supposed that child-rearing is a particular stressor for working women because they are overloaded with the demands of both roles. The same relationship between number of children and CHD rates is also present for men, however (7.9%, 15.4% and 18.5% respectively, Haynes, Eaker & Feinleib, 1983), although men do not appear to show any spillover from home to work which characterises working women (Crouter, 1984). There may be an interaction between type A behaviour and the demands of children for women in highly demanding jobs. Davidson & Cooper (1980b) have shown that women in senior jobs have higher type A scores than comparable men: of 135 senior female executives 61.5% were either type A1 or A2 and none could be classified as B4. It also appears that female managers have less domestic support from home, greater conflict between home and career, and less emotional support at home than their male counterparts (Davidson & Cooper, 1983).

If the effects of work spillover do have consequences for disease risk the spillover should also be reflected in physiological strain measures. This has been shown. Rissler (1977) reports after-effects of overtime on post-work evening urinary levels of adrenalin in a two-month longitudinal study. During a four-week block of overtime evening adrenalin levels were elevated by more than 200% over pre-overtime levels, suggesting that unwinding after work overload may be a slow process with significant biological spillover into the home. Of course, such prolonged unwinding effects would be expected to interfere with social interactions between marital partners if they are also accompanied by psychological concomitants. Cohen (1980) provides a review of the after-effects of stress on human performance and social behaviour.

If work stress can have indirect strain consequences for those who interact with the job incumbent it is useful to investigate whether they can perceive the sources of the work stress of the job incumbents. Whilst this does not preclude the possibility that non-perceived stressors have an important causal effect in determining strain levels, it would demonstrate whether the perceived work stressors are similar for both the job incumbent and those at secondary risk. There is some support for this assertion, although the topic has not received much study. Long & Voges (1987) have investigated the degree to which a wife's perception of the sources of her husband's occupational stress correlates with his perception. Their sample consisted of 301 prison officers and their wives. Over 55% of the wives had jobs outside the home. A 39-item 'Sources of Stress Questionnaire' was administered to both husbands and wives. For those items which were confined to the stressors of being a prison officer, wives were asked to complete them in terms of the level of stress they thought it had caused their husbands in the past 12 months. Factor analyses of prison officers' responses to the stressors questionnaire produced four factors: aspects of work which interfered with family life (52% of common variance), concerns about living in prison villages (18.1%), worry about the potentially violent aspects of their work (13.4%), and personality and attitude changes in them which could adversely affect their family (5.9%). The factor analysis of the wives' responses produced the same four factors, although the order of the middle two were reversed. Statistical comparison of the factor structures showed very strong correlations between the relevant factors of prison officers and their wives. The results strongly suggested that prison officers' wives did accurately perceive the source and effect of their husbands' stress. It cannot be assumed that the congruence in perceptions would be revealed in more dispersed occupational communities (over 72% of the couples lived in the prison village). The study was, however, able to show that the congruence was a result of communicated information from the prison officers: few of the wives had any direct experience of their husbands' work environment, nor did they produce responses in accordance with the prevailing stereotype of the prison officer.

DISEASE CONCORDANCE OF MARITAL PARTNERS

If significant occupational stress is partly responsible for the life expectancy of both marital partners one might expect this to be reflected in the cause of death of both partners. If this were so the psychosocial transmission of occupational stress would imply that marital partners should show related causes of death. That is, there should be a significant excess likelihood of marital partners dying from the same cause.

There is some evidence that marital partners may share similar disease risk factors. For example, in a prospective examination of 269 married couples over a 10-year period, cigarette smoking was significantly correlated among the spouse pairs with a coefficient of 0.21 when the potentially confounding effects of age and time married were partialled out. Relative body weight was similarly correlated. Sixty-six per cent of the spouse pairs were also concordant in terms of systolic blood pressure when it was dichotomised above or below 160 mmHg (Haynes, Eaker & Feinleib, 1983). This examination of Framingham inhabitants also showed spouse pairs to be concordant in terms of the degree of expressed ambitiousness, although none of the other personality characteristics of husbands and wives were related (type A, emotional lability, non-easygoing).

Research does suggests that marital partners show a significant excess likelihood of dying from the same disease, although the proviso must be made that much of the evidence has been based on small sample sizes and is often methodologically suspect. Some studies do warrant reference. Ciocco (1941) studied the death certificates of over 2500 married couples, and reports a significant concordance in the cause of death between marital partners for tuberculosis, influenza and pneumonia, cancer and heart diseases. MacMahon & Pugh (1965) report that the spouses of those who had committed suicide were themselves a high-risk suicide group for many years after suffering the bereavement. In Parkes, Benjamin & Fitzgerald's (1969) well-known study of 4486 bereaved widowers, 48 of the 213 (22.5%) widowers who died did so from the same disease as their spouses. This 40% elevation in death rates was evident for six months following the death of the spouse. Dying of a broken heart was at best a metaphorical description of the data, since there was an excess of concordance over expected rates for five of the six disease groups considered (arteriosclerotic and degenerative heart disease; other heart and circulatory disorders; pneumonia; influenza and bronchitis, cancer; and all other causes). Hirayama (1981) has also shown concordance in the lung cancer disease rates of married couples in a large Japanese study of 91 540 non-smoking wives who were followed for up to 14 years. In Japan about three out of every four men smoke, and the age-adjusted mortality rate for lung cancer in women closely parallels that of men, despite the fact that less than 15% of women smoke. Of the women in the sample 174 died of lung cancer. The non-smoking wives of smoking husbands had a 1.61 excess risk of contracting lung cancer if their husbands smoked less than 20 cigarettes a day, and 2.08 if their husbands smoked more than 20 per day. Interestingly, the relation between the husband's smoking habit and wife's risk of developing lung cancer was much more marked for those whose husbands worked in agriculture, with comparable risk ratios of 3.17 and 4.57 for a younger age group. In this study, of course, the concordance is presumed to be due to both partners sharing a common smoky environment.

It should be noted that not all studies have confirmed that there is concordance between the causes of death of marital partners. Helsing and colleagues (Helsing & Szklo, 1981; Helsing, Comstock & Szklo, 1982) report a prospective study of 4032 people (1204 male, 2828 female) aged over 18 years, who became widowed. The study matched each widowed person with a comparable married person. Observed numbers of deaths were compared to expected numbers for all causes and 11 major causes of death, for four time periods after bereavement. From their analyses they concluded that "The similarity in causes of death of the widowed and their predeceased spouses was no greater than expected to occur by chance" (Helsing, Comstock & Szklo, 1982, p. 524). It should be noted, however, that the numbers in each of the relevant cells were very small: 28 of the 48 comparisons had observed and expected numbers of spouse pairs with similar underlying causes of death of less than 1. In fact, for the time periods up to 12 months following bereavement, nine of the 10 cells in which observed and/or expected deaths were 1 or more, showed observed deaths exceeding expected numbers. The single case in which this was not true was for 'other causes of death' occurring up to five months after bereavement, and here there was 1 expected and 1 observed case.

Little is known about the influence of occupational factors on the disease risks of the workers' spouses, although it has been suggested, for example, that the excess chronic bronchitis risks for the wives of workers in dusty environments is due to the wives being directly exposed to the dust particles when handling their clothes (Fox & Adelstein, 1978; McLaughlin, 1966). Indeed in 1985 an important legal precedent was set by the death of Mrs Winifred Wilson. She was the wife of a London dock worker. The husband had died from mesothelioma, an asbestos-related cancer, eight months previously. Mrs Wilson died of mesothelioma which the coroner recorded was a result of industrial illness. Mrs Wilson never worked directly with asbestos and the cause was attributed to secondary exposure from washing her husband's dusty overalls used to load asbestos at the West India Docks (*The Times*, 23 February 1985, p. 3).

Women's cervical cancer risk has also been related to the occupation of the husband, independently of the observed social class gradient (Beral, 1974; Singer, 1982), supporting a viral risk spillover effect from work to the home environment (Beral, 1974; Jordan, Sharp & Singer, 1982; Skegg *et al.*, 1982). Beral (1974) examined cervical cancer mortality of married women from 1959 to 1963 and reported marked differences (based on husand's occupation) between occupations in the same social class. In social class IV, for example, women married to fisher-men had a cervical cancer SMR of 257, although the figure for shopkeepers' wives was only 71. (The standardised mortality ratio (SMR) is the ratio of number of actual deaths over the number of expected deaths given the age-specific mortality rates of the general population. The SMR is standardised at 100, and scores greater than that indicate excess mortality risk. The proportional mortality ratio (PMR) is similar, but uses proportions of deaths rather than numbers of deaths.) Recent figures show a similar pattern. Mortality of married women aged 20–59 from cancer of the cervix in Great Britain 1979–80 and 1982–83 also show marked differences dependent upon the husband's occupation. For example, the PMR for the wives of architects, planners and surveyors (occupation number 031) was only 27, whereas that for the wives of marketing, sales and other managers (005) was 61; the wives of paper and paper product makers (094) had a PMR of 277, against only 22 for printing workers (100); wives of bus, coach and lorry drivers (152) exhibited a PMR of 166, those married to labourers in civil engineering and building (143) produced a PMR of 188, whilst wives of general labourers (160) showed a lower risk at 130 (OPCS, 1986a). These variations between risks for different occupations within social classes neutralise the criticism that risks are due to common social class factors which one would expect given that there is considerable concordance in the social class of bride and groom (Haskey, 1983) or, by definition, in the social class of established marital partners.

Recent research by Gardner and co-workers (1990a,b) has also shown that radiation exposure of men at work may be responsible for observed excess of childhood leukaemia and lymphoma around Sellafield nuclear plant in the UK. For example, the relative risk (compared to same area controls) was 6.42 for children of fathers who received 100 mSv or higher radiation dose prior to the conception of the child, compared to 1.06 for those whose fathers received a dose of less than 50 mSv, and 0.17 for those who lived an excess of 5 km from the plant. Although the study was not able to rule out the possible confounding factors of maternal infection and maternal radiation exposure (e.g. X-rays), it is strongly suggestive that the excess risk of cancer in the children was an indirect consequence of exposure in the workplace, which must be mediated by some factor such as the effect of work radiation on the male reproductive system.

In general, previous research has concentrated on specific occupations or clusters of occupations in an attempt to isolate injurious work-based toxins. Research done by the author, however, has considered the whole gamut of occupations, and showed that the overall life expectancy of both men and married women, and their cause of death, could be predicted from the occupation of the husband (e.g. Fletcher, 1983b, 1988b). This research will be discussed below.

THE TRANSMISSION OF OCCUPATIONAL MORTALITY RISK

The basic notion in this research is that occupational stress can, in the long run, result in premature death. Premature death would be revealed by high SMR scores for specific occupational groups. There are very marked differences in the overall mortality rates of different occupations, as well as in the mortality rates for different causes of death. Table 6.3 illustrates this point. Of course, many factors influence life expectancy (e.g. social class, diet, geographical location, exposure to physical toxins in the workplace, smoking behaviour). The research presented below does, however, suggest that work stress may play a significant role in life expectancy: the variations in SMRs across different occupations cannot be explained solely in terms of these other factors. It is suggested that a husband's occupation is a predictor of the life expectancy and cause of death of married women. Why such associations exist is unclear. Indeed in the past (OPCS, 1971, 1978) it has been taken as evidence that occupational factors cannot be a major influence on the mortality rates of the job incumbents: if wives show a parallel risk when classified by their husband's occupation it has been suggested that wider social factors are responsible for the SMRs of both. A reconsideration of the potential role played by psychological factors provides an alternative explanation which accounts for more of the evidence.

The Mortality Analyses

The principal data for the occupational mortality analyses come from government statistics (OPCS, 1971, 1978, 1986a,b). Fletcher (1983) reports an analysis of the deaths of 1 088 995 people in the eight years 1959–63 and 1970–72. Fletcher (1988b) considers the deaths of 324 822 men aged 20–64 and 35 915 women aged 20–59 in Great Britain for the years 1979–80 and 1982–83. Men and single women were classified on the basis of their own occupational unit, and married women according to their husband's occupation, not their own. In the later analyses there are 166 occupational groupings, 121 of which include subsumed occupational units, making a maximum number of 556 different occupational classifications. These categorisations allow fine-grain distinctions between different types of job (see OPCS, 1980, 1986a). SMRs were not calculable for a number of the occupational classifications, particularly for single women who were not represented in large numbers in many jobs.

The first finding of importance is the association between the SMRs of men and married women both classified by the occupation of the male. Table 6.1 shows the zero-order correlations separately for each of the three time periods for death from *all causes* (ICD no. 001-999, 9th revision). The later occupational mortality statistics were also analysed according to specific causes of death to identify if there was any concordance between married partners in terms of what they died of rather than simply in terms of how long they lived overall. To this end the correlational analysis was repeated separately for *diseases of the circulatory system* (390–459), *neoplasms* (140–239), *diseases of the respiratory system* (460–519) and *external causes of injury and poisoning* (E800–E999). These disease categories produced large sample sizes in enough of the 556 occupational categories to make very sound statistical comparisons. In this sample circulatory diseases accounted for 48% of deaths of occupied men, 27% of deaths of married women, and 22% of deaths

Table 6.1.   Zero-order correlations between the occupational mortality rates (SMRs) of working-age men and single women (classified according to their own occupations) and married women (classified by their husband's occupation) across all occupations

YEARS	Men and married women (husband's occupation)		Men and single women (own occupation)	
1959–63	0.91	(203)	0.61	(67)
1970–72	0.86	(222)	0.50	(122)
1979–80 and 1982–83	0.77	(489)	0.40	(285)

The figures in parentheses are the number of occupations on which the correlation is based (the system of classification having changed over the years).

of single women. Neoplasms accounted for 29%, 49% and 41% respectively external injury and poisoning for 9%, 7% and 16%, and respiratory diseases for 7%, 6% and 7%.

Table 6.2 presents the major results from this analysis. It can be seen that the correlations are highly significant, with the exception of 'neoplasms'. One could argue that outliers, or extreme SMR scores, could have a large effect on the correlations, and that any apparent association is an artifact of this. However, when the range of SMRs is limited to those between 60 and 140, to remove the effect of extreme scores, all five correlations are statistically significant. When the range of variance was reduced further by including only SMRs between 80 and 120 the correlation for all causes of death remained significant ($r=0.36$, $p<0.001$). This suggests that the life expectancy, and the specific cause of death, of married women is significantly affected by the male's occupational mortality risk. This occupational risk does not appear to be simply a generalised disease risk since there is an excess risk, common to both men and married women, for specific causes of death. One way to show this is to partial out the contribution of all other causes of death on the association between men and married women for any specific cause of death. Table 6.2 also shows the result of partialling out 'all causes' on each of the four specific causes considered. The partial correlations show the same pattern as the zero-order correlations, with the same three out of four correlations between men and married women remaining statistically significant. The sizes of the corre lations are reduced because occupations would be expected to carry some general mortality risk, as well as the specific disease category risk for both marital partners.

Mortality risk is inversely related to social class (see Chapter 7). In order to rule out the possibility that the observed concordance of risk is a consequence of marital partners sharing similar social conditions, as has been suggested by Fox & Adelstein (1978), the correlations were done separately for each social class. Occupational units were categorised into social classes according to the OPCS criteria (1980) when this was unambiguously possible. As can be seen from Table 6.2, 29 of the 30 correlations are statistically significant. It should be noted that statistical

Table 6.2.   Zero-order and partial correlations between the SMRs of men and married women (classified by husband's occupation), and men and single women (classified by their own occupation) for the major causes of death for all occupations considered together and for occupations categorised by social class reproduced by permission (from Fletcher, 1988b)

	Men and married women					Men and single women				
	All causes	Circulatory diseases	Neoplasms	Respiratory diseases	External causes	All causes	Circulatory diseases	Neoplasms	Respiratory diseases	External causes
All occupations	0.77 (489)	0.64 (450)	NS (472)	0.50 (347)	0.67 (323)	0.40 (285)	0.27 (185)	0.38 (230)	0.29 (108)	NS (147)
All occupations (only†SMRs 60–140)	0.57 (289)	0.32 (198)	0.32 (244)	0.22* (95)	0.23* (83)	NS (109)	NS (57)	NS (96)	NS (25)	NS (31)
Partial correlations†	—	0.10** (269)	NS (274)	0.25 (224)	0.70 (217)	—	NS (181)	0.24* (226)	NS (104)	NS (143)
Social class I	0.90 (27)	0.58 (27)	0.80 (27)	0.42* (21)	0.67 (26)	NS (27)	NS (27)	NS (27)	NS (27)	NS (27)
Social class II	0.76 (65)	0.56 (63)	0.61 (65)	0.71 (57)	0.32* (57)	NS (65)	NS (65)	NS (65)	NS (62)	NS (65)
Social class IIINM	0.60 (44)	0.86 (39)	0.49 (43)	0.57 (32)	0.87 (30)	NS (46)	0.40* (45)	0.35* (43)	NS (37)	NS (40)
Social class IIIM	0.79 (267)	0.60 (237)	0.74 (253)	0.38 (159)	0.57 (138)	0.19 (278)	NS (276)	0.19 (270)	NS (225)	NS (204)
Social class IV	0.68 (63)	0.56 (61)	NS (61)	0.29* (56)	0.46 (52)	NS (63)	NS (63)	NS (62)	NS (62)	NS (62)
Social class V	0.94 (18)	0.93 (18)	0.90 (18)	0.85 (18)	0.86 (17)	NS (18)	NS (18)	NS (18)	NS (18)	NS (18)

The number of occupational units on which each correlation is based is shown in parentheses.
All correlations are positive and significant at the $p<0.001$ level except those marked * ($p<0.02$) or ** ($p<0.05$) (NS = $p>0.05$).
† Partialling out the SMRs for 'all causes' for both men and women.

manipulation diminishes the likelihood that the overall effect is due to numerator/ denominator biases which can affect the interpretation of SMRs (e.g. the problems which result from inadequate occupational descriptions on the death certificate or on the 10-yearly census forms which are used to establish baseline data). In fact, only 58 of the occupational groupings are believed to be subject to numerator/ denominator bias (OPCS, 1986a) and would only significantly affect confidence in the correlations for social class V, where most misclassifications are likely to occur.

Table 6.3 presents mortality statistics for a number of occupations from each social class. Both men and married women were classified by the male's occupation. The selection of the occupations was relatively random, although their occupational titles were required to be relatively self-explanatory to the reader without recourse to the source job descriptions. Some better-known and more interesting occupational categories were deliberately chosen, and other jobs chosen for specific comparison purposes (e.g. machine tool setters, machine tool operators). The purpose of Table 6.3 is to show in some concrete or descriptive form the points made by the statistics in the preceding sections. The statistical analyses were based on data from all occupations, if available; Table 6.3 presents only eight examples from each social class. It should be noted that the SMRs are separately standardised for men and women; therefore the scores cannot be used to compare the relative mortality rates of men and women.

It can be clearly seen in Table 6.3 that there are marked differences in mortality rates *within each social class*, as well as between classes, and that the risk is, to some extent, disease-specific. The examples reflect the statistical results shown in Table 6.2. From Table 6.3 it can be seen that there is a wide range of SMRs for men from different occupations within each social class, and that the SMRs of married women classified by their husband's occupation closely mirror them. More interestingly, however, it is clear that occupations have different mortality risks for different causes of death, and that the risks for married women are similar to those of their husband's occupation.

The importance of the husband's occupation on the mortality of women is further demonstrated by the fact that virtually all the correlations between men and single women classified by their own occupation are non-significant or considerably smaller than those between men and married women (Tables 6.1 and 6.2). This suggests a synergy between occupation and marriage, because it implies that the wife of a man in any given occupation is more likely to die of the same disease as her husband compared to a single woman employed in the same occupation as her male counterpart. Such synergy explains why the correlations between men's and married women's SMRs are significant, but not those between men and single women. Marriage could be seen as amplifying the occupational factors. Such a suggestion is consistent with previous studies of occupational mortality (Fletcher, Gowler & Payne, 1980; Fletcher, 1983b) and with research showing that married women are perceptive about the source of their husband's occupational stress (Long & Voges, 1987). It also gives credence to the view that job factors are more predictive

Table 6.3. SMRs (1979–81 and 1982–83) for all causes and major causes of death of men and married women (classified by their husband's occupation) for a range of occupations stratified by social class (reproduced by permission from Fletcher 1988b)

Occupation and OPCS no.	All causes		Neoplasms		Circulatory diseases		Respiratory diseases		External causes	
	Men	Women	Men	Women	Men	Women	Men	Women	Men	Women
Social class I										
001 Judges, barristers, advocates, solicitors	74	84	82	114	66	33	53	28	92	84
002 Accountants, valuers, finance specialists	64	67	68	83	70	40	42	46	51	69
007 National government administrators	52	59	58	75	56	45	31	30	16	21
007.01 As 007, assistant secretary and above	113	108	115	147	102	95	106	68	88	64
012.02 Education officers, school inspectors	79	93	91	95	86	98	22	—	43	36
012.03 Social & behavioural scientists	59	79	58	67	58	77	53	—	100	221
015 Medical & dental practitioners	65	78	58	85	62	45	26	25	115	151
025 Civil, structural, municipal, etc., engineers	105	95	114	107	112	74	51	89	93	71
Social class II										
002.05 Financial managers	43	53	51	65	45	23	23	28	31	89
006 Statutory and other inspectors	127	107	133	125	140	85	86	84	106	95
007.02 As 007, HEO to Senior Principal level	48	55	54	70	54	42	26	28	11	18
016 Nurse administrators, nurses	115	132	104	127	121	140	96	176	132	153
019 Authors, writers, journalists	87	96	87	107	79	68	60	76	120	155
021.01 Actors, entertainers, singers, etc.	99	83	88	87	91	51	104	148	140	125
012.02 Musicians	132	116	110	94	123	92	160	161	163	263
033.02 Building & civil engineering technicians	23	46	15	48	21	50	31	60	39	40
Social class IIINM										
022.01 Photographers, cameramen	93	82	95	87	87	75	58	64	133	143
035 Site managers, building foremen, clerk of works etc.	52	55	57	65	58	47	25	36	32	33
045.02 Supervisors of stores and despatch clerks	254	228	281	128	280	431	333	710	—	—
045.04 Supervisors of other clerks & cashiers (not retail)	142	152	149	182	162	131	93	96	51	80
049.02 Typists, secretaries, shorthand writers	19	40	16	40	22	25	13	54	19	134
057.05 Sales representatives	75	73	77	82	78	62	52	54	75	78
060 Police sergeants, fire fighting supervisors etc.	146	144	163	164	165	153	97	146	71	81
061.01 Policemen (below sergeant)	94	94	109	106	107	80	61	75	81	88

continued overleaf

177

Table 6.3. (continued)

Occupation and OPCS no.	All causes		Neoplasms		Circulatory diseases		Respiratory diseases		External causes	
	Men	Women	Men	Women	Men	Women	Men	Women	Men	Women
Social class IIIM										
064 Chefs, cooks	135	143	125	131	124	153	137	117	169	190
097.01 Rubber process workers, tyre makers etc.	111	119	140	116	104	131	136	145	46	48
112.03 Machine tool setter operators	44	49	52	48	46	44	55	68	10	55
118.02 Maintenance fitters (aircraft engines)	20	14	19	6	2	32	22	52	23	—
095.09 Foremen of rubber makers and repairers	65	34	39	43	7	31	109	76	36	—
108.01 Foremen of furnace operators (metal)	413	469	388	519	47	607	290	—	276	211
111 Foremen of engineering machinery	132	145	161	175	13	120	88	81	56	84
149.01 Foremen of railway guards	870	1117	986	1428	96	1320	—	—	—	—
Social class IV										
070.02 Hospital, ward orderlies	101	95	94	102	10	101	63	79	109	102
087.03 Winders, reelers	52	55	16	57	6	—	130	164	44	—
098.04 Textile process workers	113	132	105	108	12	162	147	187	51	81
112.04 Machine tool operators	154	182	153	177	15	178	146	211	174	224
137 Inspectors, viewers, packers, bottlers, etc.	71	72	71	72	7	74	73	65	59	52
141.02 Road surfacers, concreters	165	178	208	165	14	215	203	396	159	98
148 Deck, engineroom hands, bargemen, boatmen, etc.	304	250	292	230	23	269	421	222	499	315
157 Storekeepers, stevedores, warehousemen etc.	120	118	123	111	12	134	134	138	89	87
Social class V										
157.03 Goods porters	87	83	92	78	7	88	91	93	99	57
Labourers (Nec) in:										
160.01 Textiles (not textile goods)	216	223	187	184	22	248	242	285	198	317
160.02 Chemical & allied trades	84	66	91	58	8	61	101	65	35	80
160.03 Coke ovens & gas works	136	133	119	100	14	121	191	171	115	156
160.04 Glass & ceramics	95	86	105	80	8	86	149	89	85	19
160.05 Foundries in engineering & allied trades	142	146	123	98	13	182	223	194	134	144
160.06 Engineering & allied trades	146	141	147	119	14	177	195	198	95	83
160.07 Coal mines	228	289	200	247	22	363	359	429	279	234

Abstracted from the microfiche tables of the OPCS decennial supplement Series DS no. 6, Part 2, 1986.

of illness and behaviour than non-work factors (Karasek, Gardell & Lindell, 1987). It should be borne in mind, however, that the range of occupations in which women are employed is considerably smaller than that of men (Table 6.1 shows this to some extent). It is possible that the apparent synergy is in part an artifact of the reduction in potential error variance (although such an explanation is unlikely, given that this had no effect on other comparisons shown in Table 6.2).

In analyses which consider even more specific disease categories than those above (e.g cancers or coronary heart disease) the association between the male's occupation and wives' disease-specific mortality risk is still present. For example, Table 6.4 shows the latest, and previously unpublished, results for a number of very specific disease classifications for the 1979–82 time period. This confirms the fact that those effects reported above are not an artifact of the broad disease categories used (which might be more susceptible to hidden confounding factors). Table 6.4 presents the zero-order correlations, as above, and the partial correlations when the relationship for 'all causes' of death is removed to leave the specific disease-concordant association. As can be seen, even for specific causes of death the occupational mortality rate of the husband has predictive value for the specific cause of death of women married to men in those occupations.

Table 6.4. Correlations (zero-order and partial) between the SMRs of men and married women for specific causes of death across the whole range of occupations

	Zero-order correlation	Partial correlation
Stomach cancer	0.50	0.39
Colon cancer	0.64	0.48
Digestive and peritoneal cancer	0.61	0.34
Trachea, bronchus, lung cancer	0.64	0.25
Lymph and Haematopoietic tissue cancer	0.34	0.16
Leukaemia	0.42	0.30
Diabetes mellitus	0.57	0.48
Multiple sclerosis	0.74	0.72
Acute myocardial infarction	0.59	0.13
Cerebrovascular disease	0.64	0.32
Pneumonia	0.37	0.54
Bronchitis, emphysema	0.49	0.09(NS)
Ulcer of stomach/duodenum	0.40	0.33
Nephritis and nephrosis	0.52	0.54
Motor vehicle accidents	0.36	0.12
Suicide	0.50	0.39
Open verdicts	0.40	0.16

Men and women are both classified according to the male's occupation.

Explanations Which May Be Ruled Out

The section above has examined the mortality statistics of men and women of working age for the years 1959–63, 1970–72, 1979–80 and 1982–83. It has involved an examination of the deaths of nearly 1.4 million people from over 550 different occupations. The results and analyses have demonstrated that there is a positive association between the overall life expectancy and the disease-specific mortality risks of men and married women *when both are classified by the male's occupation.*

The explanation of these findings is difficult but some obvious alternatives can be ruled out.

Shared social class

The disease risk concordance of marital partners cannot be due to the common social conditions of both partners since the relationship is present within each social class (Table 6.2). In addition, the differences in the mortality rates across occupations *within* each social class are, in some cases, at least as large as the differences between classes (Table 6.3).

Bereavement

It is unlikely to be due to a bereavement or 'broken heart' effect: men do show at least a short-term excess mortality risk of about 40% as a consequence of the death of their spouse (Mellstrom *et al.*, 1982; Parkes, Benjamin & Fitzgerald, 1969) but for women the effects are much less, if present, and are not shown in the short term (Bowling, 1987; Clayton, 1979; Helsing & Szklo, 1981; Jacobs & Ostfeld, 1977). The bereavement effect itself has not been unequivocally demonstrated. Some writers suggest that there are shortcomings in virtually every study which purports to demonstrate the effect (Stroebe *et al.*, 1981–82). The bereavement explanation also relies on a specific temporal ordering of deaths.

Physical transmission

Previous researchers have suggested that marital partners may be exposed to the same pathogens because they may be carried from the workplace into the home. A general viral or toxic substance transmission explanation (e.g. as reported by McLaughlin, 1966; Jordan *et al.*, 1982) would seem highly implausible here, however, since the effects reported are not confined to occupations exposed to toxic substances, and they are present for each cause of death and are particularly prominent for external causes of injury and poisoning.

Stressful occupations

It has been shown that the correlations between the mortality risks of men and married women are present when the analysis was restricted to SMRs within a narrow range. This finding seems to preclude the possibility that only particularly stressful or extreme occupations demonstrate a risk transmission between marital partners.

Like marries like

It might be suggested that people with the same disease risks are likely to marry one another. For example, bride and groom are generally from the same social class (Haskey, 1983), and very early work has shown that the physical characteristics (e.g. height) of husband and wife pairs are significantly correlated (Pearson & Lee, 1903). Certain biological coronary disease risk factors are also correlated in married partners, especially the longer they have been married, although there is little evidence that they share similar personality characteristics such as type A behaviour (Haynes, Eaker & Feinleib, 1983). Men and married women are also more likely to be engaged in *broadly* similar types of work (Fletcher, 1983b; OPCS, 1978). Homogamy, shared marital environments, and broadly similar work environments might partly explain some of the results presented here. Such an explanation would seem untenable, however, in view of the fine-grain occupational differences in SMRs observed in these figures. It would seem implausible, for example, to propose that machine tool operators or machine tool setter operators marry women with totally different mortality risks to reflect their own mortality risks. Such fine-grain differences between occupations, and the specificity of the disease category risks across occupations, also rule out another class of interpretations centred on other common risks marital partners are exposed to. It might be argued, for example, that the correlations observed here are a consequence of marital partners sharing similar social conditions, despite the separate analyses for each social class reported above: perhaps the partners do share the same social conditions, but these conditions are different for each social class. Alternatively it could be argued that husband and wife may expose themselves conjointly to similar risks and, therefore, die from the same diseases; for example they may drive together and die in the same accidents. Such explanations are totally inadequate, however, in view of the marked but subtle differences between occupational SMRs which can be seen in Table 6.3.

Data limitation

A limitation of the present database should be noted. Unfortunately it has not been possible to analyse the SMRs separately for single men and married men: males have been considered as a single homogeneous category. There are at least three reasons why this should not be considered too limiting here. First, the majority of men of working age are married, or have been. Second, the *occupational* risk on mortality is probably the same for both married and single men who are directly exposed to the same work stressors, even if there is a synergy between occupation and marriage. According to the analyses outlined above it is only the women who should show a different mortality risk depending upon their marital status. Finally, if the effects of occupational factors on mortality are different for married and single men this would *reduce* the size of the statistical associations reported. Perhaps the true size of the effects is even larger.

A tentative explanation

Any explanation of the findings must be able to account for two central aspects of the data. First, it must suggest a reason for the observed generality of the associations for each cause of death and across the whole range of occupations considered. Second, it must account for the occupational specificity of effect which has been outlined. This can be achieved only by showing how occupational factors may affect the SMRs of both marital partners. None of the explanations considered above takes account of both of these aspects. The explanation which can accommodate both aspects is that occupational risks are transmitted by psychological mechanisms to spouses through their shared domestic environment. How such mechanisms operate is unknown, and the suggestion needs further empirical investigation. It is known, however, that wives can have accurate perceptions of the source of their husband's occupational demands and stressors, and such stressors have been empirically shown to be responsible for the concordance in mental health of married couples (Long & Voges, 1987).

A model to represent this explanation is shown in Figure 6.1. This hypothesises that the occupational environment in which the man is working directly affects his experience and cognitive structure. Very subtle changes occur which can have 'configural effects' (see the configural model in Chapter 1) which in turn affects his perceptions, psychological make-up, communications with others and social behaviour. These changes can lead to resultant effects on his mental and physical health.

The work experience, and his response to it, also influences his wife's attitudes and cognitive structure, beliefs and behaviour, through the domestic psychological environment. The whole ecology of the husband's occupation, and other shared environments, affects the psychological framework of both partners.

The reciprocal influence of women on men

The data presented here should not be taken as demonstrating that a male's occupation has more effect on the life expectancy of both marital partners than a female's occupation. What has been shown is that a male's occupation is *one* predictor of the death rates of both partners. In 1990 in the UK it is the case that the majority of married women and mothers are in paid employment outside the home. The statistical analyses do not exclude the possibility of a reciprocal influence of a married woman's occupation on the life expectancy of her husband. This cannot be tested with the present database. Other research is somewhat equivocal on the issue. For example, Cochrane & Stopes-Roe (1981) report that husband's employment status had a significant effect on the depression levels of wives. However, whilst a woman's employment status was a major predictor of her own mental health, there was no reciprocal effect on her husband's. Billings & Moos (1982), on the other hand, report that higher wives' occupational stress was associated with lower levels of husbands' well-being.

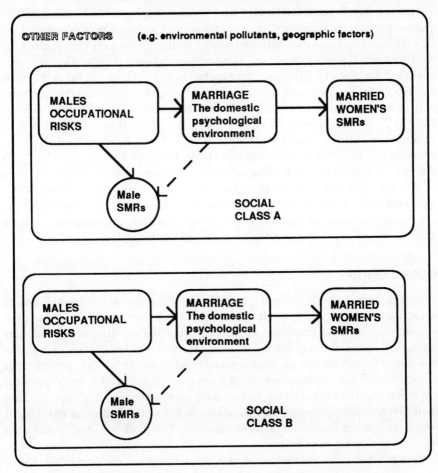

Figure 6.1   How the transmission of occupational mortality risk may occur

Non-occupational and occupational spouse characteristics have also been shown to influence the heart disease morbidity rates of married men. In the Framingham Heart Study of men aged 45–64, men married to women with 13 or more years of education (i.e. some college education) were 2.61 times more likely to develop coronary heart disease than those whose wives had only a grammar school education. Men married to women with more years of education than themselves (whatever their level) were also more likely to develop CHD. For example, men with grammar school education were 4.36 times more likely to develop CHD if their wives were more educated. In addition, men married to wives who had spent at least half their adult life in white-collar jobs were up to 5.36 times more likely to develop heart disease than if their wives were blue-collar workers (Haynes, Eaker &

Feinleib, 1983). In fact, the effect of wives' educational level on husbands' CHD mortality interacted with whether or not the women had been in employment outside the home for more than half their adult life: the effects were very marked for working women, although there was no association between the education of housewives and the rates of CHD among their husbands. Eaker, Haynes & Feinleib (1983) also report that the personality characteristics of wives seem to affect the likelihood of their husbands' developing CHD. Type B men were twice as likely to develop CHD if they were married to type A rather than type B wives. Type A men exhibited no extra risk, compared to type B men, if their wives were also type A, although type A men were 3.2 times more likely than type B men to develop CHD if they were married to type B women. The effect of type A behaviour on CHD risks of men also interacted with the type of work they did, the type of work their wives were employed in, and their wives' ambitiousness. The authors concluded that type A husbands were physiologically hyperreactive to certain characteristics of their spouses, especially if they were in blue-collar jobs themselves.

CONCLUSION

Although there is clearly a need for empirical investigation of the transmission of occupational risks hypothesis, it appears that there may be a link between the disease risks of those employed in an occupation and the disease risks of their spouses. It seems unlikely that the disease-specific mortality concordance is due to obvious factors such as the shared social conditions of both. It is possible that occupational environments carry with them a whole range of specific physical environmental risks (viruses, etc.) which are transmitted to spouses, thus affecting their disease risks in a way which is related to the worker's disease risks, but it would seem more reasonable and parsimonious to hypothesise the contribution of a psychological mechanism.

This psychological interpretation is consistent with a considerable body of research showing that psychosocial factors play an important role in the onset of human diseases and general immunological functioning (Chapters 2, 3, 4 and 5), the increasing literature implicating occupational factors in the disease process (Chapters 1 and 7), and the research showing work spillover effects (discussed in this chapter). That the psychosocial impact of work is not confined to the workplace is, of course, no surprise. That its effects may be so far-reaching gives a wry twist to the phrase 'work as a way of life'.

Chapter 7
The Epidemiology of Work Stress

This final chapter is a consideration of the epidemiology of physical health and well-being of job incumbents. It is be primarily concerned with disease states and their possible precursors (physiological and psychological) with little, if any, reference to job satisfaction/dissatisfaction, and non-validated self-report measures of work strain. The title of this chapter, 'the epidemiology of work stress', would not traditionally imply a major role for consideration of psychological variables in the causal chain because this steps outside the realm of the 'casually documented' or 'theoretically neutral' sets of variables usually considered. We have seen in Chapter 1, however, that occupational psychological stressors are important dimensions of some models of stress. Subsequent chapters have highlighted the need to consider psychological factors in the disease process, with Chapter 6 making a case that they are implicated in life expectancy. This suggests that psychological factors should be an integral aspect of epidemiological studies of disease. The first part of this chapter will consider the case for including occupational psychological factors in epidemiological studies.

Behavioural epidemiology attempts to take account of behaviours which may be injurious to health by showing that they are linked to morbidity or mortality outcomes. Behaviours considered in the past include such factors as eating excessive saturated fats, smoking, inadequate exercise, inadequate dietary fibre, excessive dietary sodium, alcohol, calorie intake, non-use of seat belts, and sexual habits (Sexton, 1979). *Descriptive epidemiology* is the investigation of the relative frequencies of outcome variables (e.g. psychological or physical ill-health) classified according to broad categories such as geographic location, age, biological characteristics, living habits, occupational types and other social and economic characteristics. *Analytic epidemiology* aims to study the causes of disease patterns by trying to account for the relative frequencies with reference to the categories of analysis utilised (see Lilienfield, 1980). The epidemiological research considered here is primarily of the latter nature, and includes an analysis of occupational factors which affect the biological and psychological precursors of actual clinical disease states.

It is becoming necessary for epidemiological methods to take a wider account of the possible role of psychological causes if its methods are to provide useful insights about the etiology of disease. At one level there is now a considerable corpus of documented evidence in the occupational stress and health literature to make such exercises worthwhile. Kasl (1978), in his review of epidemiological contributions to the study of work stress, saw the necessity to trawl the literature with a wider net than provided for by traditional epidemiological tools.

There are a number of reasons for suggesting that greater emphasis should be placed on psychological factors in epidemiological investigations. First, since the time of Kasl's review there has been an increasing number of studies of occupational stress which have utilised epidemiological methods (comparative observation, case-controlled or experimental epidemiology, prospective studies, etc.).

Second, more recent models of occupational stress outlined in Chapter 1 take it as axiomatic that strain must be predicted by taking account of intra-individual perceptions of work stressors. Failure to do so will result in little of the predictable variance being accounted for, and the subsequent failure of important psychological factors in strain being revealed. The person–environment fit models (e.g. Cox, 1978; French *et al.*, 1982), for example, require the measurement of a person's perception of their own abilities to meet the perceived environmental job demands. Measurement of environmental demands alone is insufficient, especially since under-demand or under-utilisation of ability is one of the better predictors of work strain (Margolis, Kroes & Quinn, 1974) when no account is taken of the individual's needs and capabilities. The demands–supports–constraints model (Payne, 1979; Payne & Fletcher, 1983) also proposes that it is necessary to measure the balance of these three variables for each individual, or at least for a group of individuals who do very similar work. The configural or catastrophe model (see Chapter 1) takes it as axiomatic that minor psychological perturbations may have major and unattributed health consequences. Models derived from large population samples, which fail to take adequate account of psychological factors, may be misleading. For example, Karasek's (1979) influential job demands–discretion model, which has been successfully applied to the prediction of a range of physical and psychological strains, may be picking up social class differences, rather than occupational differences, due to the large heterogeneous samples he has used (for example, lower social class jobs tend to be those which are associated with little discretion). These factors can make it difficult to assess the contribution of occupational stressors on strain, even in studies which circumvent the contamination of using self-report measures. In the Alfredsson *et al.* (1982) study, for example, psychosocially relevant aspects of 118 different occupations were identified by conducting a nationwide interview survey of 3876 working men. These results were then used to attempt to discriminate 334 myocardial infarct cases from double case-control men matched for age, sex and area of residence. A number of 'occupational' psychosocial characteristics were significant discriminators, including shift work, monotony, low autonomy over work tempo, not learning new things, and heavy lifting. However, it would be dangerous to conclude that these factors are occupational risks because the study is effectively comparing one occupation with another (only major characteristics of jobs are noted) and not one psychosocial factor with another. The study does not, therefore, compare otherwise homogeneous jobs, but probably picks up a package of other non-work variables which become subsumed under the psycho-social variable.

Using samples which are relatively homogeneous with respect to potentially important non-work factors may have the effect of reducing variance in the measures. Occupational homogeneity of the subject population may partly account for some failures to find that occupational factors have a direct impact on physiological indicators of strain, such as cholesterol ratio (Hendrix, Ovalle & Troxler, 1985).

Third, establishing differences in the patterns of morbidity and mortality by occupational classifications, and then searching for possible work-based explanations, is unlikely to be very helpful in determining etiology. Kasl (1978) suggests a number of difficulties which would scupper such attempts including (a) self-selection; (b) company selection; (c) health reasons; (d) determining exposure; (e) inadequate documentation or record; (f) bias in follow-up; (g) other confounding variables such as smoking, diet and exercise; (h) small case numbers. As Kasl notes, such an epidemiological paradigm "is probably too simple to be a methodological guide to the study of work stress" (p. 11). More important, perhaps, is the need to realise that 'occupation' may be too crude a variable to provide causally useful data. French *et al.* (1982), for example, in their stress and health study of 2010 people from 23 occupations, perceived that the term 'occupation' "is really a surrogate for a variety of characteristics of the job and of the person" (p. 88). It is more important to determine what *job factors* produce strain than to consider the pattern of strain across occupations. French *et al.* (1982) give two overriding reasons for favouring this approach: (a) symptoms do not reveal causes—knowing that some occupations have high strain levels does not provide information about the stressors, (b) occupations reflect a whole constellation of factors, only some of which affect strain. Traditional epidemiology leaves us the problems of isolating those work factors that are stressful, as well as being generally unhelpful about the role played by non-work stressors both on the effects of work, and directly on strain itself (Fletcher & Payne, 1980a). French *et al.* report that occupational psychological factors predicted between 14% and 45% of the variance in predicting strain, compared to only 2–6% of the variance when occupation was used as the predictor. Shifting the emphasis away from 'occupations' to 'occupational factors' does not, of course, remove the burden of proof. Such factors may be considered relevant only if they have been determined by scientific (and preferably experimental) techniques.

Fourth, if occupational psychological factors are important causal agents in the ontogenesis of disease, ignoring them may well lead to models with poor predictive power, fruitless searches for other causal factors, and incomplete understanding of the disease process. There is, however, as we have seen, considerable controversy in the biomedical field about the potential role psychological factors may play in disease. Psychological theories are generally not predictive at the level of the individual, although they are at the group level (a point well made for the occupational stress area by Payne, Jick & Burke, 1982). This cannot be taken as a criticism, nor does it reduce the power of psychological phenomena in the disease process: it should not be forgotten that, in general, psychology shares with medicine a probabilistic framework for diagnosis and empirical research which sits uncomfortably with deterministic or mechanistic models (Fletcher, 1980). Whilst the research outlined in this book contains many controversies and inconsistencies it should be remembered that such research is attempting to link a complex constellation of poorly understood variables with crude measuring tools to determine influences that are dynamic and generally chronic, may have occurred in the past, with less-than-optimal research designs, using all kinds of people, only a small number of whom will exhibit the outcome under consideration, and then perhaps will do so primarily as a consequence of other reasons.

The Size of the Work Stress Problem

It is difficult to estimate the size of any problem when the outcome variables have multifactorial 'causes' and one is particularly interested in one aspect of etiology. This is not an issue peculiar to the psychological investigation of disease. It is even more difficult when there is little consensus about the measurement of the relevant variables. This is often the case with psychological variables as is evident in, for example, the assessment of psychological factors in epidemiological studies of cardiovascular disease (e.g. Ostfeld & Eaker, 1985). Occupational strain is no exception in this respect, although it does present the additional difficulty, probably related to the often-mentioned 'lack of definition of stress', that strain may manifest itself in many forms.

The definitional difficulty is compounded by the potentially multifaceted manifestations of stress. Cox (1978), for example, lists multiple examples of six categories of work strain: cognitive, physiological, health, organisational, behavioural and subjective. Each strain (blood pressure, absence, smoking behaviour, heart disease, etc.) has numerous contributing causes, which makes it difficult to apportion the contribution, if any, of work stressors. Little is gained by an examination of those epidemiological studies which attempt to estimate the contribution work stressors make to any strain (as, for example, in the Framingham Heart Study discussed in Chapter 5). Multiple regression and other multiple logistic risk assessment techniques are not utilised as often as they might be, perhaps partly because large numbers are required for the subpopulations under examination, and because the contribution of psychological work factors is itself difficult and, to some extent, dependent upon a conceptual clarity which is not present in the discipline.

There is a sense in which the very nature of epidemiological research excludes adequate measurement of psychological factors in the workplace. Unless studies tap a large proportion of the universe of potentially contributing occupational factors, it would be surprising if the few factors measured (or implied) did account for much of the observed variance in the outcome measures. The standard physiological and medical risk factors for coronary heart disease or cancer are not good predictors of the degree or incidence of the clinical manifestation of the diseases. A critical reading of the epidemiological literature would soon convince the reader that trad-itional risk factors (e.g. smoking behaviour, blood pressure, obesity, cholesterol levels, etc., in coronary heart disease) themselves account for only a small proportion of the predictable variance, that relative and attributable risks from combined risk variables often show synergistic relationships exist (making the measurement of their combinations necessary), that single risk factors do not predict disease outcomes with unequivocal consistency, and that it is the weight of evidence, not absolute proof, that needs consideration.

It has been fashionable to question the contribution psychology may make in epistemological investigations of disease by referring to the small correlations often reported. For example, in occupational stress the stressor–strain relationships are commonly around 0.2. Some commentators (e.g. Fletcher & Payne, 1980a; Kasl, 1978) have suggested this indicates the relative non-importance of the stressor in strain etiology. It is true, as Cohen (1977) has described, that a correlation of this size accounts for only 4% of the predictable variance, and should be considered small. It will, however, be reliably detected in large sample studies. A number of other points should be borne in mind when considering such results. Frese (1985), for example, suggests that small correlations may mask results of considerable clinical importance. In his study, workers in the highest rather than the lowest stressor had up to *nine times* the excess risk of being psychosomatically impaired, even though stressor–strain relationships were around 0.2. Methodological reasons may also mitigate against obtaining high correlations (poor measuring tools which increase the error variance, the use of homogeneous samples [e.g. from similar occupations] which restrict the variance, etc.).

What is required is studies that truly attempt to examine causal models of work stressor–strain, against alternatives. Such studies are rare, but do support the contention that occupational factors are true causes of strain. Frese (1985), for example, examined a series of four hypotheses commonly offered as alternatives to the causal view that work stressors produce strain. His study of blue-collar workers took account of subjective self-report stressor assessment by including stressor assessment by colleagues and independent observers, it involved a longitudinal component to investigate whether being under strain was the cause of the stressors, it assessed whether the work stressor–strain relationship was present only for a subsample of the population by considering the difference for 'overestimators' and 'underestimators', and it enabled the partialling out of some factors which are often considered to intervene between the stressor–strain relationship such as job insecurity, age, socio-economic status (SES), the financial situation and political factors. The resulting analyses supported the contention that stressors in the workplace were independent causal contributors to strain (psychosomatic complaints). Such studies also demonstrate the need to account for a multitude of factors in order to provide a realistically convincing argument that work stressors have important medical consequences. Unfortunately, similar studies utilising disease-based measures of strain, rather than psychometrically assessed strain, are methodologically and pragmatically unfeasible.

A third reason for small work stressor–strain relationships is, of course, that work is only one of many contributing factors to strain. The interface between the domestic and occupational environments, as well the interaction of both with personality or individual perceptions, requires careful investigation.

Stress has Financial as well as Human Costs

The multifaceted effects of stress, and the problems inherent in this field of research, make the estimation of the costs of stress virtually impossible. Nonetheless, attempts have been made. For example, I have estimated that for every 1000 employees a company will be losing around £1.6 million per annum due to stress, assuming an average gross salary cost of £20 000 per person/annum. Moreover, if stress plays any role in absenteeism and labour turnover, reductions in these indicators would produce massive savings. Kearns (1986) suggests that 60% of absence from work is caused by stress-related disorders, and that in the UK alone 100 million working days are lost each year because people cannot face going to work. A company with a 5% absenteeism rate per annum, and a wage bill of £20 million per annum, would benefit to the tune of £200 000 per annum if it could reduce absenteeism by just 1%. If it costs £20 000 to replace someone who leaves, a reduction in labour turnover of 1% would produce a saving of £200 000 per annum/1000 employees. Cooper (1986) presents financial statistics indicating that £1.3 billion per annum is lost as a result of alcoholism in industry, and that American employers spend some $700 million per annum replacing men below retiring age due to CHD incapacity. In addition to these payoffs, there is also the benefit gained in productivity and well-being from reducing stress for the majority of workers who do not show strain in any of these ways (i.e. those who appear to be healthy). It is, of course, difficult to know what savings would be made (and at what cost) if work could be made physically and psychologically healthy. Certainly some practitioners believe that instituting better work practices, essentially better management, would probably reduce the problem (Stone, 1985), as would trends to redesign jobs to increase either group or individual autonomy, feedback, task identity, variety and significance (e.g. Wall, 1980). The fact that many large companies are investing money to help reduce the stress problems for their employees (e.g. Cooper, 1986; Fletcher & Hall, 1984) is probably a significant indicator that they believe it is more than mental health that is improved by such exercises. Companies are also investing more money in examining the psychological micro-culture of the workplace, and various tools (e.g. Fletcher, 1989) can be used to identify the psychological factors which are associated with various work outcomes such as absenteeism, labour turnover, organisational commitment, psychological and physical well-being.

Just as pathogens do not necessarily result in clinical manifestations of disease, stressors do not invariably produce strain. Occupational stressors are factors in the work environment which increase the *probability* of strain reactions. In the same way mediators (such as individual differences) are factors which increase the likelihood that a change in the normal stressor–strain relationship will occur. The degree of strain which is actually exhibited provides only the tip of the underlying problem. This is one reason it makes no sense to concentrate investigations of the cause of stress by close examination of those individuals with strain (whatever the strain). The answers derived from such investigations will be contaminated by what I have called 'secondary stressors' (see the configural model in Chapter 1). These factors are associated with the strain measures only because the organism is under strain as a result of 'primary stressors' which are the true causes of the strain.

The reliance on *exhibited strain* is an inbuilt limitation to epidemiological studies. Indeed, epidemiological research expends considerable resources on attempting to limit the possible contaminations due to such factors. It is a commonly held view, for example, that prospective designs are superior for determining cause–effect relationships (e.g. Fox, 1978; Kasl, 1983) because they are necessary to show that observed case-control differences are not a consequence of the illness itself. 'Cause' is not, however, a solely time-based concept and can, depending on the context, be better revealed by cross-sectional designs which provide a richer examination of psychosocial issues with a larger usable sample pool. Traditional epidemiological studies can never remove the fundamental limitation. What is needed, perhaps, is an understanding of how much of a limitation it is.

Levels of Stressors in the Workplace

Table 7.1 provides population data relating to a number of the occupational stressors depicted in Figure 1.1. The data are taken from Fletcher, Glendon & Stone (1987). The figures provided here are from a random sample of people taken from the Electoral Registers of England, Scotland and Wales ($n=820$). Respondents were asked to rate each of 129 work factors according to how they impinged upon themselves or their work on a 1–5 scale, ranging from 'never' to 'all the time'. A 'not relevant to my job' category was also provided. No mention was made of the word 'stress'. The *psychosocial factors* were rated in terms of the extent to which "they happen in your job"; the *individual factors* the extent to which they were "personally concerned" about them; the *objective environment factors* the extent to which the things "affect your work performance"; the *physical environment factors* the extent to which they "make your work difficult"; and *organisational factors* the extent to which they "affect your relationship with your employer". It should be noted that almost all the ratings for the 129 factors were significantly correlated with scores obtained on both the depression and free-floating anxiety scales of the Crown–Crisp Experiential Index (Crisp, Gaynor-Jones & Slater, 1978; Crown & Crisp, 1979). This supports the view that such occupational factors contribute to minor psychiatric morbidity. Of the 258 possible correlations 249 were significant (235 at $p<0.001$).

Work, Stress, Disease and Life Expectancy

Table 7.1. Job stressors in a random population sample

	Present 'all the time' (%)	Present 'often' (%)	Mean score (1–5 scale)
Psychological factors			
Not paid enough	34	9	4.0
No career prospects	23	12	3.7
Much work in bursts	14	35	3.6
Irregular work load	15	22	3.5
Being undervalued	17	17	3.4
Sudden panics of work	9	21	3.3
Capabilities not fully used	12	19	3.4
No participation in decisions	10	14	3.2
Conflicting information issued	5	15	3.0
No support from supervision	6	13	3.1
Conflicting instructions given	6	13	3.0
Authority is poorly defined	5	12	3.0
Job lacks security	10	7	3.2
Job lacks variety	8	9	3.1
Responsibilities poorly defined	5	11	3.0
Responsibility for people problems	4	10	3.0
Job poorly defined	4	7	2.9
Problems with status	4	7	2.9
Job gives no pleasure	4	7	2.8
No discretion or control of work	3	8	2.8
Individual factors			
Feels taken for granted	17	20	3.4
Working too many hours	13	14	3.3
No opportunity to learn	12	12	3.3
No time to relax	10	19	3.2
There is nothing to achieve	9	7	3.2
Fear of redundancy	9	7	3.2
No other jobs in line of work	7	8	3.2
Poor working conditions	7	9	3.1
Others keep changing their minds	7	19	3.1
Little time for family life	7	12	3.1
Insufficient responsibility	7	10	3.1
Too much pressure from above	6	12	3.0
Difficult to hear at work	4	12	2.9
Conditions of work keep changing	6	10	2.9
Trouble with supervision	4	9	2.8
Insufficient competition at work	4	6	2.9
Do not like the work	4	6	2.8
Objective environment			
Work accuracy	16	12	3.5
Pay rates	15	13	3.5
Management policies	11	17	3.4
Working in public	11	7	3.4
Unpaid overtime affects work	8	6	3.4

Table 7.1.   (*continued*)

	Present 'all the time' (%)	Present 'often' (%)	Mean score (1–5 scale)
Unsociable work hours	12	10	3.3
Working alone	8	10	3.3
Work requiring quick reactions	10	13	3.2
The work organisation	7	16	3.2
Dirty work	7	7	3.2
Excessive work hours	7	9	3.1
Physically demanding work	7	8	3.1
Fast work	5	10	3.1
Lack of encouragement	8	15	3.1
Frustrating work	6	16	3.1
Too much to do	6	14	3.1
Unsupervised work	8	9	3.1
Working conditions	7	11	3.0
Work requiring rapid choice	5	12	3.0
Emotionally demanding work	6	8	3.0
Monotony of work	5	9	3.0
Physical environment			
Poorly ventilated workplace	8	10	3.2
Affected by toxic fumes or dust	6	8	3.2
Workplace layout	8	12	3.1
Working in draughts	5	9	3.0
Inadequate rest periods	4	9	3.0
Poor machine design	2	4	3.0
Too much noise at work	4	9	2.9
Too hot at work	4	9	2.9
Difficult travelling to and from work	5	7	2.9
Pitch of noise	3	8	2.9
Too cold at work	3	8	2.9
Poor lighting	4	6	2.9
Affected by intermittent noise	2	4	2.9
Insufficient protective equipment	2	4	2.9
Organisational factors			
Poor fringe benefits provided	17	13	3.6
Given little information	8	18	3.2
Poor communications	8	16	3.2
Poor management	8	16	3.2
No performance feedback	7	16	3.2
Promotions unfairly handled	8	9	3.1
Little contact with management	6	11	3.1
Changing work targets	5	11	3.0
Poor social or welfare contacts	6	5	3.0
Too much work	3	9	2.9
Little contact with supervision	2	9	2.8
Too much labour turnover	3	4	2.8

A number of aspects of the data are reported. The first two columns show the percentage of the sample who reported each factor as affecting them 'all of the time' and 'often', ranked in descending order of conjoint frequency. The third column presents the mean score (on the 1–5 scale) for all respondents *who perceived the factors as being relevant to their job*. Only a sample of factors is shown.

From Table 7.1 it can be seen that a large percentage of the working population report being significantly affected (i.e. at least 'often') by a range of occupational factors. Almost 50% feel that much of their work is in bursts, 37% having irregular work loads, 35% feel they have no career prospects, 34% that they are undervalued, 31% that their capabilities are not utilised, 28% that poor management policies affect their performance, as does the lack of encouragement they receive (23%)—indeed poor management in a number of respects is perceived to affect employee relations and work performance (e.g. 26% are affected by being given little information, 23% no performance feedback). It is somewhat concerning that physical environmental factors are reported by significant proportions of the populations. For example, as many as 14% feel their work is affected by toxic fumes or dust, and that 18% report poor ventilation.

The percentages shown in Table 7.1 give a relatively theoretically neutral account of how people perceive various aspects of their work environment and the aspects of it that impinge upon them in various ways. Whether or not these potential stressors produce strain is another question. The fact that each of the stressors correlates with the psychoneurotic scales suggests that they may be actual stressors (i.e. they are predictive of health outcomes). Other researchers who have measured a large number of work stressors (e.g. Caplan *et al.*, 1975 measured some 19 work factors) have concluded that a more theoretically positive stance is justified. French *et al.* (1982), for example, view stressors as those factors which produce a misfit between a person's perception of their work environment and their perception of their own abilities and motives (see the P-E fit model in Chapter 1). Viewed in this way, a considerable minority of their working male sample (*n*=300) showed a large degree of misfit on some occupational factors (defined as 1½ standard deviations or more from perfect fit): income, 33%; responsibility for persons, 16%; workload, 14%; role ambiguity, 14%; job complexity, 13%; education, 10%; overtime, 9%. To be useful in epidemiological study, however, it is necessary to demonstrate in more scientific ways that these occupational factors are related to disease outcomes. Before considering some of this evidence, however, we should consider both how much strain or ill-health there is in a typical workforce, and which sectors of the workforce suffer more than others.

HOW MUCH STRAIN IS THERE?

There are many possible metrics of the extent of strain in the working population. The remainder of this chapter will provide data on the extent of the stress problem for a few of these.

Psychological Strain

In a random sample of 3077 British adults 14% of men and 19% of women reported having experienced unpleasant emotional strain for at least half of yesterday (weekday) (Warr & Payne, 1982a). Forty-four per cent of full-time employed men and 28% of similar women attributed the cause of the strain to their job—the single most important cause. People who reported pleasure yesterday generally attributed the cause to themselves or their family, not their job. In the same study 15% of men and 20% of women had suffered the strain for more than one month. Whilst work may produce negative affect for some, however, it may contribute positively to health too. Warr & Payne (1983), for example, found that over 15% of employed men and women derived pleasure from their jobs for at least half of yesterday.

In a longitudinal study of coping behaviour in young engineers (Newton & Keenan, 1985) 33% had suffered a stress incident at work within the past 14 days. Whilst most individuals attempted to cope in positive ways (e.g. 30% talked to others, 18% took direct action for resolution, 11% took preparatory action) a significant proportion (30%) expressed either helplessness, resentment or withdrawal behaviour.

In the Framingham Heart Study of men and women over 45 years old, over 48% of the sample described themselves as being "often troubled by feelings of tenseness, tightness, restlessness, or inability to relax", and 37% as being "usually pressed for time" (Haynes *et al.*, 1978b). High-stress jobs have also been associated with higher rates of nervousness. For example, in a comparison of high-risk jobs with controls Johansson, Aronsson & Lindström (1978) observed that "slight nervous disturbance" was reported by 36% more of the individuals in the former than the latter group.

In an examination of a sample of 1% of physically healthy community residents aged 15–69 in a large city Finlay-Jones & Burvill (1977) report some 13.6% of men and 18.9% of women have General Health Questionnaire (GHQ) scores indicating a growing need for medical and psychiatric treatment. Stone's (1985) randomised survey revealed that 14% had case levels of anxiety and 12% case levels of depression. Dohrenwend *et al.* (1980), from an analysis of epidemiological studies done in North America and Europe since 1945, have estimated that the prevalence (for a few months to a year) of functional mental disorders is between 16% and 25%. In addition, another 13% would have severe psychological/somatic illness not accompanied by recognisable mental disorder.

A large study of 8700 full-time members of a major Swedish labour federation has also enabled an assessment of the extent of psychological ill-health (Karasek, Gardell & Lindell, 1987). It was found that 40% of men and 45% of women were suffering from exhaustion; 15% and 23% respectively from depression. Nearly one in five of all workers were markedly dissatisfied with their job.

Examinations of particular occupational groups have also revealed levels of minor psychiatric morbidity levels which should give some cause for concern. Pratt (1978) reports that 21% of his teacher sample had elevated GHQ scores. Over 21% of student nurses scored at case levels on the MHQ in Parkes' (1982) study. Fletcher & Payne (1982), using the Crown–Crisp index, found 19% of teachers to be depressed beyond the level of psychiatric outpatients. In addition, 22% had felt as if they were going to have a nervous breakdown, of which 53% attributed the cause primarily to their job.

In a prospective National Survey of Health and Development of 1415 26-year-old men, Cherry (1978) reports that 38% of the sample said they were under some or severe nervous strain at work, whereas only 8% were under some or severe strain at home or in their personal lives. Almost 50% of those under severe strain also reported physical health symptoms. Of the 13 work causes considered, 36% reported 'pressure of work' as the cause of the strain, 24% 'responsibility' and 12% 'contact with people'. In a follow up 6 years later Cherry (1984) questions whether the strain symptoms related to pre-existing indicators of susceptibility rather than to the apparently stressful nature of their jobs. MacIver (1969) suggests that it has not been difficult for industrial psychiatrists to accept that 25% of the industrial population have significant emotional problems. He suggests that these problems will be exhibited in the form of neuroses (including depression) in about 5%, personality disorders in 5%, alcoholism in 3%, and psychophysiological disorders in around 10%. Even this estimate, however, seems to underestimate the size of the problem. As long ago as 1947, for example, Fraser's excellent work for the Industrial Health Research Board of the Medical Research Council revealed that some 9% of men and 13% of women in light and medium engineering factories had exhibited definite and disabling neurosis (anxiety, depression, obsessionality, hysteria, psychosis, etc.) in the six months of the study. A further 19% of men and 23% of women had suffered from minor neuroses (which included psychosomatic illness). Such neuroses were responsible for up to one-third of all absences from work, causing a loss, for the workforce as a whole, of 1.1% (men) and 2.4% (women) of possible working days. For example, women exhibiting definite neuroses (without physical illness) were absent on 13% of possible working days as a result of the neuroses. A number of work factors were found to be associated with more than the usual incidence of neurosis including working in excess of 75 hours per week, work found boring or disliked, light or sedentary work, work requiring skill inappropriate to the worker's intelligence, work requiring constant attention, especially allied with constrained scope or responsibility and work offering little variety. Fraser's (1947) work can be seen to have predated much of the modern impetus in stress research (including the 'Life Events' work of Holmes & Rahe *et al.* in Chapter 2, the emphasis on low demand and lack of autonomy, and the person–environment fit model in Chapter 1).

A number of studies have examined the prevalence rates of stress reactions in large work organisations. For example, Zaleznik, Kets de Vries & Howard (1977) report the results of an analysis of 2131 employees in the middle and high occupational brackets of a large company. Since they estimated that 15% of the employees did not complete the questionnaires due to illness or schedule conflicts the prevalence rates they report are likely to underestimate the degree of strain. Nonetheless, 24% reported suffering insomnia, 21% restlessness and agitation, 19% fatigue, 16% felt their work adversely affected their health, 13% felt the need to withdraw and 11% were worried about having a nervous breakdown. Ferguson (1973), in a study of 516 telegraphists, reports that 33% had or have had disabling neurosis as determined by medical interview/examination (neurosis was defined as anxiety state, neurasthenia, nervous exhaustion or debility, or nervous dyspepsia).

Such estimates of emotional distress may have important implications for absence behaviour, labour turnover, and efficiency at work, as well as indicating that a significant proportion of the workforce is unhappy. Perhaps more important for epidemiology, however, is that such mental ill-health predisposes employees to physical manifestations of ill-health too. In Russek's well-known early research of 89 infarction and 11 angina-on-effort patients with case-controls, for example, he says that "prolonged emotional strain associated with job responsibility...preceded the attack in 91% of the patients as compared with an occurrence of similar strain in only 20% of normal control subjects" (Russek, 1965, p. 189; see also Russek & Zohman, 1958). (Job responsibility is here defined in terms of the amount or volume of work being done, not the level of the person in the organisation. Job responsibility was considered high for those with two or more jobs or those working in excess of 60 hours/week.) In a more recent study Maschewsky (1982) compared 313 infarction survivors with 220 controls. All subjects were employed and aged between 30 and 64. Of 48 psychologically relevant dimensions only having "nervous strain in the last 10 years" discriminated between the groups at better than the 5% level.

Physiological Risk Factors and Physical Illness

Fraser's (1947) early work with 3500 factory workers showed that 14% of men and 18% of women had suffered a definite disabling physical illness causing seven days or more absence in the preceding six months. A further 24% of men and 22% of women had suffered more minor physical illness necessitating absence of less than seven days. Clearly, many types of physical illness would contribute to the absence behaviour and the prevalence and incidence of some these will be considered.

In the International Cooperative Study of some 8841 Dutch male workers over 39 years old Reeder, Schrama & Dirken (1973) found that 14.3% of the workforce showed abnormal electrocardiograms and 23.7% had serum cholesterol levels in excess of 279 mg%. Other studies of specific occupational groups have also been done. Cooper, Mallinger & Kahn (1978) report that 16.7% of their dentist sample showed ECG abnormalities. Marmot *et al.* (1978) report that 12.6% of administrative grade civil servants had elevated plasma cholesterol levels. Zaleznik, Kets de Vries & Howard (1977), in their study of managers, found that 8.4% of them reported having had 10 days or more off recently due to cardiovascular problems. In addition, 8% reported presently having rapid heart beats, and 7% having suffered them. In the Swiss part of the International Study the male population over 30 years of age of a Zurich factory were examined (*n*=885) (Schar, Reeder & Dirken, 1973). Ninety four per cent of the sample were blue-collar workers. Because of the type of work required, the workforce was quite selected, and showed a low prevalence of elevated cholesterol, glucosurea, proteinurea and cardiovascular pathology. Nonetheless their health history showed that 36.6% had a severe illness or accident, 6.9% some cardiovascular–renal disease and 6.4% a cerebrovascular stroke, infarction or pathological hypertension.

The prevalence rates of ischaemic heart disease derived from major recent studies reveal that a sizeable minority of the working population suffer from significant coronary conditions. For example, the French–Belgian Collaborative Group (1982) examined men aged 40–60. The study showed that factory workers in Brussels–Ghent had prevalence rates between 16% and 24%, depending upon the age group, and civil servants in Marseilles 7–22% (diagnostic criteria used the Rose questionnaire and Minnesota Codes for the ECGs). In the Framingham Heart Study the prevalence of total CHD (myocardial infarction and angina) was some 9% (Haynes *et al.*, 1978a). That CHD prevalence varies with the stressfulness of work was suggested in an early study by Russek (1962). The stressfulness of particular professions was assessed independently of the case sample by qualified specialists. In the three professional groups considered (medicine, dentistry and law) the so-called high-stress occupations within each profession were associated with considerably higher prevalence rates of CHD. For example, GPs and anaesthesiologists (high stress) showed an age-adjusted rate of 12%, which was 2.7 times that of pathologists and dermatologists (low stress).

In addition to occupational differences there are large international differences. In a comparison of the CHD mortality rates of 27 industrialised countries, for example, the highest rates were 2.7 (men)/3.8 (women) times those of the lowest rate (Uemura & Pisa, 1985). These international league tables place both France and Belgium in the lowest quartile, the United States of America in the middle of the table, and the United Kingdom nearer the top.

Incidence rates are derived from prospective studies of populations initially free of manifest CHD. The prospective phase of the British Regional Heart Study (Shaper *et al.*, 1985) examined a random sample of 7735 men aged 40–59. The average annual incidence rate of major ischaemic heart disease was 6.2/1000 (ICD 410–414). In a five-year prospective study of Israeli civil servants and municipal workers an annual incidence rate of 5.2/1000 was observed for clinical myocardial infarction (Goldbourt, Medalie & Neufeld, 1975) and 5.7/1000 for angina pectoris without infarction (Medalie & Goldbourt, 1976). Since it has been estimated that more than $700 million/annum is spent by American companies alone to replace premature CHD employees (Cooper, 1986), such incidence rates in the working population can be very costly.

Some estimates of the prevalence of hypertension suggest that as many as 18% of the population have blood pressures exceeding 160/95 mmHg (Health and Nutrition Examination Survey, 1977). Both systolic and diastolic pressures have been shown to predict CHD mortality (e.g. Lichtenstein, Shipley & Rose, 1985). Studies of working populations indicate prevalence rates rather lower than this. Charlesworth, Williams & Baer (1984), for example, found that 10% of a corporation's workforce had blood pressures over 140/90 mmHg, or were under treatment for essential hypertension. Fletcher & Jones (1990), in a blood pressure screening study (n=3095), report that 14% of working men and 21% of employed women had high blood pressure (in excess of 140/90 up to 45 years old, or 150/90 for older people). In a study of 17 530 male civil servants 12.8% had systolic pressures in excess of 159 mmHg (Marmot *et al.*, 1978). Clearly, since high blood pressure is largely asymptomatic and poorly monitored by health services, self-report studies suggest even lower rates. In such a study of a managerial workforce, for example, Zaleznik, Kets de Vries & Howard (1977) found that only 6.2% reported currently having high blood pressure. Males are, of course, more likely to have high blood pressure, particularly when they are younger. Wadsworth *et al.* (1985), in a birth cohort study of 36-year-olds, report 17.3% of men and 9.5% of women had diastolic pressures above 90 mmHg, and 12.3% of men and 6.2% of women had systolic pressures above 140 mmHg.

The extent of pill consumption has been linked with job stressors such as job demands and lack of job discretion (Karasek, 1979). Pill consumption is common. In the Zaleznik, Kets de Vries & Howard (1977) study over 21% took vitamin pills, 3% took sleeping pills, and 10% took other types of pill. Ferguson (1973) reported that 12% of his telegraphist sample took some form of sedative, and 13% took analgesics. Although alcohol consumption shows occupationally linked patterns (e.g. Plant, 1977) the rates appear to be related more to access, armed forces and old social traditions than to occupational stressors. It has been shown, however, that 9% of employed men and 7% of employed women cope with the unpleasant emotional strain they felt yesterday by drinking more alcohol than usual (Warr & Payne, 1982b). Six per cent of employed men cope by taking medicine or tablets, 15% smoke more, and 6% eat more than usual (the comparable figures for employed women were 15%, 9% and 17%).

Headaches have also been associated with occupational stress. For example, Johansson, Aronson & Lindstrom (1978) found that individuals in high-stress risk jobs in a saw-mill had prevalence rates 36% higher than the control groups. Turner & Stone (1979), in a random sample survey, found that 88% of people report having headaches, of whom 23% suffer between one and three per week. Green (1977), in a sample of 14 893 people, reports 19% of men and 26% of women suffered from migraine which necessitated an average of four days' absence from work per year. Waters (1970), on the basis of a postal survey, reports that as many as 28% of men and 41% of women will have had a unilateral headache in the preceding year, although proper clinical diagnoses reduce these prevalence estimates somewhat (Waters & Conners, 1971).

In Karasek *et al.*'s (1987) large Swedish study, the analyses of physical ill-health amongst the full-time workers revealed sizeable proportions of both men and women exhibiting strain. Some of their findings are shown in Table 7.2.

Table 7.2.   The percentage of the workforce affected by physical ill-health (data obtained from Karasek, Gardell & Lindell, 1987)

	Men	Women
Physical ill-health		
Muscular skeletal aches	19.0	25.3
Gastrointestinal problems	17.4	19.7
Heart disease (factor-analytic based)	13.9	13.7
Respiratory illness	9.4	13.3
Headaches (at least 'often')	8.8	20.0
Dizziness	5.1	12.8
Heart disease (theoretical definition)	5.1	4.6
Health-related behaviours		
Absenteeism (4+ sick periods/year)	7.1	17.0

Occupational factors are clearly not entirely responsible for the patterns of morbidity and mortality. Work may, for example, have positive health benefits as well as negative ones. Unemployment and retirement from work are associated with excess risk of psychological dysfunction (Jackson & Warr, 1984; Warr, 1983; Cobb & Kasl, 1977; Kasl, 1980) although the evidence that loss of a job leads to increased risk of cardiovascular disease is, at best, equivocal (Kasl & Cobb, 1980).

Specific occupational factors may be beneficial to health. Energy expenditure *at work* is one such protective factor. In a 22-year follow-up of 3686 longshoremen from a birth-cohort study, Paffenbarger *et al.* (1977) classified jobs into those requiring high energy output (an average of 1876 kcal over basal output per eight-hour working day), intermediate (1473 kcal) and light (865 kcal). The age-adjusted rates of fatal heart attacks for each cohort showed that high energy expenditure at work was associated with the lowest incidence rates, although obesity, abnormal glucose metabolism and high serum cholesterol did not add to the risk. For example, the adjusted rates per 1000 were 4.3 for high, and 7.69 for intermediate energy expenditure. Sudden death within one hour of an infarction was also less likely amongst the high energy output group. More recent epidemiological work by Paffenbarger *et al.* (1984) has confirmed that habitual leisure-time exercise among those who are likely to do more sedentary work (a study of 16 936 Harvard alumni) is associated with improved lifestyle, cardiovascular health and longevity. An important point to remember is that energy expenditure is likely to have important psychological benefits that may be at least partly responsible for the protective benefits. For example, Schar *et al.* (1973) found that higher energy expenditure was correlated with higher work satisfaction and lower social stress, neuroticism and subjective work strain.

Work and Type A 'Coronary-prone Work Behaviour'

As we saw in Chapter 5, type A or 'coronary-prone behaviour' is characterised by sustained drive towards poorly defined goals, preoccupation with deadlines, competitiveness and desire for advancement and achievement, mental and behavioural alertness or aggressiveness, chronic haste and impatience. Such behaviours are seen as being promoted by environmental factors (Friedman & Rosenman, 1974) and it is from this perspective that the work environment may be important. Typically more than 50% of a workforce would be classified as type A by one of the commonly used validated measures. There is some evidence that companies with a higher proportion of type A individuals show more profitable sales trends and a higher return on investment (Boyd, 1984). In a study of managers from 12 different companies Howard, Cunningham & Rechnitzer (1976) report that 61% were type A, 44% of whom exhibited the more extreme type A1 behaviour. High growth companies also tended to have more type A managers—up to 76% in one company. Women managers also appear to have to demonstrate high degrees of type A behaviour in order to succeed. In a sample of 135 female executives Davidson & Cooper (1980b) found 61.5% were type A with no type B4 (who are defined as those who show the complete absence of type A behaviours) in the sample at all.

Type A behaviour is by no means confined to the managerial levels. Hurrell (1985), for example, examined 2803 paced letter sorters and 2715 non-paced postal service workers. Some 54% of the workforce (men and women) were classified as type A with a disproportionately high representation among paced male workers. Those prospective studies, which include sufficient numbers of blue- and white-collar workers to enable sound comparisons, do suggest that white-collar workers score more highly on type A scales (e.g. Haynes & Feinleib, 1982; Johnston, Cook & Shaper, 1987).

As Kasl (1978) has pointed out, however, it is unclear what this psychosocial risk factor implies about the occupational environment. The majority of the research has been derived from primarily white-collar managerial samples, although there is evidence from blue-collar workers that the type A/B distinction has a direct influence on some mood states (e.g. tension–anxiety, anger–hostility) (Hurrell, 1985). There is also evidence that shows that type A individuals achieve their higher levels of occupational status because they devote more of their discretionary time to work (Byrne & Reinhart, 1989). It does appear that type A individuals are more likely to smoke (e.g. Haynes & Feinleib, 1982; Howard *et al.*, 1986) and less likely to give up smoking than type B individuals (Caplan *et al.*, 1975). Smoking behaviour has been associated with work stressors such as objective quantitative work load (e.g. number of office visits, phone calls, meetings per unit time) responsibility for the work of others, equipment and others' futures (French & Caplan, 1970), ambiguity about one's future, role ambiguity (Caplan *et al.*, 1975), job complexity and workload variance (French *et al.*, 1982). It is likely, therefore, that work factors may promote injurious behaviours, particularly for type A individuals.

The work environment will, of course, affect different individuals in different ways, and if type A behaviour were shown to moderate the effects of work stressors, this would have important implications for work and health. Some researchers have proposed that the behavioural distinction does indeed moderate the work stressor–strain relationship, and present models to this effect (e.g. Davidson & Cooper, 1980b), although some empirical work (e.g. Hurrell, 1985) would not support this view. Certainly, however, type A people exhibit a number of effects which are of relevance to the work environment. Howard *et al.* (1986), for example, report a two-year prospective study of 278 managerial staff, who were classified as type A or type B individuals. They were particularly interested in how changes in the work stressor role ambiguity (Kahn *et al.*, 1964; Van Sell, Brief & Schuler, 1981) were affected by behaviour type and job satisfaction, and the relationship of these variables to coronary risk factors. For type A managers the multiple regressions showed that changes in ambiguity were significantly related to systolic blood pressure, diastolic blood pressure and triglyceride levels. These effects were also moderated by intrinsic satisfaction such that larger changes were present for those with initially higher or lower levels of satisfaction. Other analyses also showed cholesterol level changes were related to changes in role ambiguity. A totally different picture was obtained for type B managers. The regression showed that only systolic blood pressure was related to ambiguity changes, and that the effect was in the opposite direction: increases in ambiguity were associated with decreases in blood pressure. Other research has shown that type A individuals respond to stressors at work in a different way to type B. Newton & Keenan (1985), for example, demonstrate that type A individuals are less likely to use potentially helpful coping strategies in response to a work stress incident: instead they tend to show greater helplessness and resentment.

Laboratory studies also demonstrate type A/B differences in response to stressors which are of relevance to the work environment (see also Chapter 5). For example, on a treadmill task type A people will do more work than type B, although they will not admit to being as fatigued (Carver *et al.*, 1976). They also appear to deny distress more than type B individuals under conditions of physiological arousal, which led Pittner & Houston (1980) to conclude that they are more likely consciously to try to cope with a difficult situation.

Occupation, Morbidity and Mortality

In the final section of the chapter some detailed occupational mortality data will be presented and discussed. The purpose of this section is to present, in broad terms, some data on what sectors of a workforce suffer most from strain. It may have been noted from the above discussion of the French–Belgian Collaborative Group study (1982) that the prevalence and incidence rates of heart disease of the factory workers were larger than those of the civil servants. This was true for both hard events and angina pectoris, and for each of the four age bands considered. For the 40–44-year-olds, for example, the incidence rate of hard coronary event and angina was 4.35 times higher for the factory workers. The relationship between broad occupationally derived social variables and mortality and morbidity rates is the subject of considerable debate. The relevance of such a debate to occupational stress is that it has become increasingly clear that purely physical environmental agents/facilities cannot adequately account for the disease patterns. Berkman & Syme (1979)—in their review of social class, susceptibility and sickness, for example—state that poor housing, crowding, racial factors, low income, poor education, unemployment, poor nutrition, poor use and availability of medical services, strenuous employment, non-hygienic settings, and increased exposure to toxic agents are all inadequate to explain the associations which have been observed between a large number of diseases and social class. Improvements in such factors, for example, do not appear to affect the social class gradient markedly. It is suggested that at least some of the relationship between occupational and social categories and disease is due to psychological factors which compromise the disease defences and affect general susceptibility.

In the past there has been considerable controversy over the relationship between illness/mortality rates and occupational category, particularly when the latter forms the basis of socioeconomic classifications (e.g. Biorck, Blomqvist & Sievers, 1958; Stamler *et al.*, 1960; Lee & Schneider, 1958; Pell & D'Alonzo, 1963). Antonovsky (1968), in his well-known review of social class and the major cardio-vascular diseases, concluded that for cardiovascular diseases, circulatory diseases, hypertensive heart disease, diseases of the heart, arteriosclerotic and degenerative heart disease, or coronary heart disease, "no fewer studies report inverse class gradients than direct gradients, and both are outnumbered by the number of studies showing no clear gradient" (p. 102). Cerebral haemorrhage (ICD 330–334) and "other myocardial degeneration" (422) did show consistent inverse class gradients. There is some evidence that the relationships have probably changed over time (e.g. Jenkins, 1982; Morgenstern, 1985), which suggests that more attention should be paid to more recent studies.

One reason for many of these early inconsistencies may have been that many different ways of measuring socioeconomic variables were employed (Lehman, 1967; Morgenstern, 1985) and some of the confusion is probably due to failures to compare like with like. When epidemiological studies have adopted two different classificatory procedures the results have not always been consistent (e.g. Finlay-Jones & Burvill, 1977).

The difficulty of assessing the true role of occupational factors in mortality and morbidity as revealed by social class gradients is greatly confounded by the degree to which the occupation determines the classification. The Edwards scale (1934), commonly used in the USA, is weighted by average income and educational level to produce six categories: professional and technical, managers, administrators and proprietors, sales and clerical, skilled craftsmen and foremen, semi-skilled operatives, and unskilled labourers. The Duncan Index and its derivatives (Duncan, 1961; Blau & Duncan, 1967; Stevens & Featherman, 1981) include accounts of prestige ratings, whilst the Warner Index (Warner, Meeker & Eells, 1949) includes reference to other social aspects besides occupational status, such as source of income and quality of domicile. Hollingshead & Redlich's (1958) index did include reference to educational level and quality of neighbourhood, as well as occupational status, although the neighbourhood dimension does not add much predictability to the scale (Hollingshead, 1971).

The British Registrar General's Social Class Scale divides occupations into six different categories: professional and similar (A or I), intermediate (B or II), non-manual skilled (C1 or IIIN), manual skilled (C2 or IIIM), partly skilled (D or IV), and unskilled occupations (E or V). The basis of this scale is the level of work skill required by the job:

> The occupation groups included in each of these categories have been selected in such a way as to bring together, so far as is possible, people with similar levels of occupational skill...and no account is taken of differences between individuals in the same occupation group e.g. differences of education or level of remuneration (OPCS *Classification of Occupations*, 1900, p. xi).

Other scales (e.g. Wright & Perrone's (1977) Class Typology) are concerned more with the degree of authority and control in the workplace. Whilst each of these scales categorises workers according to different criteria (the value of which may change with time) such broad groupings do have a limited value in assessing the impact of broad-spectrum stressors on health. All schemes which attempt to categorise a group of occupational descriptions or labels under common characteristics are bound to have limitations, especially when the descriptions are themselves dubious catchers of reality (e.g. the description 'company director'). The use of 'social class' descriptors can also be particularly problematic when using standardised statistics of morbidity and mortality, such as the Standardised Mortality Ratio (SMR), because of numerator/denominator bias, as revealed by longitudinal study (OPCS *Decennial Supplement*, 1986a) although such bias is particularly problematic only for the unskilled category. Such problems with statistics like the SMR are considerably outweighed by their advantages.

In addition, it has been suggested that some of the discrepancies in the literature may be a result of previous failures to take account of such factors as 'social mobility' and 'status discordance' (see Jenkins, 1971; Kasl, 1978). More recent reviews, however, provide a more sceptical view (Berkman, 1980; Jenkins, 1976a,b), and it has been suggested that if there are health effects of such factors they are probably dependent on individual and situational factors (Morgenstern, 1985).

Socioeconomic variables do represent one of the most commonly measured psychosocial factors in epidemiology, and it is necessary to attempt to dissect what contribution occupational psychological factors may play in these observed patterns of disease. This can be difficult, because the different scales weight occupational factors to different degrees. It has been suggested, for example, that when occupational rank is related to (e.g.) risk of coronary heart disease within an organisational context, the relationship is likely to be an inverse one. Using broader community and regional settings, however, changes the nature of the relationship (Lehman, 1967). A consideration of recent evidence strongly supports the contention that, for almost any significant measure of strain, the higher a worker is up the occupational ladder, the less likely they are to suffer significant illness (Fletcher, 1979; Fletcher & Payne, 1980a; Fletcher *et al.*, 1979). Some of this evidence will be considered below, considering a range of strains from biomedical risks, through morbidity rates, to life expectancy. Whilst there are exceptions to the inverse gradient between occupational level and strain, and each occupational classification and strain measure has its own associated limitations, the weight of evidence is relatively consistent. As to what the pattern means, that is another question.

Psychological Strain

Kornhauser's (1965) famous work with Detroit car workers showed clearly that "The higher the occupation the better the mental health on the average" (p. 56). He found that when the workers were classified into job levels by reference to work skill, variety, responsibility and pay, mental health scores (which were relatively assessed) showed a consistent correlation with the occupational gradient. For example, considering only middle-aged blue-collar workers, the proportions in each occupational group with good mental health were: skilled workers 56%, high semi-skilled 41%, ordinary semiskilled 38%, repetitive semiskilled 26%, repetitive machine-paced 26%. These occupational differences were present when a number of other factors were partialled out, including age, education level, job satisfaction, perceived utilisation of ability and opportunity for advancement, income level in boyhood, and a range of other childhood variables including deprivation, anxiety, happiness and aspirations. Kornhauser thus concludes that "they still show group differences in mental health corresponding to their occupational level—differences roughly comparable in size to those for the total occupational group" (p. 73). This supported the view that the job was a major contributing cause to the level of mental health of the workers.

Warr & Payne's (1982a) survey of experiences of strain and pleasure among adults also revealed significant relationships with socioeconomic status. Men (19%) and women (23%) from socioeconomic groups DE were more likely to have experienced emotional strain for at least half of yesterday than those of C2 status (13% men, 19% women) or ABC1 (11% men, 11% women). In addition, they were considerably more likely to have experienced the strain for at least one month. The DE women were also more likely to react to the strain by smoking more, compared to the C2 and ABC1 women (20%, 15%, 10% respectively) (Warr & Payne, 1982b).

When considering validated indices of mental health a similar pattern is revealed. Crown & Crisp (1979), in their normative data for the CCEI, demonstrate that those in social classes A and B have lower scores than those from C and D for the scales of free-floating anxiety, phobic anxiety, obsessionality (women), depression (men), and somatic anxiety (men and women). Finlay-Jones & Burvill (1977), in their 1% 'healthy' community sample, showed that the lowest two occupational groupings had a greater prevalence of minor psychiatric cases than the top four (18.5% vs.

11.2%). It should be borne in mind, however, that different measures of socio-economic status have been shown to produce inconsistent patterns (e.g. Finlay-Jones & Burvill, 1977; Goldberg, 1972). Some studies also show a J-shaped relationship between socioeconomic status and mental health, such that the highest levels show an increase, not a decrease, in ill-health (e.g. Goldberg, 1972, Appendix 7; Hepworth, 1980). Hepworth (1980), for example, reports General Health Questionnaire (GHQ) scores of unemployed men, categorised by the Registrar General's classification of their former occupations. The GHQ scores obtained (and percentage of samples above the cut-off point indicating at least minor morbidity) were: managerial, 3.2 (46%); skilled non-manual, 2.8 (25%); skilled manual, 4.0 (61%); partly skilled, 6.2 (80%); unskilled 6.5 (70%) (but see Payne, Warr & Hartley, 1984). Using an earlier version of the same socioeconomic scale, Finlay-Jones & Burvill (1977) also observed an increased case prevalence in the 'professional and similar' workers (15.6%), compared to the 'intermediate' (primarily managerial) group (11.5%). A similar effect has been observed for the prevalence of arteriosclerotic diseases amongst white-collar males in a large organisation (Lee & Schneider, 1958), with five-year rates of 11.8% for 'top executives', 7.7% for 'executives', 6.6% for 'minor executives' and 15.3% for non-executives (see also Holme *et al.*, 1982).

The broadly negative relationship between occupational or social position and psychological distress which has been consistently documented in epidemiological surveys may not be simply due to the lower strata being exposed to a greater level of stressors. Kessler & Cleary (1980), for example, suggest that statistical adjustment for differential exposure to stressors does not account for much of the variance. Instead one needs to consider that a significant aspect of the relationship is due to differences in responsiveness to stressors. According to this view those in the lower occupational levels are more likely to develop symptoms when exposed to a stressor: their general psychological defences (and biological defences) are weaker than those higher up the ladder. Such possibilities imply that minor differences in stressor levels (which might be difficult to detect reliably) would be amplified in strain manifestations.

Whatever the reason for these patterns of psychiatric morbidity, there is some evidence that the higher the status of the workers the more likely they are to admit or believe they have stress problems. Cherry (1978) reports that 54% of professional workers admitted suffering from nervous strain, compared to only 10% of unskilled manual workers: the myth of executive stress in action. Perhaps this is why the majority of stress courses are for managerial employees! In view of this it is not too surprising to find examples of studies which show that those higher up the occupational ladder are more likely to use professional help for personal problems. Kulka, Veroff & Douvan (1979), for example, report the results of two national surveys of the American adult population, done in 1957 and 1976. They found that the higher the income or educational level the more likely a person was to show "readiness for self-referral". They also report that help-seeking behaviour was largely independent of psychological symptom levels.

Disease Risk Factors

Uric acid in high levels may lead to crystallisation in the joints or the urinary tract, leading to gout or kidney stones. Evidence suggests that uric acid levels rise with occupational and social class. Dunn *et al.* (1963), for example, found that 43% of executives had a serum urate level of greater than 6 mg%, compared to 12% of craftsmen. The uric acid levels also showed a monotonic increase with number of years of schooling. Other factors (e.g. diet, aspirin consumption, obesity) could not account for the observed relationship. These early findings have been replicated and extended. There is also other evidence that levels are related to achievement and achievement-oriented behaviour, and are affected by work stress and losing one's job (see a review by Mueller *et al.*, 1970).

Other biochemical indices have also been shown to be lower among low level jobs. Caplan *et al.* (1975), for example, showed marked occupational differences in serum cortisol levels, a stress hormone of the adrenal–cortical axis. Low levels were observed in machine assemblers, with significantly elevated levels in scientists and administrators. Payne *et al.* (1985) have also reported that members of a cardiac surgery firm showed cortisol levels above the normal range on 72% of measurements, with mean levels higher the more senior the doctor.

Some studies have also observed plasma cholesterol levels to be higher in those higher up the occupational ladder. Marmot *et al.* (1978) reported that the higher the civil service grade, the more likely a person was to have cholesterol levels above 260 mg% (12.6% of the highest grade, and 7.8% for the lowest), and the higher the mean level (201 vs. 192 mg%). The authors attributed this to the richer fat diet of the higher administrative grades. Other studies, however, have not found a direct relationship between occupational level and cholesterol levels. The Oslo Study, in which 14 677 men aged between 40 and 49 were screened for coronary risk factors, observed an inverse gradient between levels and socioeconomic class (Holme *et al.*, 1977). This discrepancy is not simply a function of the crudeness of the social class scale in the latter study, since the same data broken down into specific occupational groups show that, for symptom-free men, lower status occupations such as tram drivers, metal foundry workers, construction machinery operators and taxi drivers are associated with the highest plasma cholesterol levels (Holme *et al.*, 1977). It should also not be thought that the discrepancy is necessarily a function of specific occupational stressors being appropriate to white-collar jobs, and not blue-collar jobs (although the reverse may be true). Low-level jobs (defined by the Duncan Scale or by specific job title) are characterised by underutilisation of abilities, low participation, flexibility and autonomy, but occupational level is also inversely correlated with 'executive stressors' such as role conflict, role ambiguity and ambiguity over one's future (Caplan *et al.*, 1975). The existing data are, however, inadequate to make anything but the broadest of generalisations.

When other coronary risk factors are considered the literature would support the contention that, on the whole, there is an inverse gradient between occupational level and coronary risk. Obviously, the more marked the differences between occupational levels, the more clearly this picture is shown.

In their study of employment grade and CHD in British civil servants, Marmot *et al.*, (1978) show that a man's grade was a strong predictor of the presence of the major coronary risk factors in their seven-and-a-half-year longitudinal study. Four grades were considered: messengers/unskilled personnel, clericals, professionals/executives, and administrators (in order of grade). For the risk factors of systolic blood pressure, smoking behaviour, obesity, and physical inactivity the higher the grade the lower the age-adjusted means and the lower the percentage of cases showing 'elevated' values. For example, the mean systolic pressure of administrators was 134 mmHg, with 11% showing elevated values (above 159 mmHg). The figures obtained for messengers were 138 mmHg and 17%. The differences were present for those in the under 40 and 40–49-year-old age bands (Marmot & Khaw, 1982). In addition, 61% of messenger grade men smoked and only 15% had never smoked, compared to 29% and 33% for the administrators. Fifty-six per cent of the messenger grades were physically inactive compared to only 26% of the administrators (Marmot *et al.*, 1978). Similar patterns have been demonstrated in other studies of coronary risk. In the Oslo Study, for example, data for 43 occupational groups are presented (Holme *et al.*, 1977). In general, those in the blue-collar occupations exhibited considerably higher multiplicative coronary risk scores (based on factors such as blood pressure, serum cholesterol, triglycerides and smoking behaviour) than those in white-collar jobs. Those in pedagogical work (e.g. university lecturers and professors) showed the lowest risk. Executives and managers had relatively low risk, clerical and sales personnel medium risk, higher risks for transport workers (e.g. bus and taxi drivers), and considerably raised risks for metal foundry workers and machinery operators. For example, the levels of risk factors for "leading administrators & executive officials" were: 29% smoked, triglycerides 2.0 mmol/l, blood pressure 131/83 mmHg, cholesterol 272 mg/dl. For "administrative, executive & managerial workers" the relative figures were 37%, 2.12 mmol/l, 134/86 mmHg, 266 mg/dl; and for metal foundry workers, 58%, 2.5 mmol/l, 141/89 mmHg, 280 mg/dl.

As part of the study of coronary heart disease in civil servants Markowe *et al.* (1985) measured several haemostatic variables in 29 lower grade and 45 higher grade men. They found a significant difference in the clotting factor plasma fibrinogen between the groups (3.39 g/l vs. 2.95 g/l), although none of the other measures showed the same pattern (clotting factors II, VII, VIII and X, % antithrombin III, platelet aggregation, etc.). Of additional relevance here was that fibrinogen concentration was significantly related to a measure of job stress, and was consistent with data on clinical CHD rates. Several studies have suggested that fibrinogen concentrations are important in the development of CHD (e.g. Meade *et al.*, 1985; Smith & Staples, 1981).

Disease and Life Expectancy

In their massive study of 270 000 employees of Bell Telephone Company, Hinkle *et al.* (1968) report the results of a three-year study in which 6347 events of disability or death were due to coronary heart disease. The age-standardised incidence rates of first events of disabling coronary heart disease were inversely related to occupational level. The rates/1000 were 1.85 for executives, 2.85 for general area managers, 3.91 for local area managers and supervisors, 4.52 for foremen, and 4.33 for skilled manual workers. Although educational level at the time of hiring was shown to have a marked effect on these rates, those at the lowest level (workers) were still about twice as likely to suffer a coronary event, compared to executives, whether one considers only the population with college education (4.15/1000 vs. 1.65/1000), or only those without college education (4.46/1000 vs. 2.46/1000).

The study by Hinkle *et al.* (1968) clearly demonstrated the importance of educational factors in affecting the likelihood of a person suffering a coronary event which "has been approximately 30 per cent lower among college men than among no-college men under all circumstances.... Up to now we have not encountered any exception to this rule" (p. 243), which suggests that factors outside the workplace play a major role in determining coronary risk (Hinkle *et al.* even proposed that the workforce could be divided into two populations with notably different biological features). One should not, however, ignore the interaction between the work environment and the pre-existing personal characteristics. The Framingham Study, for example, has shown that type A coronary risk is not exhibited in a greater incidence of CHD for blue-collar workers, although among white-collar workers the excess risk for type A individuals is over 2.4 that of type B (Haynes & Feinleib, 1982). It should also be borne in mind that the occupational/social status gradient generally observed for CHD is not explicable solely in terms of differences in the risk factor gradients discussed in the previous section. A number of studies have shown that, even when traditional risk factors are controlled for, the gradient does not change appreciably (Holme *et al.*, 1982; Marmot *et al.*, 1978; Rose & Marmot, 1981). In the Marmot *et al.* (1978) longitudinal study of civil servants, for example, the messengers in the lowest grades had 3.6 times the CHD mortality of those in the highest administrative grades. Although men in the lower grades tended to show higher risks in terms of most of the traditional risk factors (see above), the excess risk accounted for by such factors was minimal, leaving a large part of the inter-grade differences in CHD mortality rates unexplained. The authors suggested that "psychosocial differences between the grades" (p. 249) may have been the major discriminating risk factor.

What occupational psychosocial factors may be responsible for the pattern of CHD observed is a contentious issue. The factors shown to be associated with increased risk include work overload (e.g. Jenkins, 1982; Russek, 1965; Theorell & Floderus-Myrhed, 1977), although it is also clear that the low-level jobs are associated with strain indicators because of factors related to work underload. In a study by Margolis, Kroes & Quinn (1974) underutilisation of abilities correlated with overall strain more strongly than did most other stressors. Kritsikis, Heinemann & Eitner (1968) observed that workers on conveyor-line systems had a particularly high prevalence of angina pectoris. The job redesign literature emphasises, at a theoretical and pragmatic level, that changes in the work environment which increase worker autonomy, task identity, significance, variety and feedback all serve to increase mental health, even if these changes are made only at the level of the work group, leaving the basic work processes of the individual largely undisturbed (Wall & Clegg, 1981; Kemp *et al.*, 1983). It seems likely that the occupational factors relating to overload and underload, although both affecting the endocrinal systems in similar ways, may have their influence through separate psychological mechanisms. If one considers overload and underload as being separate unipolar dimensions (each being stressors) rather than a single bipolar dimension, a good degree of sense can be made of the literature. The way in which models of stress have accounted for the incidence and prevalence rates of CHD and other chronic and acute strains was considered in Chapter 1.

The relationship obtained between occupational status and disease, discussed above, is not just present for CHD. Table 7.3 presents mortality statistics (Fletcher, 1988a) for all the major causes of death for occupied men aged 20–64 years, and single women aged 20–59 classified according to their own occupation (based on the OPCS *Classification of Occupations*, 1980). The figures relate to deaths in the years 1979–80 and 1982–83, and have been abstracted from the OPCS *Occupational Mortality Decennial Supplement* microfiche tables (1986b). Perusal of Table 7.3 shows that for almost every major cause of death the higher the occupational class the lower the SMRs. The relationship is not confined to infectious diseases and those (such as respiratory diseases) for which there may be relatively clear physical environmental agents responsible. Nor should it be flippantly suggested that such factors as diet and smoking behaviour are the major discriminating variables. Not only do these factors fail to explain the whole pattern shown here, but such explanations naively ignore the role psychological work stressors play in determining the presence of such risk factors themselves. It is perhaps worth pointing out that patients in lower socioeconomic categories do not have a higher perception of pain or neuroticism about illness than those in higher classes (Larson & Marcer, 1984). Recent research has also confirmed that there are similar social class gradients for cancer *survival* rates once diagnosis has been made and not merely in overall cancer mortality. This was so for 11 out of the 13 specific cancer sites considered for men, and 12 out of 15 for women.

There are, of course, many factors involved in good health and life expectancy, and it would be extreme to assert that all (or even many) of these factors are occupationally and psychologically determined. There is a direct gradient, for example,

Table 7.3. Deaths in Great Britain from major causes, 1979–80 and 1982–3 for occupied men 20–64, married women (classified by husband's occupation) and single women aged 20–59

Cause of death (ICD no. 9th Revision)	Percentage deaths, occupied men	Percentage deaths, married women	Percentage deaths, single women	SMRs for men						SMRs for married women						SMRs for single women					
				I	II	IIIN	IIIM	IV	V	I	II	IIIN	IIIM	IV	V	I	II	IIIN	IIIM	IV	V
Diseases of circulatory system (390–459)	48	27	22	69	80	102	108	113	151	54	68	84	119	140	191	60	57	81	128	123	128
Ischaemic heart disease (410–414)	37	14	10	70	82	104	109	112	144	46	63	80	122	144	194	51	57	82	153	127	142
Acute myocardial infarction (410)	28	10	7	71	83	105	109	111	143	43	62	83	122	145	192	64	56	88	157	121	140
Neoplasms (140–239)	29	49	41	69	77	89	113	117	154	89	95	101	110	117	132	108	94	96	133	117	112
Trachea, bronchus, lung (162)	11	7	4	43	63	80	120	126	178	50	73	81	122	138	170	94	72	85	168	157	158
Digestive organs and peritoneum (150–159)	8	9	7	80	83	92	110	115	141	91	93	101	110	120	130	84	75	94	130	136	132
Stomach (151)	2	2	1	50	67	83	119	127	158	77	79	86	118	128	161	43	78	82	154	135	181
Colon (153)	2	3	2	114	99	105	103	101	116	104	104	116	108	105	98	122	79	94	141	146	90
Lymphatic and haematopoietic tissue (200–208)	2	3	3	107	97	98	105	104	121	95	104	98	106	115	119	32	96	104	151	114	113
Female breast (174)	—	5	13	—	—	—	—	—	—	109	105	114	104	107	104	140	110	99	126	101	100
External causes of injury and poisoning (E800–E999)	9	7	16	67	70	78	93	121	226	75	81	91	79	105	150	103	84	81	79	103	154
Motor vehicle accidents (E810–E825)	3	2	5	65	79	81	106	118	181	89	85	96	75	103	123	126	113	99	105	106	159
Suicide and self inflicted injury (E950–E959)	3	3	5	89	80	95	86	114	198	91	91	111	77	94	123	153	83	85	65	109	111
Disease of respiratory system (460–519)	7	6	7	36	50	83	102	129	210	47	64	76	118	143	220	19	32	54	83	93	97
Diseases of digestive system (520–579)	3	3	3	67	79	91	92	112	204	70	85	76	112	116	196	9	52	72	97	89	126
Stomach and duodenum ulcer (531–533)	0.6	0.5	0.6	39	55	80	94	124	261	54	58	79	114	136	280	—	45	82	87	86	135
Diseases of nervous system and sense organs (320–389)	1	2	3	69	61	100	80	109	185	98	85	92	110	128	132	49	37	61	95	66	88
Endocrinal, nutritional and metabolic diseases and immunity disorders (240–279)	1	1	2	72	76	110	99	118	156	49	60	88	114	145	242	88	43	79	141	84	96
Diabetes mellitus (250)	0.7	0.8	1	67	76	113	100	123	155	47	59	92	114	147	247	94	51	75	130	86	113
Diseases of genitourinary system (580–629)	0.6	1	1	43	69	106	94	116	185	45	63	105	113	134	241	24	50	56	98	93	139
Infectious and parasitic diseases (001–139)	0.5	0.7	0.9	65	62	93	89	117	215	68	86	73	112	128	187	76	61	89	94	64	85
Mental disorders (290–319)	0.4	0.4	0.7	35	48	55	84	97	342	63	66	83	95	116	227	67	44	76	41	65	61
All causes (001–999)	n=326573	n=90713	n=10209	66	76	94	106	116	165	75	83	93	111	125	160	75	68	80	111	107	117

Data reproduced by permission from Fletcher, 1988a.
The percentage of deaths attributable to each cause and SMRs according to social class . According to OPCS *Classification of Occupations*, 1980, HMSO;
Abstracted from OPCS *Occupational Mortality Decennial Supplement*, DS6, Part 2 (microfiche), 1986, HMSO.

between occupational status, or number of years of formal education completed, and the number of common surgical operations a person is likely to have undergone (Coulter & McPherson, 1985). Such findings are independent of known morbidity rates by socioeconomic status, and clearly imply that broader factors are responsible for surgical contact rates. What is needed, however, is a sympathetic consideration of the possible role of psychological (and particularly occupational) factors in disease and death. This book has attempted to do this in the preceding chapters.

References

Abse, D. W., Wilkins, M. M., Kirschner, G., Weston, D. L., Brown, R. S. & Buxton W. D. (1972). Self frustration, nighttime smoking and lung cancer, *Psychosomatic Medicine*, **34**, 395–404.

Achterberg, J., Lawlis, G. F., Simonton, O. C. & Mathews-Simonton, S. (1977). Psychological factors, blood factors and blood chemistries as disease outcome predictors for cancer patients, *Multivariate Experimental and Clinical Research*, **3**, 107–22.

Ader, R. (ed.) (1981). *Psychoneuroimmunology*, Academic Press, New York.

Ader, R. & Cohen, N. (1975). Behaviourally conditioned immunosuppression, *Psychosomatic Medicine*, **37**, 333–40.

Ader, R. & Cohen, N. (1981). Conditioned immunopharmacologic responses. In R. Ader (ed.), *Psychoneuroimmunology*, Academic Press, New York.

Ader, R. & Cohen, N. (1984). Behaviour and the immune system. In D. Gentry (ed.), *Handbook of Behavioural Medicine*, Guilford Press, New York.

Ader, R. & Cohen, N. (1985). CNS–Immune system interactions: conditioning phenomena, *Behavioural and Brain Sciences*, **8**, 379–94.

Ader, R. & Friedman, S. B. (1965). Differential early experiences and susceptibility to transplanted tumour in the rat, *Journal of Comparative and Physiological Psychology*, **59**, 361–4.

Ader, R., Cohen, N. & Bovbjerg, D. (1982). Conditioned suppression of humoral immunity in the rat, *Journal of Comparative and Physiological Psychology*, **96**, 517–21.

Agras, S. & Jacob, R. (1979). Hypertension. In O. F. Pomerlean and J. P. Brady (eds) *Behavioural Medicine: Theory and Practice*, Williams and Wilkins, Baltimore.

Ahnve, S., Faire, U., Orth-Gomer, K. & Theorell, T. (1979). Type-A behaviour in patients with non-coronary chest pain admitted to a coronary care unit, *Journal of Psychosomatic Research*, **23**, 219–23.

Albert, Z. (1967). Effect of number of animals per cage on the development of spontaneous neoplasms. In M. L. Conalty (ed.), *Husbandry of Laboratory Animals*, Academic Press, New York.

Alexander, F. (1939). Emotional factors in essential hypertension: presentation of a tentative hypothesis. *Psychosomatic Medicine*, **1**, 173–9.

Alexander, F. (1950). *Psychosomatic Medicine*, Norton, New York.

Alfredsson, L., Karasek, R. A. & Theorell, T. (1982). Myocardial infarction risk and psychosocial environment—An analysis of the male Swedish working force, *Social Science and Medicine*, **16**, 463–7.

Amkraut, A. & Solomon, G. F. (1972). Stress and murine sarcoma virus (Maloney) induced tumours, *Cancer Research*, **32**, 1428–33.

Anderson, T. W. (1978). Re-examination of some of the Framingham blood pressure data, *The Lancet*, **ii**, 1139–41.

Andervont, E. B. (1944). Influence of environment on mammary cancer in mice, *Journal of the National Cancer Institute*, **4**, 579–81.

214   *References*

Andrews, G. & Tennant, C. (1978). Being upset and becoming ill: an appraisal of the relation between life events and physical illness, *Medical Journal of Australia*, 1, 324–27.
Anisman, H. & Sklar, L. S. (1984). Psychological insults and pathology. Contribution of neurochemical, hormonal and immunological mechanisms. In A. Steptoe & A. Mathews (eds.), *Health Care and Human Behaviour*, Academic Press, New York.
Anisman, H. & Zacharko, R. M. (1982). Depression: the predisposing influence of stress, *Behavioural and Brain Sciences*, 5, 89–137.
Anisman, H. & Zacharko, R. M. (1985). Brain and the immune system: multiple sites of interaction, *Behavioural and Brain Sciences*, 8(3), 397–8.
Antonovsky, A. (1968). Social class and the major cardiovacular diseases, *Journal of Chronic Diseases*, 21, 65–106.
Ardlie, N. G., Glew, G. & Schwartz, C. J. (1966). Influence of catecholamines on nucleotide-induced platelet aggregation. *Nature*, 2, 415–17.
Bacon, C. L., Renneker, R. & Cutler, M. (1952). A psychosomatic survey of cancer of the breast, *Psychosomatic Medicine*, 14, 453–60.
Baer, P., Collins, F. H., Bourianoff, G. G. & Ketchele, M. F. (1979). Assessing personality factors in essential hypertension with a brief self-report instrument, *Psychosomatic Medicine*, 41, 321–30.
Bahnson, C. B. (1979). An historical family systems approach to coronary heart disease and cancer. In K. E. Schaefer, U. Stave & W. Blankenburg (eds), *A New Image of Man in Medicine*, Futura, Mount Kisco, NY.
Bahnson, C. B. (1981). Stress and cancer: the state of the art. Part 2. *Psychosomatics*, 22(3), 207–20.
Bahnson, C. B. & Bahnson, M. B. (1964). Career as an alternative to psychosis. In D. M. Kirsen & I. Leshan (eds), *Psychosomatic Aspects of Neoplastic Disease*, J. B. Lippincott, Philadelphia, PA.
Baker, D. G. & Jahn, A. (1976). The influence of a chronic environment stress on radiation carcinogenesis, *Radiation Research*, 68, 449–58.
Bakker, C. B. & Levenson, R. M. (1967). Determinants of angina pectoris, *Psychosomatic Medicine*, 29, 621–33.
Ballieux, R. E. & Heijnen, C. J. (1985). The seven veils of immune conditioning, *Behavioural and Brain Sciences*, 8(3), 396.
Bammer, K. (1982). Stress, spread and cancer. In K. Bammer & B. H. Newberry (eds), *Stress and Cancer*, C. J. Hogrefe, Toronto.
Bartrop, R. W., Lazarus, L., Luckhurst, E. & Kiloh, L. G. (1977). Depressed lymphocyte function after bereavement, *The Lancet*, 16 April, i, 834–6.
Bassett, J. R., Strand, F. L. & Carincross, K. D. (1978). Glucocorticoids, adrenocorticotrophic hormone and related polypeptides in myocardial sensitivity to noradrenaline, *European Journal of Pharmacology*, 49, 243–9.
Battacharyya, A. K. & Pradhan, S. N. (1979). Effects of stress on DMBA-induced tumor growth, plasma corticosterone, and brain biogenic amines in rats, *Research Communications in Chemical Pathology and Pharmacology*, 23, 107–16.
Bech, K. & Hilden, T. (1975). The frequency of secondary hypertension, *Acta Medica Scandinavica*, 197, 65–9.
Bennett, P. & Carroll, D. (1990). Stress management approaches to the prevention of coronary heart disease, *British Journal of Clinical Psychology*, 29, 1–12.
Benton, D. & Roberts, G. (1988). Effect of vitamin and mineral supplement on intelligence of a sample of school children, *The Lancet*, i, 140–3.
Beral, V. (1974). Cancer of the cervix: a sexually transmitted infection?, *The Lancet*, i, 1037–40.
Berkman, L. F. (1980). Physical health and the social environment: a social epidemiological

perspective. In L. Eisenberg & A. Kleinman (eds), *The Relevance of Social Science for Medicine*, Reidel, New York.

Berkman, L. F. (1982). Social networks and analysis of coronary heart disease, *Advances in Cardiology*, **29**, 37–49.

Berkman, L. F. (1985). Measures of social networks and social support: evidence and measurement. In A. M. Ostfeld & E. D. Eaker (eds), *Measuring Psychosocial Variables in Epidemiologic Studies of Cardiovascular Disease: Proceedings of a Workshop*, US Department of Health and Human Sciences.

Berkman, L. & Breslow, L. (1983). *Health and Ways of Living: Findings from the Alameda County Study*, Oxford University Press, New York.

Berkman, L. F. & Syme, S. L. (1979). Social networks, lost resistance, and mortality: a nine-year follow-up study of Alameda County residents, *American Journal of Epidemiology*, **109**(2), 186–204.

Berndt, K., Gunther, H. & Rothe, G. (1980). Personlichkeits struktur nach Eysenck bei Kranken mit Brustdusenund Bronchizekrebs und Diagnoseverzogerung durch den Patienten, *Archiv für Gewulstforschung*, **50**, 359–68.

Betz, B. J. & Thomas, C. B. (1979). Individual temperament as a predictor of health or premature disease, *Johns Hopkins Medical Journal*, **144**, 81–9.

Bevan, A. T., Honour, A. J. & Stott, F. H. (1967). Direct arterial pressure recording in unrestricted man, *Physiological Review*, **47**, 178–213.

Bhagat, R. S., McQuaid, S. J., Lindholm, H. & Segovis, J. (1985). Total life stress: a multimethod validation of the construct and its effects on organisationally valued outcomes and withdrawal behaviours, *Journal of Applied Psychology*, **70**, 202–14.

Bieliauskas, L. A. & Garron, D. C. (1982). Psychological depression and cancer, *General Hospital Psychiatry*, **4**, 187–95.

Billings, A. G. & Moos, R. H. (1982). Work stress and the stress-buffering roles of work and family resources, *Journal of Occupational Behaviour*, **3**, 215–32.

Biondi, M. & Pancheri, P. (1985). Stress, personality, immunity, and cancer: a challenge for psychosomatic medicine. In R. M. Kaplan & M. H. Criqui (eds), *Behavioural Epidemiology and Disease Prevention*, Plenum, New York and London.

Biorck, G., Blomqvist, M. K. & Sievers, J. (1958). Studies on myocardial infarction in Malmo, 1935–1954. II. Infarction rate by occupational group, *Acta Medica Scandinavica*, **161**(1), 21–32.

Blalock, J. E. (1984). The immune system as a sensory organ. *Journal of Immunology*, **132**, 1067.

Blau, P. & Duncan, O. D. (1967). *The American Occupational Structure*, John Wiley & Sons, New York.

Bloom, B. L., Asher, S. J. & White, S. W. (1978). Marital disruption as a stressor, *Psychological Bulletin*, **85**, 867–94.

Blumenthal, J. A., Williams, R., Kong, Y., Schanberg, S. M. & Thomson, L. W. (1978). Type A behavior and angiographically documented coronary disease, *Circulation*, **58**, 634–9.

Booth, G. (1964). Cancer and culture: psychological disposition and environment (a Rorschach study) (Unpublished).

Booth-Kewley, S. & Friedman, H. S. (1987). Psychological predictors of heart disease: a quantitative review, *Psychological Bulletin*, **101**, 343–62.

Bortner, R. W. (1969). A short rating scale as a potential measure of pattern A behaviour, *Journal of Chronic Diseases*, **22**, 87–91.

Bourne, H. R., Lichtenstein, L. M., Melmon, K. L., Henney, C. S., Weinstein, Y. & Shearer, G. M. (1974). Modulation of inflammation and immunity by cyclic AMP, *Science*, **84**, 19–28.

Bourque, L. B. & Back, K. W. (1977). Life graphs and life events, *Journal of Gerontology*, **32**, 669–74.

Bovbjerg, D., Ader, R. & Cohen, N. (1982). Behaviorally conditioned immunosuppression of a graft-vs-host response, *Proceedings of the National Academy of Sciences, USA,* **79**, 583–5.

Bowling, A. (1987). Mortality after bereavement: a review of the literature on survival periods and factors affecting survival, *Social Science and Medicine,* **24**, 117–24.

Boyd, D. P. (1984). Type A behaviour, financial performance and organizational growth in small business firms, *Journal of Occupational Psychology,* **57**, 137–40.

Broadbent, D. E. & Gath, D. (1979). Chronic effects of repetitive and non-repetitive work. In C. J. Mackay & T. Cox (eds), *Response to Stress: Occupational Aspects,* Independent Publishing Company, London.

Brown, G. W. (1974). Meaning, measurement and stress of life events. In B. S. Dohrenwend & B. P. Dohrenwend (eds), *Stressful Life Events: their Nature and Effects,* John Wiley & Sons, New York.

Brown, G. W. (1981). Life events, psychiatric disorder and physical illness. *Journal of Psychosomatic Research,* **25**, 461–73.

Brown, G. W. (1984). Social conditions related to the life stress process: contextual measures of life events. In B. S. Dohrenwend & B. P. Dohrenwend (eds), *Stressful Life Events and their Contexts,* Rutgers University Press, New York.

Brown, G. W. & Harris, T. (1978). *Social Origins of Depression: a Study of Psychiatric Disorder in Women,* Tavistock, London.

Brown, G. W. & Harris, T. (1982). Fall-off in the reporting of life events, *Social Psychiatry,* **17**, 23–8.

Brown, G. W., Sklair, F., Harris, T. O. & Birley, J. L. T. (1973). Life events and psychiatric disorders. Part 1: Some methodological issues, *Psychosomatic Medicine,* **3**, 74–87.

Bruhn, J. G., Chandler, B., Miller, M. C., Wolf, S. & Lynn, T. N. (1966). Social aspects of coronary heart disease in two adjacent, ethnically different communities, *American Journal of Public Health,* **56**, 1493–1506.

Bruhn, J. G., Chandler, B. & Wolf, S. (1969). A psychological study of survivors and non-survivors of myocardial infarction. *Psychosomatic Medicine,* **31**, 8–19.

Bulloch, K. & Moore, R. Y. (1981). Innervation of the thymus gland by brainstem and spinal cord in mouse and rat, *American Journal of Anatomy,* **162**, 157–66.

Burke, R. J., Weir, T. & Duwors, R. E. Jr (1979). Type A behavior of administrators and wives' reports of mental satisfaction and well-being, *Journal of Applied Psychology,* **64**, 57–65.

Burke, R. J., Weir, T. & Duwors, R. E. Jr (1980). Work demands on administrators and spouse well-being, *Human Relations,* **33**, 253–278.

Burnet, F. M. (1970). *Immunological Surveillance,* Pergamon Press, London.

Burnet, F. M. (1971). Immunological surveillance in neoplasia, *Transplantation Reviews,* **7**, 3–25.

Byers, S. O., Friedman, M., Rosenman, R. H. & Freed, S. C. (1962). Excretion of 3-methoxy-4-hydroxymandelic acid in men with behaviour pattern associated with high incidence of coronary artery disease, *Federation Proceedings, Federation of American Social Experimental Biology,* **21** (Suppl. 11), 99–101.

Byrne, D. G. (1980). Attributed responsibility for life events in survivors of myocardial infarction, *Psychotherapy and Psychosomatics,* **33**, 7–13.

Byrne, D. G. & Reinhart, M. I. (1989). Work characteristics, occupational achievement and the Type A behaviour pattern, *Journal of Occupational Psychology,* **62**, 123–134.

Byrne, D. G. & White, H. M. (1980). Life events and myocardial infarction revisited: the role of measures of individual impact, *Psychosomatic Medicine,* **42**, 1–10.

Caine, T. M. & Foulds, G. A. (1967). *Personality Questionnaire (HDHQ),* University of London Press, London.

Caine, T. M., Foulds, G. A. & Hope, K. (1967). *Manual of the Hostility and Direction of Hostility Questionnaire*, University of London Press, London.

Caplan, R. D., Cobb, S., French, J. R. P., Van Harrison, R. & Pinneay, S. R. (1975). *Job Demands and Worker Health*, HEW Publication No. (N10SH) 75–160, US Government Printing Office, Washington.

Cappuccio, F. P., Markandu, N. D., Beynon, G. W., Shore, A. C., Sampson, B. & MacGregor, G. A. (1985). Lack of effect of oral magnesium on high blood pressure: a double-blind study, *British Medical Journal*, **291**, 235–8.

Carruthers, M. E. (1969). Aggression and atheroma, *The Lancet*, **ii**, 1170–1.

Carver, C. S., Coleman, A. E. & Glass, D. C. (1976). The coronary-prone behaviour pattern and suppression of fatigue on a treadmill test, *Journal of Personality and Social Psychology*, **33**, 460–6.

Case, R. B., Heller, S. S., Case, N. B., Moss, A. J. and the Multicenter Post-Infarction Research Group. (1985). Type A behaviour and survival after acute myocardial infarction, *New England Journal of Medicine*, **312**, 737–41.

Cassel, J. (1976). The contribution of the social environment to host resistance, *American Journal of Epidemiology*, **104**, 107–23.

Castro, J. E. (1978). An overview of tumour immunology and immunotherapy. In J. E. Castro (ed.), *Immunological Aspects of Cancer*, MTP Press, Lancaster.

Charlesworth, E. A., Williams, B. J. & Baer, P. E. (1984). Stress management at the worksite for hypertension: compliance, cost-benefit, health care and hypertension-related variables, *Psychosomatic Medicine*, **46**(5), 387–97.

Cherry, N. (1978). Stress, anxiety and work: a longitudinal study, *Journal of Occupational Psychology*, **51**, 259–70.

Cherry, N. (1984). Nervous strain, anxiety and symptoms amongst 32-year-old men at work in Britain, *Journal of Occupational Psychology*, **57**, 95–105.

Ciocco, A. (1941). On the interdependence of the length of life of husband and wife, *Human Biology*, **13**, 505–25.

Clark, R. A., Nye, F. I. & Gecas, V. (1978). Work involvement and marital role performance, *Journal of Marriage and the Family*, **40**, 9–22.

Clayton, P. J. (1979). The sequelae and nonsequelae of conjugal bereavement, *American Journal of Psychiatry*, **136**, 1530–4.

Cobb, B. (1952). A socio-psychological study of the cancer patient. Unpublished thesis. University of Texas, Austin, Texas.

Cobb, S. (1976). Social support as a moderator of life stress, *Psychosomatic Medicine*, **38**, 300–13.

Cobb, S. & Kasl, S. V. (1977). *Termination: the Consequences of Job Loss*, US Department of Health, Education and Welfare, Cincinatti, OH.

Cochrane, R. & Stopes-Roe, M. (1981). Women, marriage, employment and mental health, *British Journal of Psychiatry*, **139**, 373–81.

Cohen, F. (1981). Stress and bodily illness, *Psychiatric Clinics of North America*, **4**, 269–86.

Cohen, J. (1977). *Statistical Power Analysis for the Behavioural Sciences*, Academic Press, New York.

Cohen, J. B., Syme, S. L., Jenkins, C. D., Kagan, A. & Zyzanski, S. J. (1979). Cultural context of Type A behaviour and risk for CHD: a study of Japanese-American males. *Journal of Behavioural Medicine*, **2**, 375–84.

Cohen, S. (1980). After-effects of stress on human performance and social behaviour: a review of research and theory. *Psychological Bulletin*, **88**, 82–108.

Cohen, S. & McKay, G. (1984). Social support, stress and the buffering hyupothesis: a theoretical analysis. In A. Baum, J. E. Singer & S. E. Taylor (eds), *Handbook of Psychology and Health*, Vol. 4, Erlbaum, Hillsdale, NJ.

Cohen, S. & Wills, T. A. (1989). Stress, social support and the buffering hypothesis, *Psychological Bulletin*, **98**, 310–57.

Comsa, J., Leonhardt, H. & Wekerle, H. (1982). Hormonal co-ordination of the immune response, *Reviews of Physiology, Biochemistry and Pharmacology*, **92**, 115–89.

Connolly, J. (1976). Life events before myocardial infarction, *Journal of Human Stress*, **2**, 3–17.

Cook, T. D. & Campbell, D. T. (1979). *Quasi-experimentation. Design and Analysis Issues for Field Settings*. Houghton-Mifflin, Boston, MA.

Cooke, R. A. & Rousseau, D. M. (1984). Stress and strain from family roles and work-role expectations, *Journal of Applied Psychology*, **69**, 252–60.

Cooper, C. L. (1979). *The Executive Gypsy: The Quality of Managerial Life*, Macmillan, London.

Cooper, C. L. (1986). Job distress: recent research and the emerging role of the clinical occupational psychologist, *Bulletin of the British Psychological Society*, **39**, 325–31.

Cooper, C. L. (ed.) (1988). *Stress and Breast Cancer*, John Wiley & Sons, Chichester.

Cooper, C. L. & Marshall, J. (1976). Occupational sources of stress. a review of the literature relating to coronary heart disease and mental ill-health, *Journal of Occupational Psychology*, **49**, 11–28.

Cooper, C. L., Mallinger, M. & Kahn, R. (1978). Identifying sources of occupational stress among dentists, *Journal of Occupational Psychology*, **51**, 227–34.

Coppen, A. & Metcalfe, M. (1963). Cancer and extraversion, *British Medical Journal*, July 6th, 18–19.

Coulter, A. & McPherson, K. (1985). Socioeconomic variations in the use of common surgical operations, *British Medical Journal*, **295**, 183–7.

Cox, T. (1978). *Stress*, University Park Press, Baltimore, MD.

Cox, T. (1984). Stress: a psychophysiological approach to cancer. In C. L. Cooper (ed.), *Psychosocial Stress and Cancer*, John Wiley & Sons, Chichester.

Cox, T. & MacKay, C. (1982). Psychosocial factors and psychophysiological mechanisms in the aetiology and development of cancers, *Social Science and Medicine*, **16**, 381–96.

Craig, T. K. J. & Brown, G. W. (1984). Life events, meaning and physical illness: a review. In A. Steptoe & A. Matthews (eds), *Health Care and Human Behavior*, Harcourt & Brace Jovanovich, London.

Cramer, I., Blohmke, M., Bahnson, C. B. *et al.* (1977). Psychosoziale Faktoren und Krebs: Untersuchung von 80 Frauen mit einem psychosozialen Fragebogen. *Munch Med Wochenschr.*, **119**(43), 1387–92.

Crisp, A. H., Gaynor-Jones, M. & Slater, P. (1978). The Middlesex Hospital Questionnaire: a validity study, *British Journal of Medical Psychology*, **51**, 269–80.

Crouter, A. C. (1984). Spillover from family to work: the neglected side of the work-family interface, *Human Relations*, **37**, 425–44.

Crown, S. & Crisp, A. H. (1979). *Manual of the Crown–Crisp Experiential Index*, Hodder & Stoughton, London.

Culbert, S. A. & Renshaw, J. R. (1972). Coping with the stresses of travel as an opportunity for improving the quality of work and family life, *Family Process*, **11**, 321–7.

Cunningham, A. J. (1985). Conditioned immunosuppression: an important but probably non-specific phenomenon, *Behavioral and Brain Sciences*, **8**(3), 397.

Dattore, P., Shontz, F. & Coyne, L. (1980). Premorbid personality differentiation of cancer and non-cancer groups, *Journal of Consulting and Clinical Psychology*, **48**(3), 388–94.

Davidson, M. J. & Cooper, C. L. (1980a). The extra pressures of women executives, *Personnel Management*, June, pp. 48–51.

Davidson, M. J. & Cooper, C. L. (1980b). Type A coronary prone behaviour and stress in senior female managers and administrators, *Journal of Occupational Medicine*, **22**, 801–6.

Davidson, M. J. & Cooper, C. L. (1983), *Stress and the Woman Manager*, Martin Robertson, Oxford.

Davis, H., Porter, J. W., Livingstone, J., Herrman, T., MacFadden, L. & Levine, S. (1977). Pituitary–adrenal activity and leverpress shock escape behaviour, *Physiological Psychology*, **5**, 280–4.

Dean, A. & Lin, N. (1977). The stress-buffering role of social support, *Journal of Nervous and Mental Disease*, **165**, 403–17.

Deanfield, J. E., Shea, M., Kensett, M., Horlock, P., Wilson, R. A., de Landsheere, C. M. & Selwyn, A. P. (1984). Silent myocardial ischaemia due to mental stress, *The Lancet*, **ii**, 1001–5.

DeBacker, G., Kornitzer, M., Kittel, F., Bogaert, M., Van Durme, J. P., Vincke, J., Rustin, R. M., Degre, C. & De Shaepdrijver, A. (1979). Relation between coronary-prone behavior pattern, excretions of urinary catecholamines, heart rate and heart rhythm, *Preventive Medicine*, **8**, 14–22.

Dechambre, R. P. (1981). Psychosocial stress and cancer in mice. In K. Bammer & B. H. Newberry (eds), *Stress and Cancer*, C. J. Hogrefe, Toronto.

Dechambre, R. P. & Gosse, C. (1968). Influence of population density on mortality in mice bearing transplanted tumors. *Comptes Rendues de l'Academie des Sciences*, **267**, 2200–2.

Dechambre, R. P. & Gosse, C. (1971). Influence of an isolation stress on the development of transplanted ascites tumors in mice. Role of the adrenals. *Comptes Rendues de l'Academie des Sciences*, **272**, 2720–2.

Dembroski, T. M. & MacDougall, J. M. (1983). Behavioral and psychophysiological perspectives on coronary prone behavior. In T. M. Dembrowski, T. H. Schmidt & G. Blumchen (eds), *Biobehavioral Bases of Coronary Heart Disease*, Karger, Basel.

Dembroski, T. M., MacDougall, J. M., Shields, J. L., Petitto, J. & Lushene R. (1978). Components of the Type A coronary-prone behavior pattern and cardiovascular responses to psychomotor performance challenge, *Journal of Behavioral Medicine*, **1**, 159–76.

Dembroski, T. M., MacDougall, J. M., Herd, J. A. & Shields, J. L. (1979a). Effects of level of challenge on pressor and heart rate responses in Type A and B subjects, *Journal of Applied Social Psychology*, **9**, 209–28.

Dembroski, T. M., MacDougall, J. M. & Lushene, R. (1979b). Interpersonal interaction and cardiovascular response in Type A subjects and coronary patients, *Journal of Human Stress*, **5**, 28–36.

Dembroski, T. M., MacDougall, J. M., Herd, J. A. & Shields, J. L. (1983). Perspectives on coronary-prone behavior. In D. S., Krantz, A. Baum & J. E. Singer (eds), *Handbook of Psychology and Health*, Lawrence Erlbaum, London.

Denney, D. R. & Frisch, M. B. (1981). The role of neuroticism in relation to life stress and illness, *Journal of Psychosomatic Research*, **25**, 303–7.

Derogatis, L. R., Abeloff, M. D. & Melisaratos, N. (1979). Psychological coping mechanisms and survival time in metastatic breast cancer, *Journal of the American Medical Association*, **242**, 1504–8.

Dimsdale, J. E. (1985). Methodology discussion: neuroendocrine reactivity. In A. M. Ostfeld & E. D. Eaker (eds), *Measuring Psychosocial Variables in Epidemiologic Studies of Cardiovascular Disease: Proceedings of a Workshop*, US Department of Health and Human Services.

Dimsdale, J. & Moss, J. (1980). Plasma catecholamines in stress and exercise, *Journal of the American Medical Association*, **243**, 340–2.

Dimsdale, J. E., Hackett, T. P., Hutter, A. M., Block, P. C. & Catanzano, D. M. (1978). Type A personality and extent of coronary atherosclerosis, *American Journal of Cardiology*, **42**, 583–6.

Dimsdale, J. E., Hackett, T. P., Hutter, A. M., Block, P. C. & Catanzano, D. M. (1979).

Type A behavior and angiographic findings, *Journal of Psychosomatic Research*, **23**, 273–6.

Dohrenwend, B. P., Dohrenwend, B. S., Gould, M. S., Link, B., Neugebaner, R. & Wunsch-Hitzig, R. (1980), *Mental Illness in the United States: Epidemiological Estimates*, Praeger, New York.

Dohrenwend, B. P. & Shrout, P. E. (1985). Hassles in the conceptualization and measurements of life stress variables, *American Psychologist*, **40**, 780–5.

Dohrenwend, B. S. (1973a). Life events as stressors: a methodological inquiry, *Journal of Health and Social Behavior*, **14**, 167–75.

Dohrenwend, B. S. (1973b). Social status and stressful life events, *Journal of Personality and Social Psychology*, **28**, 225–35.

Dohrenwend, B. S. & Dohrenwend, B. P. (1984). Life stress and illness: formulation of the issues. In B Dohrenwend & B. P. Dohrenwend (eds), *Stressful Life Events and their Contexts*, Rutgers University Press, New York.

Dohrenwend, B. S., Krasnoff, L., Askenasy, A. R. & Dohrenwend, B. P. (1978). Exemplification of a method for scaling life events: the PERI life events scale, *Journal of Health and Social Behavior*, **19**, 205–29.

Dooley, D., Rook, K. & Catalano, R. (1987). Job and non-job stressors and their moderators, *Journal of Occupational Psychology*, **60**, 115–32.

Dorian, B. J., Keystone, E., Garfinkel, P. E. & Brown, G. M. (1982). Aberrations in lymphocyte subpopulations and functions during psychological stress, *Clinical and Experimental Immunology*, **50**, 132–8.

Drechsler, I., Bruner, D. and Kreitler, S. (1987). Cognitive antecedents of coronary heart disease, *Social Science and Medicine*, **23**, 581–8.

Duncan, O. D. (1961). A socioeconomic index for all occupations. In A. J. Reiss (ed.), *Occupation and Social Status*, Free Press, New York.

Dunn, J. P., Brooks, G. W., Maysner, J., Rodnan, G. P. & Cobb, S. (1963). Social class gradient of serum uric acid levels in males, *Journal of the American Medical Association*, **185**, 431–6.

Duszyuski, K. R., Shaffer, J. W. & Thomas, C. B. (1981). Neoplasm and traumatic events in childhood: how are they related? *Archives of General Psychiatry*, **38**, 327–31.

Eaker, E. D., Haynes, S. G. & Feinleib, M. (1983). Spouse behaviour and coronary heart disease in men: prospective results from the Framingham Heart Study. II. Modification of risk in type A husbands according to the social and psychological status of their wives, *American Journal of Epidemiology*, **118**, 23–41.

Eaves, L. & Eysenck, H. J. (1980). The genetics of smoking. In H. J. Eysenck (ed.), *The Causes and Effects of Smoking*, Part II, Maurice Temple Smith, London.

Edwards, E. A. & Dean, L. M. (1977). Effects of crowding mice on humoral antibody formation and protection to lethal antigenic challenge, *Psychosomatic Medicine*, **39**, 19–24.

Edwards, J. R., Baglioni, A. J. Jr. & Cooper, C. L. (1990). The psychometric properties of the Bortaer Type A scale. *British Journal of Psychology*, **81**(3), 315–34.

Elias, M. F., Robbins, M. A., Blow, F. C., Rice, A. D. & Edgecombe, J. L. (1982. A behavioral study of middle-aged chest pain patients: physical symptom reporting, anxiety, and depression, *Experimental Ageing Research*, **8**, 45–51.

Elliot, G. R. & Eisendorfer, C. (eds) (1982). *Stress and Human Health: Analysis and Implications of Research*. Springer, New York.

Engel, B. T. (1977). Operant conditioning of cardiovascular function: a behavioural analysis. In S. Rachman (ed), *Contributions to Medical Psychology*, pp. 75–89. Pergamon Press, London.

Engel, B. T. (1985). Immune behaviour, *Brain and Behavioural Sciences*, **8**, 399–400.

Engel, B. T. (1986). An essay on circulation as behaviour, *The Behavioural and Brain Sciences*, **9**, 285–318.

Engel, B. T. & Bickford, A. F. (1961). Response specificity: stimulus–response and individual–response specificity in essential hypertensives, *Archives of General Psychiatry*, **5**, 47779–84.

Engel, G. L. (1968). A life setting conducive to illness: the giving-up–given-up complex, *Bulletin of the Menninger Clinic*, **32**, 355–65.

Ericsson, K. A. & Simon, H. A. (1980). Verbal reports as data, *Psychological Review*, **87**, 215–51.

Ernst, F. (1979). Learned control of coronary blood flow, *Psychosomatic Medicine*, **41**, 79–85.

Ernster, V. L., Sacks, S. T., Selvin, S. & Petrakis, N. L. (1979). Cancer incidence by marital status: US third national cancer survey, *Journal of the National Cancer Institute*, **63**, 567–85.

Esler, M., Julius, S., Zweifler, A., Randall, O., Harburg, E., Gardiner, H. & DeQuattro, V. (1977). Mild high-renin essential hypertension: neurogenic human hypertension?, *New England Journal of Medicine*, **296**, 405–11.

Evans, P. D. (1990). Type A behaviour and coronary heart disease: When will the jury return? *British Journal of Psychology*, **81**, 147–57.

Eysenck, H. J. (1980). *The Causes and Effects of Smoking*. Maurice Temple Smith, and Sage, Los Angeles.

Eysenck, H. J. (1981). Personality and psychosomatic diseases, *Activitas Nervosa Superior*, **23**, 112–29.

Eysenck, H. J. (1983). Stress, disease and personality: the 'inoculation effect'. In C. L. Cooper (ed.), *Stress Research*, John Wiley & Sons, New York.

Eysenck, H. J. (1984). Personality, stress and lung cancer. In S. Rachman (ed.), *Contributions to Medical Psychology*, Vol. 3, Pergamon Press, Oxford.

Eysenck, H. J. (1988). Personality, stress and cancer: prediction and prophylaxis, *British Journal of Medical Psychology*, **61**, 57–75.

Eysenck, H. J. & Grossarth-Maticek, R. (1991). Creative novation behaviour therapy as a prophylactic treatment for cancer and coronary heart disease: Part II—Effects of treatment, *Behavioural Research & Therapy*, **29**(1), 17–31.

Fairbank, D. T. & Hough, R. L. (1984). Cross-cultural differences in perceptions of life events. In B. S. Dohrenwend & B. P. Dorhenwend (eds), *Stressful Life Events and their Contexts*, Rutgers University Press, New York.

Ferguson, D. (1973). A study of neurosis and occupation, *British Journal of Industrial Medicine*, **30**, 187–98.

Finlay-Jones, R. A. & Burvill, P. W. (1977). The prevalence of minor psychiatric morbidity in the community, *Psychological Medicine*, **7**, 474–89.

Fischer, C. L., Daniels, J. C., Levin, S. L., Kimzey, S. L., Cobb, E. K. & Ritzman, W. E. (1972). Effects of the spaceflight environment on man's immune system: II. Lymphocyte counts and reactivity, *Aerospace Medicine*, **43**, 1122–5.

Fisher, S. (1984). *Stress and the Perception of Control*, Lawrence Erlbaum, London and New Jersey.

Fisher, S. (1990). *Homesickness, Cognition and Health*, Lawrence Erlbaum, London and New Jersey.

Fleming, R., Baum, A. & Singer, J. E. (1984). Toward an interactive approach to the study of stress, *Journal of Personality and Social Psychology*, **46**, 939–49.

Fletcher, B. (C) (1979). Stress, illness and social class, *Occupational Health*, **31**(9), 405–11.

Fletcher, B. (C) (1980). Commentary. In A. J. Chapman & D. M. Jones (eds), *Models of Man*, BPS Publications, Leicester.

Fletcher, B. (C) (1983a). The role of category information in word identification: a parallel decision model, *Memory and Cognition*, **11**, 237–50.

Fletcher, B. (C) (1983b). Marital relationships as a cause of death: an analysis of occupational mortality and the hidden consequences of marriage—some UK data, *Human Relations*, **36**(2), 123–34.

Fletcher, B. (C) (1988a). The epidemiology of occupational stress. In C. L. Cooper & R. L. Payne (eds), *Causes, Coping and Consequences of Stress at Work*, John Wiley & Sons, Chichester.

Fletcher, B. (C) (1988b). Occupation, marriage and disease-specific mortality concordance, *Social Science and Medicine*, **27**(6), 615–22.

Fletcher, B. (C) (1989). *The Cultural Audit: an Individual and Organisation Investigation*, PSI, Cambridge.

Fletcher, B. (C) (1990). *Clergy Under Stress*, Mowbray, London.

Fletcher, B. (C) & Hall, J. (1984). Coping with personal problems at work, *Personnel Management*, 1984, February, 30–33.

Fletcher, B. (C) & Jones, F. (1990). The role of occupational factors in casual blood pressure: some unexpected findings. 4th European Health Psychology Conference, Oxford University, July.

Fletcher, B. (C) & Jones, F. (1991). Karasek's demand–discretion model: some confirmations and some major concerns. Presented to British Psychological Society, Occupational Division Annual Conference, January, Cardiff.

Fletcher, B. (C) & MacPherson, D. A. J. (1989). Stressors and strains in Church of England parochial clergy. Presented to British Psychological Society, London.

Fletcher, B. (C) & Morris, D. (1988). The health of London licensed taxi drivers: evidence obtained using the Crown–Crisp Experiential Index, the Job Diagnostic Survey, and the Demands, Supports & Constraints Questionnaire. Presented to British Psychological Society, London.

Fletcher, B. (C) & Payne, R. L. (1980a). Stress at work: a review and theoretical framework: Part 1, *Personnel Review*, **9**(1), 19–29.

Fletcher, B. (C) & Payne, R. L. (1980b). Stress at work: a review and theoretical framework: Part 2, *Personnel Review*, **9**(2), 4–8.

Fletcher, B. (C) & Payne, R. L. (1982). Levels of reported stressors and strains amongst schoolteachers: some UK data. *Educational Review*, **34**, 267–78.

Fletcher, B. (C), Gowler, D. & Payne, R. L. (1979). Exploding the myth of executive stress, *Personnel Management*, **11**(5), 30–5.

Fletcher, B. (C), Gowler, D. & Payne, R. L. (1980). Transmitting occupational risks, *The Lancet*, ii, 1193.

Fletcher, B. (C), Glendon, I. & Stone, F. (1987). The epidemiology of 129 occupational stressors, depression and free-floating anxiety: a national random sample survey. Unpublished manuscript.

Fobair, P. & Cordoba, C. S. (1982). Scope and magnitude of the cancer problem in psychosocial research. In J. Cohen, J. W. Cullen and L. R. Martin (eds), *Psychosocial Aspects of Cancer*, Raven Press, New York.

Folkow, B. (1982). Physiological aspects of primary hypertension, *Physiological Review*, **62**, 347–504.

Fox, A. J. & Adelstein, A. M. (1978). Occupational mortality: work or a way of life?, *Journal of Epidemiology and Community Health*, **32**, 73–8.

Fox, B. H. (1978). Premorbid psychological factors as related to cancer incidence, *Journal of Behavioral Medicine*, **1**(1), 45–133.

Fox, B. H. (1981). Psychosocial factors in the immune system in cancer. In R. Ader (ed.), *Psychoneuroimmunology*, pp. 103–58, Academic Press, New York.

Fox, B. H. (1982). A psychosocial measure as a predictor of cancer. In J. Cohen, J. W. Cullen & L. R. Martin (eds), *Psychosocial Aspects of Cancer*, Raven Press, New York.

Frankenhaeuser, M., Lundberg, U. & Forsman, L. (1980a). Dissociation between sympathetic–adrenal and pituitary–adrenal responses to an achievement situation characterised by high controllability: comparison between Type A and Type B males and females, *Biological Psychology*, **10**, 79–91.

Frankenhaeuser, M., Lundberg, U. & Forsman, L. (1980b). Note on arousing Type A persons by depriving them of work, *Journal of Psychosomatic Research*, **24**, 45–7.

Fraser, R. (1947). The incidence of neurosis among factory workers, *Medical Research Council Industrial Health Research Board Report No. 90*, HMSO, London.

French–Belgian Collaborative Group (1982). Ischemic heart disease and psychological patterns: prevalence and incidence studies in Belgium and France, *Advanced Cardiology*, **29**, 25–31.

French, J. R. P. & Caplan, R. D. (1970). Psychosocial factors in coronary heart disease, *Industrial Medicine*, **39**(9), 383–97.

French, J. R. P., Caplan, R. D. & Van Harrison, R. (1982). *The Mechanisms of Job Stress and Strain*, John Wiley & Sons, Chichester.

French, J. R. P., Rogers, W. & Cobb, S. (1974). A model of person–environment fit. In G. V. Coelho, D. A. Hamburgh & J. E. Adams (eds), *Coping and Adaptation*, Basic Books, New York.

Frese, M. (1985). Stress at work and psychosomatic complaints: a causal interpretation, *Journal of Applied Psychology*, **70**, 314–28.

Fried, Y., Rowland, K. M. & Ferris, G. R. (1984). The physiological measurement of work stress: a critique, *Personnel Psychology*, **37**, 583–615.

Friedman, G. D., Ury, H. K., Klatsky, A. L. & Siegelaub, A. B. (1974). A psychological questionnaire predictive of myocardial infarction: results from the Kaiser–Permanente Epidemiologic Study of Myocardial Infarction, *Psychosomatic Medicine*, **36**, 327–43.

Friedman, H. S. & Booth-Kewley, S. (1988). Validity of the type A construct: a reprise, *Psychological Bulletin*, **104**(3), 381–4.

Friedman, M. & Rosenman, R. H. (1959). Association of specific overt behaviour pattern with blood and cardiovascular findings: blood cholesterol level, blood clotting time, incidence of arcus senilis, and clinical coronary artery disease, *Journal of the American Medical Association*, **169**, 1286.

Friedman, M. & Rosenman, R. H. (1974). *Type A Behaviour and Your Heart*, Alfred A. Knopf, New York.

Friedman, M., St George, S., Byers, S. O. & Rosenman, R. H. (1960). Excretion of catecholamines, 17-ketosteroids, 17-hydroxycorticoids and 5-hydroxyindole in men exhibiting a particular behavior pattern (A) associated with high incidence of clinical coronary artery disease, *Journal of Clinical Investigation*, **39**, 758–64.

Friedman, S. B., Ader, R. & Grota, L. J. (1973). Protective effect of noxious stimulation in mice infected with rodent malaria, *Psychosomatic Medicine*, **35**, 533–7.

Friedman, M., Thorsesen, C. E., Gill, J. J., Ulmer, D., Thompson, L., Powell, L., Price, V., Elek, S. R., Rabin, D. D., Breall, W. S., Piaget, G., Dixon, T., Bourg, E., Levy, R. A. & Tasto, D. L. (1982). Feasibility of altering type A behavior pattern after myocrdial infarction, *Circulation*, **66**, 83–92.

Frone, M. R. & Rice, R. W. (1987). Work–family conflict: the effect of job and family involvement, *Journal of Occupational Behaviour*, **8**, 45–53.

Fulker, D. W. (1981). The genetic and environmental architecture of psychoticism, extraversion and neuroticism. In H. J. Eysenck (ed.), *A Model for Personality*, Springer Verlag, Berlin and New York.

Fuller, R. H., Brown, E. .& Mills, C. A. (1941). Environmental temperatures and spontaneous tumors in mice, *Cancer Research*, **1**, 130–3.

Ganster, D. C. & Victor, B. (1988). The impact of social support on mental and physical health, *British Journal of Medical Psychology*, **61**(1), 17–37.

Gantt, W. H. (1960). Cardiovascular components of the conditioned reflex to pain, food and other stimuli, *Physiological Review*, **40**, 266–91.

Gardner, M. J., Snee, M. P., Hall, A. J., Powell, C. A., Downes, S. & Terrell, J. D. (1990a). Results of case-control study of leukaemia and lymphoma among young people near Sellafield nuclear plant in West Cumbria, *British Medical Journal*, **300**, 423–9.

Gardner, M. J., Hall, A. J., Snee, M. P., Downes, S., Powell, C. A. & Terrell, J. D. (1990b). Methods and basic data of case-control study of leukaemia and lymphoma among young people near Sellafield nuclear plant in West Cumbria, *British Medical Journal*, **300**, 429–34.

Garrity, T. F., Somes, G. W. & Marx, M. B. (1977). The relationship of personality, life change, psycho-physiological strain and health status in a college population, *Social Science and Medicine*, **11**, 251–263.

Gentry, W. D., Chesney, A. P., Gary, H. E., Hall, R. P. & Harburg, E. (1982). Habitual anger-coping styles. I. Effect on mean blood pressure and risk for essential hypertension, *Psychosomatic Medicine*, **44**, 195–202.

Gergen, K. J. & Gergen, M. M. (1982). Explaining human conduct: form and function. In P. Secord (ed.), *Explaining Human Behaviour: Consciousness, Human Action, and Social Structure*, Sage, Beverley Hills.

Gersten, J. C., Langner, T. S., Eisenberg, J. G. & Simcha-Fagan, O. (1977). An evaluation of the etiologic role of stressful life-change events in psychological disorders, *Journal of Health and Social Behaviour*, **18**, 228–44.

Gesell, A. & Ilg, F. L. (1943). *Infant and Child in the Culture of Today*, Harper & Bros., New York.

Gillum, R., Leon, G. R., Kamp, J. & Becerra-Aldama, J. (1980). Prediction of cardiovascular and other disease onset and mortality from 30-year longitudinal MMPI data, *Journal of Consulting and Clinical Psychology*, **48**, 405–6.

Glass, D. C. (1977). *Behaviour Patterns, Stress and Coronary Disease*, Lawrence Erlbaum, Hillsdale, NJ.

Glass, D. C. (1983). Psychosocial influences and the pathogenesis of arteriosclerosis. In J. A. Herd & S. M. Weiss (eds), *Behaviour and Arteriosclerosis*, Plenum Press, New York and London.

Glass, D. C. (1985). Acute physiologic reactivity: working group summary. In A. M. Ostfeld & E. D. Easker (eds), *Measuring Psychosocial Variables in Epidemiologic Studies of Cardiovascular Disease: Proceedings of a Workshop*, US Department of Health and Human Services.

Glass, D. C. & Contrada, R. (1983). Type A behaviour and catecholamines: a critical review. In C. R. Lake & M. Ziegler (eds), *Norepinephrine: Clinical Aspects*, Williams & Wilkins, Baltimore.

Glass, D. C., Krakoff, L. R., Contrada, R., Hilton, W., Kehoe, K., Mannucci, E. G., Collins, C., Snow, B. & Elting, E. (1980). Effect of harassment and competition upon cardio-vascular and plasma catecholamine responses in type A and type B individuals, *Psychophysiology*, **17**, 453–63.

Gliner, J. A. (1972). Predictable vs. unpredictable shock: preference behaviour and stomach ulceration, *Physiological Behaviour*, **9**, 693–98.

Goldberg, A. (1972). *The Detection of Psychiatric Illness by Questionnaire*, Maudsley Monograph No. 21, Oxford University Press, Oxford.

Goldberg, E. L. & Comstock, G. W. (1980). Epidemiology of life events: frequency in general populations, *American Journal of Epidemiology*, **3**, 736–52.

Goldbourt, U., Medalie, J. H. & Neufeld, H. N. (1975). Clinical myocardial infarction over a five-year period. III. A multivariate analysis of incidence, the Israel ischemic heart disease study, *Journal of Chronic Diseases*, **28**, 217–37.

Goldstein, I. B., Shapiro, D. & Thanopavaran, C. (1984). Home relaxation techniques for essential hypertension, *Psychosomatic Medicine*, **46**, 398–414.

Gorczynski, R. M., MacRae, S. & Kennedy, M. (1982). Conditional immune response associated with allogeneic skin grafts in mice, *Journal of Immunology*, **129**, 704–9.

Gorczynski, R. M., MacRae, S. & Kennedy, M. (1984). Factors involved in the classical conditioning of antibody responses in mice. In R. Ballieux, J. Fielding & A. L'Abbatte (eds), *Breakdown in Human Adaptation to Stress: Towards a Multi-disciplinary Approach*, Martinue Nijhoff, The Hague.

Gore, S. (1984). Stress buffering functions of social support: an appraisal and clarification of research models. In B. S. Dohrenwend & B. P. Dohrenwend (eds), *Stressful Life Events and their Contexts*, Rutgers University Press, New York.

Graham, D. T. (1972). Psychosomatic medicine. In N S Greenfield & R. A. Sternbach (eds), *Handbook of Psychophysiology*, Holt, Rinehart & Winston, New York.

Graham, S., Snell, L. M., Graham, J. B. & Ford, L. (1971). Social trauma in the epidemiology of cancer of the cervix, *Journal of Chronic Diseases*, **24**, 711–25.

Green, J. E. (1977). Migraine abroad: a survey of migraine in England, 1975–1976, *Headache*, **17**, 67–8.

Greene, W. A. (1966). The psychosocial setting of the development of leukaemia and lymphoma, *Annals of the New York Academy of Sciences*, **125**, 794–801.

Greene, W. A. & Miller, G. (1958). Psychological factors and reticuloendothelial disease, *Psychosomatic Medicine*, **20**, 124–44.

Greene, W. A. & Swisher, S. N. (1969). Psychological and somatic variables associated with the development and course of monozygotic twins discordant for leukaemia, *Annals of the New York Academy of Sciences*, **164**, 394–408.

Greene, W. A., Betts, R. F., Ochitill, H. N., Iker, H. P. & Douglas, R. G. (1978). Psychosocial factors and immunity: preliminary report, *Psychosomatic Medicine*, **40**, 87 (abstract).

Greenspan, A. M., Kay, H. R., Berger, B. C., Greenberg, R. M., Greenspan, A. J. & Gangan, M. J. S. (1988). Incidence of unwarranted implantation of permanent pacemakers in a large medical population, *New England Journal of Medicine*, **318**, 158–63.

Greer, S. & Morris, T. (1975). Psychological attributes of women who develop breast cancer: a controlled study, *Journal of Psychosomatic Research*, **19**, 147–53.

Greer, S. & Morris, T. (1978). The study of psychological factors in breast cancer: problems of method, *Social Science and Medicine*, **12**, 129–34.

Greer, S., Morris, T. & Pettingdale, K. W. (1979). Psychological response to breast cancer: effect on outcome, *The Lancet*, **ii**, 785–7.

Grissom, M., Weiner, B. & Weiner, E. (1975). Psychological correlates of cancer, *Journal of Consulting and Clinical Psychology*, **43**, 113.

Grossarth-Maticek, R. (1980). Synergistic effects of cigarette smoking, systolic blood pressure and psychosocial risk factors for lung cancer, cardiac infarct and apoplexy cerebri, *Psychotherapy and Psychosomatics*, **34**, 267–72.

Grossarth-Maticek, R. & Eysenck, H. J. (1990). Personality, stress and disease: Description and validation of a new inventory, *Psychological Reports*, **66**, 355–73.

Grossarth-Maticek, R. & Eysenck, H. J. (1991). Creative novation behaviour therapy as a prophylactic treatment for cancer and heart disease: Part 1—Description of treatment, *Behavioural Research and Therapy*, **29**(1), 1–16.

Grossarth-Maticek, R., Siegrist, J. & Vetter, H. (1982). Interpersonal repression as a predictor of cancer, *Social Science and Medicine*, **16**, 493–8.

Grossarth-Maticek, R., Kanazir, D. S., Schmidt, P. & Vetter, H. (1982). Psychosomatic factors in the process of cancerogenesis, *Psychotherapy and Psychosomatics*, **38**, 284–302.

Grossarth-Maticek, R., Bastiaans, J. & Kanazir, D. T. (1985). Psychosocial factors as strong predictors of mortality from cancer, ischaemic heart disease and stroke: the Yugoslav prospective study, *Journal of Psychosomatic Research*, **29**, 167–76.

Guyton, A. A. (ed.) (1980). *Circulatory Physiology*, Vol. III: *Arterial Pressure and Hypertension*, W. B. Saunders, Philadelphia, PA.

Hackman, J. R. & Oldham, G. R. (1976). Motivation through the design of work: test of a theory, *Organisational Behavior and Human Performance*, **16**, 250–79.

Haft, J. J. (1974). Cardiovascular injury induced by sympathetic catecholamines, *Progress in Cardiovascular Diseases*, **17**, 73–86.

Hagnell, O. (1966). The premorbid personality of persons who develop cancer in a total population investigated in 1947 and 1957, *Annals of the New York Academy of Sciences*, **125**, 846–55.

Hamilton, D. R. (1974). Immunosuppressive effects of predator-induced stress in mice with acquired immunity to *Hymenolepsis nana*, *Journal of Psychosomatic Research*, **18**, 143–50.

Harburg, E., Julius, S., McGinn, N. F., McLeod, J. & Hoobler, S. W. (1964). Personality traits and behavioral patterns associated with systolic blood pressure levels in college males, *Journal of Chronic Disability*, **17**, 405–14.

Harrower, M., Thomas, C. B. & Altman, A. (1975). Human figure drawings in a prospective study of six disorders: hypertension, coronary heart disease, malignant tumour, suicide, mental illness and emotional disturbance, *Journal of Nervous and Mental Disease*, **161**, 191–9.

Harsh, J. & Badia, P. (1975). Choice of signalled over unsignalled shock as a function of shock intensity, *Journal of the Experimental Analysis of Behaviour*, **23**, 349–55.

Hartel, U., Keil, U. & Cairns, V. (1985). Medical care utilisation and self-reported health of hypertensives: results of the Munich blood pressure study. In R. M. Caplan & M. H. Criqui, (eds), *Behavioural Epidemiology and Disease Prevention*, Plenum Press, New York & London.

Haskey, J. (1983). Social class patterns of marriage, *Population Trends*, **34**, 12–19.

Hattori, T., Hamai, Y., Ikeda, T., Takiyama, W., Hirai, T. & Miyoshi, Y. (1982). Inhibitory effects of immunopotentiators on the enhancement of lung metastases induced by operative stress in rats, *Gann*, **73**, 132–5.

Haw, M. A. (1982). Women, work and stress: a review and agenda for the future, *Journal of Health and Social Behavior*, **23**, 132–44.

Haynes, S. G. & Feinleib, M. (1980). Women, work and coronary heart disease: prospective findings from the Framingham Heart Study, *American Journal of Public Health*, **70**, 133–41.

Haynes, S. G. & Feinleib, M. (1982). Type A behaviour and the incidence of coronary heart disease in the Framingham Heart Study, *Advanced Cardiology*, **29**, 85–95.

Haynes, S. G., Feinleib, M. & Kannel, W. B. (1980). The relationship of psychosocial factors to coronary heart disease in the Framingham Study. III. Eight-year incidence of coronary heart disease, *American Journal of Epidemiology*, **111**, 37–58.

Haynes, S. G., Eaker, E. D. & Feinleib, M. (1983). Spouse behaviour and coronary heart disease in men: prospective results from the Framingham Heart Study, *American Journal of Epidemiology*, **118**, 1–41.

Haynes, S. G., Levine, S., Scotch, N., Feinleib, M. & Kannel, W. B. (1978a). The relationship of psychosocial factors to coronary heart disease in the Framingham Study, *American Journal of Epidemiology*, **107**, 362–83.

Haynes, S. G., Feinleib, M., Levine, S., Scotch, N. & Kannel, W. B. (1978b). The relationship of psychosocial factors to coronary heart disease in the Framingham Study. II. Prevalence of coronary heart disease, *American Journal of Epidemiology*, **107**(5), 384–402.

Health and Nutrition Examination Survey (1977). *Public Health Reports*, **92**(1), 91.

Helsing, K. J. & Szklo, M. (1981). Mortality after bereavement, *American Journal of Epidemiology*, **114**, 41–52.

Helsing, K., Comstock, G. W. & Szklo, M. (1982). Causes of death in a widowed population, *American Journal of Epidemiology*, **116**, 524–32.

Hendrix, W. H., Ovalle, N. K. & Troxler, R. G. (1985). Behavioral and physiological consequences of stress and its antecedent factors, *Journal of Applied Psychology*, **70**(1), 188–201.

Henry, J. P. (1976). Mechanisms of psychosomatic disease in animals, *Advances in Veterinary Science and Comparative Medicine*, **20**, 115–45.

Henry, J. P. (1982). The relation of social to biological processes in disease, *Social Science and Medicine*, **16**, 369–80.

Henry, J. P. & Stephens, P. M. (1977). *Stress, Health and the Social Environment: A Sociobiologic Approach to Medicine*, Springer, New York.

Henry, J. P., Stephens, P. M. & Watson, F. M. C. (1975). Forced breeding, social disorder and mammary tumor formation in CBA/USC mouse colonies: a pilot study, *Psychosomatic Medicine*, **33**, 277–83.

Hepworth, S. (1980). Moderating factors of the psychological impact of unemployment, *Journal of Occupational Psychology*, **53**, 139–45.

Herzberg, F. (1966). *Work and the Nature of Man*, World, Cleveland.

Hewitt, H. B., Blake, E. R. & Walder, A. S. (1976). A critique of the evidence for active host defence against cancer, based on personal studies of twenty-seven murine tumours of spontaneous origin, *British Journal of Cancer*, **33**, 241–58.

Hilderman, J. H. & Strom, T. B. (1978). Specific insulin binding site on T and B lymphocytes as a marker of cell activation, *Nature*, **274**, 62–3.

Hinkle, L. E. & Plummer, M. D. (1952). Life stress and industrial absenteeism, *Industrial Medicine and Surgery*, **21**, 363–75.

Hinkle, L. E. & Wolff, H. G. (1957). The nature of man's adaptation to his total environment and the relation of this to illness, *Archives of Internal Medicine*, **99**, 442–60.

Hinkle, L. E., Christenson, W., Kane, F., Ostfeld, A., Thetford, W. N. & Wolff, H. G. (1958). An investigation of the relation between life experience, personality characteristics and general susceptibility to illness, *Psychosomatic Medicine*, **20**, 278–95.

Hinkle, L. E. Jr, Whitney, L. H., Lehman, E. W., Dunn, J., Benjamin, B., King, R., Plakun, A. & Fehinger, B. (1968). Occupation, education and coronary heart disease, *Science*, **161**, 238–46.

Hirayama, T. (1981). Non-smoking wives of heavy smokers have a higher risk of lung-cancer: a study from Japan, *British Medical Journal*, **282**, 183–5.

Hokanson, J. E. (1961). The effects of frustration and anxiety on overt aggression, *Journal of Abnormal and Social Psychology*, **62**, 346–51.

Hollingshead, A. B. (1971). Comment on the indiscriminate state of social class measurement, *Social Forces*, **49**, 563–7.

Hollingshead, A. B. & Redlich, R. (1958). *Social Class and Mental Illness: A Community Study*, John Wiley & Sons, New York.

Holme, I., Helgeland, A., Hjerman, I., Leren, P. & Lund-Larsen, P. G. (1977). Coronary risk factors in various occupational groups: the Oslo Study, *British Journal of Preventative and Social Medicine*, **31**, 96–100.

Holme, I., Helgeland, A., Hjermann, I. & Leren, P. (1982). Socio-economic status as a coronary risk factor: the Oslo Study, *Acta Medica Scandinavica (Suppl.)*, **660**, 147–51.

Holmes, T. H. & Masuda, M. (1970). Life change and illness susceptibility. In B. S. Dohrenwend & B. P. Dohrenwend (eds), *Stressful Life Events: their Nature and Effects*, John Wiley & Sons, New York.

Holmes, T. H. & Rahe, R. H. (1967). The social readjustment rating scale, *Journal of Psychosomatic Research*, **11**, 213–18.

References

Holmes, T. S. & Homes, T. H. (1970). Short-term intrusions into the life style routine, *Journal of Psychosomatic Research*, **14**, 121–32.

Hood, J. & Golden, S. (1984). Beating time/making time: the impact of work scheduling on men's family roles. In P. Voydaneff (ed.), *Work and Family: Changing Roles of Men and Women*, Mayfield, Palo Alto, California.

Horan, P. M. & Gray, B. H. (1974). Status inconsistency, mobility and coronary heart disease, *Journal of Health and Social Behavior*, **15**, 300–10.

Horne, R. L. & Picard, R. S. (1979). Psychosocial risk factors for lung cancer, *Psychosomatic Medicine*, **41**, 503–14.

Hough, R. L., Fairbank, D. T. & Garcia, A. M. (1976). Problems in the ratio measurements of the life stress, *Journal of Health and Social Behavior*, **17**, 70–80.

House, J. S., McMichael, A. J., Wells, J. A., Kaplan, B. H. & Landerman, L. R. (1979). Occupational stress and health among factory workers, *Journal of Health and Social Behavior*, **20**, 139–60.

House, J., Robbins, C. & Metzner, H. (1982). The association of social relationships and activities with mortality: prospective evidence from the Tecumsch Community Health Study, *American Journal of Epidemiology*, **116**, 123–40.

Houston, B. K. (1983). Psychophysiological responsivity and the type A behaviour pattern, *Journal of Research in Personality*, **17**, 22–39.

Howard, J. H., Cunningham, D. A. & Rechnitzer, P. A. (1986). Health patterns associated with type A behaviour: a managerial population, *Journal of Human Stress*, **2**, 24–31.

Hudgens, R. W. (1974). Personal catastrophe and depression: a consideration of the subject with respect to medically ill adolescents and a requiem for retrospective life-event studies. In B. S. Dohrenwend & B. P. Dohrenwend (eds), *Stressful Life Events: their Nature and Effects*, John Wiley & Sons, New York.

Huggan, R. E. (1968). A critique and possible reinterpretation of the observed low neuroticism scores of male patients with lung cancer, *British Journal of Social and Clinical Psychology*, **7**, 122–8.

Hunter, S. M., Wolf, T. M., Sklov, M. C. *et al.* (1982). Type A coronary-prone behaviour patterns and cardiovascular risk factor variables in children and adolescents: the Bogalusa heart study, *Journal of Chronic Diseases*, **35**, 613–21.

Hurrell, J. J. (1985). Machine-paced work and the type A behaviour pattern, *Journal of Occupational Psychology*, **58**, 15–25.

Hypertension Detection and Follow-up Program Co-operative Group (1979a). Five-year findings of the Hypertension Detection and Follow-up Program. I. Reduction in mortality of persons with high blood pressure, including mild hypertension, *Journal of the American Medical Association*, **242**, 2562–71.

Hypertension Detection and Follow-up Program Cooperative Group (1979b). Five year findings of the Hypertension Detection and Follow-up Program. II. Mortality by race, sex and age, *Journal of the American Medical Association*, **242**, 2572–87.

Insull, W. Jr (1973). *Coronary Risk Handbook: Estimating Risk of Coronary Heart Disease in Daily Practice*, American Heart Association, Washington, DC.

Inter-Society Commission for Heart Disease Resources (1972). Primary Prevention of the atherosclerotic diseases, *Circulation*, **42**, 1–44.

Irwin, J. & Anisman, H. (1984). Stress and pathology: immunological and central nervous system interactions. In C. L. Cooper (ed.), *Psychosocial Stress and Cancer*, John Wiley & Sons, New York.

Ivancevich, J. M. & Matteson, M. T. (1988). Type A behaviour and the healthy individual, *British Journal of Medical Psychology*, **61**, 37–56.

Jackson, P. R. & Warr, P. B. (1984). Unemployment and psychological ill-health: the moderating role of duration and age, *Psychological Medicine*, **14**, 605–14.

Jackson, S. E. & Maslach, C. (1982). After-effects of job-related stress: families as victims, *Journal of Occupational Behaviour*, **3**, 63–77.

Jacobs, S. & Ostfeld, A. (1977). An epidemiological review of bereavement, *Psychosomatic Medicine*, **39**, 344–57.

Jacobs, S., Prusoff, B. A. & Paykel, E. S. (1974). Recent life events in schizophrenia and depression, *Psychological Medicine*, **4**, 444–53.

Jacobs, T. J. & Charles, E. (1980). Life events and the occurrence of cancer in children, *Psychosomatic Medicine*, **42**, 11–42.

Jamasbi, R. J. & Nettsheim, P. (1977). Non-immunological enhancement of tumour transplantability in x-irradiated host animals, *British Journal of Cancer*, **36**, 723–9.

Jarvikoski, A. & Harkapaa, K. (1988). Type A behavior and life events, *British Journal of Medical Psychology*, **61**, 353–63.

Jemmott, J. B. & Locke, S. E. (1984). Psychosocial factors, immunologic mediation and human susceptibility to infectious diseases: how much do we know?, *Psychological Bulletin*, **95**(1), 78–108.

Jemmott, J. B., Borysenko, J. Z., Borysenko, M., McClelland, D. C., Chapman, R., Meyer, D. & Benson, H. (1983). Academic stress, power motivation and decrease in secretion rate of salivary secretory immunoglobulin A, *The Lancet*, **i**, 25.

Jenkins, C. D. (1971). Psychologic and social precursors of coronary disease, *New England Journal of Medicine*, **284**, 244–55, 307–17.

Jenkins, C. D. (1976a). Recent evidence supporting psychologic and social precursors of coronary disease, *New England Journal of Medicine*, **294**, 987–94.

Jenkins, C. D. (1976b). Recent evidence supporting psychologic and social risk factors for coronary disease, *New England Journal of Medicine*, **294**, 1033–38.

Jenkins, C. D. (1978). A comparative review of the interview and questionnaire methods in the assessment of the coronary-prone behavior pattern. In T. M. Dembrowski, S. M. Weiss, J. L. Shields, S. G. Haynes & M. Feinleib (eds), *Coronary Prone Behavior*, Springer, New York.

Jenkins, C. D. (1982). Psychosocial risk factors for coronary heart disease, *Acta Medica Scandinavica (Suppl.)*, **660**, 123–36.

Jenkins, C. D., Rosenman, R. H. & Friedman, M. (1967). Development of an objective psychological test for the determination of the coronary-prone behavior pattern in employed men, *Journal of Chronic Diseases*, **20**, 371–9.

Jenkins, C. D., Rosenman, R. H. & Friedman, M. (1968). Replicability of rating the coronary-prone behavior pattern, *British Journal of Preventive and Social Medicine*, **22**, 16–22.

Jenkins, C. D., Rosenman, R. H. & Zyzanski, S. J. (1974). Prediction of clinical coronary heart disease by a test for the coronary-prone behavior pattern, *New England Journal of Medicine*, **290**, 1271–5.

Jenkins, C. D., Zyzanski, S. J. & Rosenman, R. H. (1971). Progress toward vaidation of a computer-scored test for type A coronary-prone behaviour pattern, *Psychosomatic Medicine*, **33**, 193–202.

Jenkins, C. D., Zyzanski, S. J. & Rosenman, R. H. (1976). Risk of new myocardial infarction in middle-aged men with manifest coronary heart disease, *Circulation*, **53**, 342–7.

Jenkins, C. D., Zyzanski, S. J. & Rosenman, R. H. (1978). Coronary-prone behavior: one pattern or several?, *Psychosomatic Medicine*, **40**, 25–43.

Jenkins, C. D., Zyzanski, S. J. & Rosenman, R. H. (1979). *Jenkins Activity Survey Manual*, Psychological Corporation, New York.

Jenkins, C. D., Stanton, B. A., Klein, M. D., Savageau, J. A. & Harken, D. E. (1983). Correlates of angina pectoris among men awaiting coronary by-pass surgery, *Psychosomatic Medicine*, **45**, 141–53.

Johansson, G., Aronsson, G. & Lindström, B. O. (1978). Social psychological and neuroendocrine stress reactions in highly mechanised work, *Ergonomics*, **21**, 583–99.

Johnson, J. H. & Sarason, I. G. (1978). Life stress, depression, and anxiety: internal–external control as a moderator variable, *Journal of Psychosomatic Research*, **22**, 205–8.

Johnson, J. H., Sarason, I. G. & Siegel, J. M. (1978). Arousal Seeking as a Moderator of Life Stress, Unpublished manuscript, University of Washington.

Johnston, D. W. & Shaper, A. G. (1983). Type A behaviour in British men: reliability and intercorrelation of two measures, *Journal of Chronic Diseases*, **36**, 203–7.

Johnston, D. W., Cook, D. G. & Shaper, A. G. (1987). Type A behaviour and ischaemic heart disease in middle aged British men, *British Medical Journal*, **295**, 86–9.

Jones, F., Fletcher, B. (C) & Ibbetson, K. (1991). Stressors and strains amongst social workers: demands, supports, constraints and psychological health, *British Journal of Social Work*, **21**.

Jordan, J. A., Sharp, F. & Singer, A. (1982). *Pre-clinical Neoplasia of the Cervix*, Royal College of Obstetricians and Gynaecologists, London.

Joseph, J. G. & Syme, S. L. (1982). Social connection and the etiology of cancer: an epidemiological review and discussion. In J. Cohen, J. W. Cullen & L. R. Martin (eds), *Psychosocial Aspects of Cancer*, Raven Press, New York.

Julius, S. (1977). Borderline hypertension: epidemiologic and clinical implications. In J. Genest, E. Koiw & O. Kuchel (eds), *Hypertension*, McGraw-Hill, New York.

Julius, S. (1981). The psychophysiology of borderline hypertension. In H. Weiner, M. A. Hofer & A. J. Stunkard (eds), *Brain, Behavior and Bodily Disease*, Raven Press, New York.

Julius, S. (1982). Psychophysiological evidence for the role of the nervous system in hypertension. In A. Amery, R. Fagard, P. Lijmen & J. O. Staessen (eds), *Hypertensive Cardiovascular Disease: Pathophysiology and Treatment*, Martinus Nijhoff, The Hague.

Julius, S. & Esler, M. (1975). Autonomic nervous cardiovascular regulation in borderline hypertension, *American Journal of Cardiology*, **36**, 685–96.

Kagan, A. R. & Levi, L. (1974). Health and environment—psychosocial stimuli: a review, *Social Science and Medicine*, **8**, 225–41.

Kahn, J. P., Kornfeld, D. S., Frank, K. A., Heller, S. S. & Hoar, P. F. (1980). Type A behaviour and blood pressure during coronary artery byass surgery, *Psychosomatic Medicine*, **42**, 407–14.

Kahn, R. L., Rolfe, D. M., Quinn, R. P., Snoek, J. D. & Rosenthal, R. A. (1964). *Organisational Stress: Studies in Role Conflict and Ambiguity*, John Wiley & Sons, New York.

Kakihana, R., Noble, E. P. & Butte, J. C. (1968). Corticosterone response to ethanol in inbred strains of mice, *Nature*, **218**, 360–1.

Kamerman, S. B. (1980). *Parenting in an Unresponsive Society*, Free Press, New York.

Kannel, W. B. & Sorlie, P. (1975). Hypertension in Framingham. In O. Paul (ed.), *Epidemiology and Control of Hypertension*, Stratten Intercontinental Medical Books, New York.

Kanner, A. D., Coyne, J. C., Schaefer, C. & Lazarus, R. S. (1981). Comparison of two modes of stress measurement: daily hassles and uplift versus major life events, *Journal of Behavioral Medicine*, **4**, 1–39.

Kaplan, G. A. (1985). Psychosocial aspects of chronic illness: direct and indirect associations with ischemic heart disease mortality. In R. M. Kaplan & M. H. Criqui (eds). *Behavioural Epidemiology and Disease Prevention*, Plenum Press, New York and London.

Kaplan, S. M. (1961). Hostility in verbal productions and hypnotic dreams of hypertensive patients, *Psychosomatic Medicine*, **23**, 311–22.

Karasek, R. (1978). Job socialisation, a longitudinal study of work, political and leisure activity in Sweden. *IX World Congress of Sociology (RC30)*, 15 August, Swedish Institute for Social Research, Stockholm University.

Karasek, R. A. (1979). Job demands, job decision latitude and mental strain: implications for job design, *Administrative Science Quarterly*, **24**, 285–308.

Karasek, R. A. (1990). Lower health risk with incresed job control among white-collar workers, *Journal of Organisational Behaviour*, **11**, 171–85.

Karasek, R., Gardell, B. & Lindell, J. (1987). Work and non-work correlates of illness and behaviour in male and female Swedish white-collar workers, *Journal of Occupational Behaviour*, **8**, 187–207.

Karasek, R. A., Russell, R. S. & Theorell, T. (1982). Physiology of stress and regeneration in job-related cardiovascular illness, *Journal of Human Stress*, **8**(1), 29–42.

Karasek, R. A., Theovell, T. G. T., Schwartz, J., Pieper, C. & Alfredsson, L. (1982). Job, psychological factors and coronary heart disease, *Advanced Cardiology*, **29**, 62–7.

Kasl, S. V. (1978). Epidemiological contributions to the study of work stress. In C. L. Cooper & R. L. Payne (eds), *Stress at Work*, John Wiley & Sons, New York.

Kasl, S. V. (1980). The impact of retirement. In C. L. Cooper & R. L. Payne (eds), *Current Concerns in Occupational Stress*, John Wiley & Sons, Chichester.

Kasl, S. V. (1983). Pursuing the link between stressful life experience and disease: a time for reappraisal. In C. L. Cooper (ed.), *Stress Research: Issues for the Eighties*, John Wiley & Sons, Chichester.

Kasl, S. V. & Cobb, S. (1980). The experience of losing a job: some effects on cardiovascular functioning, *Psychotherapy and Psychosomatics*, **34**, 88–109.

Kearns, J. (1986). Stress at work: the challenge of change, BUPA Series: *The Management of Health. 1: Stress and the City*, BUPA, London.

Keast, D. (1981). Immune surveillance and cancer. In K. Bammer & B. H. Newberry (eds), *Stress and Cancer*, C. J. Hogrefe, Ontario.

Keith, R. A., Lown, B. & Stare, F. J. (1965). Coronary heart disease and behavior patterns, *Psychosomatic Medicine*, **27**, 424–34.

Kellam, S. G. (1984). Stressful life events and illness: a research area in need of conceptual development. In B. S. Dohrenwend & B. P. Dohrenwend (eds), *Stressful Life Events: their Nature and Effects*, John Wiley & Sons, New York.

Kemeny, M. E., Cohen, F., Zegans, L. S. & Conant, M. A. (1989). Psychological and immunological predictors of genital herpes recurrence, *Psychosomatic Medicine*, **51**, 195–208.

Kemp, N. J., Wall, T. D., Clegg, C. W. & Cordery, J. L. (1983). Autonomous work groups in a greenfield site: a comparative study, *Journal of Occupational Psychology*, **56**, 271–88.

Kennedy, S., Kiecolt-Glaser, J. K. & Glaser, R. (1988). Immunological consequences of acute and chronic stressors: mediating role of interpersonal relationships, *British Journal of Medical Psychology*, **61**(1), 77–87.

Kessler, R. C. & Cleary, P. D. (1980). Social class and psychological distress, *American Sociological Review*, **45**, 463–78.

Kessler, R. C. & McLeod, J. D. (1985). Social support and mental health in community samples. In S. Cohen & S. L. Syme (eds), *Social Support and Health*, Academic Press, New York.

Keys, A., Taylor, H. L., Blackburn, H., Brozek, J., Anderson, J. T. & Simonson, E. (1971). Mortality and coronary heart disease among men studied for 23 years, *Archives of Internal Medicine*, **128**, 201–14.

Keys, A., Araranes, C., Blackburn, H., Van Buckem, F. S. P., Buzina, R., Djordjevic, B. S., Fidanza, F., Karvonen, M. J., Menotti, A., Puddu, V. & Taylor, H. L. (1972). Probability of middle-aged men developing coronary heart disease in 5 years, *Circulation*, **45**, 815–28.

Kidson, M. A. (1973). Personality and hypertension, *Journal of Psychosomatic Research*, **17**, 35–41.

Kiecolt-Glaser, J. K., Garner, W., Speicher, C., Penn, G. M., Holliday, J. & Glaser, R. (1984a). Psychosocial modifiers of immunocompetence in medical students, *Psychosomatic Medicine*, **46**, 7–14.

Kiecolt-Glaser, J. K., Speicher, C. E., Holliday, J. E. & Glaser, R. (1984b). Stress and the transformation of lymphocytes by Epstein–Barr virus, *Journal of Behavioral Medicine*, **7**, 1–12.

Kimmel, H. D. (1985). Conditioning of immunosuppression in the treatment of transplant tissue rejection, *Behavioural and Brain Sciences*, **8**(3), 404.

Kimzey, S. L., Johnson, P. C., Ritzman, S. E. & Mengel, C. E. (1976). Hematology and immunology studies: the second manned Skylab mission, *Aviation, Space and Environmental Medicine*, April, pp. 383–90.

Kirschner, M. A. (1977). The role of hormones in the etiology of human breast cancer, *Cancer*, **39**, 2716–26.

Kissen, D. (1963). Personality characteristics in males conducive to lung cancer, *British Journal of Medical Psychology*, **36**, 27–36.

Kissen, D. M. (1964). Lung cancer, inhalation and personality. In D. M. Kissen & C. L. Leshan (eds), *Aspects of Neoplastic Disease*, Pitman, London.

Kissen, D. M. (1966). Psychosocial factors, personality and prevention of lung cancer, *Medical Officer*, **116**, 135–8.

Kissen, D. (1969). The present state of psychosomatic cancer research, *Geriatrics*, **24**, 129.

Kissen, D. M. & Eysenck, H. J. (1962). Personality in male lung cancer patients, *Journal of Psychosomatic Research*, **6**, 123–37.

Kittel, F., Kornitzer, M., Zyzanski, S. J., Jenkins, C. D., Rustin, R. M. & Degre, C. (1978). Two methods of assessing the Type A coronary-prone behavior pattern in Belgium, *Journal of Chronic Disability*, **31**, 147–155.

Koenig, R., Levin, S. M. & Brennan, M. J. (1967). The emotional status of cancer patients as measured by a psychological test, *Journal of Chronic Diseases*, **20**, 923–30.

Kornhauser, A. (1965). *Mental Health of the Industrial Worker: A Detroit Study*, John Wiley & Sons, New York.

Krantz, D. S. & Durel, L. A. (1983). Psychobiological substrates of the type A behaviour pattern, *Health Psychology*, **2**, 393–411.

Krantz, D. S. & Glass, D. C. (1984). Personality, behavior patterns and physical illness: conceptual and methodological issues. In W. D. Gentry (ed.), *Handbook of Behavioral Medicines*, Guilford Press, New York.

Krantz, D. S. & Manuck, S. B. (1984). Acute psychophysiologic reactivity and risk of cardiovascular disease: a review and methodological critique, *Psychological Bulletin*, **96**(3), 435–64.

Krantz, D. S. & Manuck, S. B. (1985). Measures of acute physiologic reactivity to behavioural stimuli: assessment and critique. In A. M. Ostfeld & E. D. Eaker (eds), *Measuring Psychosocial Variables in Epidemiologic Studies of Cardiovascular Disease*, US Department of Health and Human Services. NIH Publication No. 85–2270.

Krantz D. S. & Raisen, S. E. (1988). Environmental, stress, reactivity and ischaemic heart disease, *British Journal of Medical Psychology*, **61**, 3–16.

Krantz, D. S., Arabian, J. M., Davia, J. E. & Parker, J. S. (1982a). Type A behaviour and coronary bypass surgery: intraoperative blood pressure and perioperative complications, *Psychosomatic Medicine*, **44**(3), 273–84.

Krantz, D. S., Durel, L. A., Davia, J. E., Shaffer, R. T., Arabian, J. M., Dembrowski, T. M. & MacDoughall, J. M. (1982b). Propranolol medication among coronary patients: relationship to Type A behavior and cardiovascular response, *Journal of Human Stress*, **8**, 4–12.

Kreitler, H. & Kreitler, S. (1976). *Cognitive Orientation and Behavior*, Springer, New York.

Kreitler, H. & Kreitler, S. (1982). The theory of cognitive orientation: widening the scope of behaviour prediction. In B. A. Maher & W. B. Maher, *Progress in Experimental Personality Research*, Vol. II, Academic Press, New York.

Kreyberg, L. (1962). *Histological Lung Cancer Types*, Norwegian Universities Press, Oslo.

Kritsikis, S. P., Heinemann, A. L. & Eitner, S. (1968). Die Angina Pectoris im Aspekt ihrer Korrelation mit biologischer Disposition, psychologischen und soziologischen Emmussfaktoren, *Deutsch Gesundheit*, **23**, 1878–85.

Krug, V., Krug, F. & Cuatrecasas, P. (1974). Emergence of insulin receptors on human lymphocytes during in vitro transformation, *Proceedings of the National Academy of Sciences, USA*, **71**, 1330–3.

Kulka, R. A., Veroff, J. & Douvan, E. (1979). Social class and use of professional help for personal problems: 1957 and 1976, *Journal of Health and Social Behaviour*, **20**, 2–17.

Kuller, L. (1966). Sudden and unexpected nontraumatic death in adults: a review of epidemiological and clinical studies, *Journal of Chronic Diseases*, **19**, 1165–92.

Kuller, L., Lilienfield, A. & Fischer, R. (1966). Epidemiological study of sudden and unexpected deaths due to arteriosclerotic heart disease, *Circulation*, **34**, 1056–68.

LaBarba, R. C. & White, J. L. (1971). Maternal deprivation and the response to Ehrlich carcinoma in BALB/C mice, *Psychosomatic Medicine*, **33**, 458–60.

Labarthe, D. R. (1985). The rationale for treatment of 'mild' hypertension. In R. M. Caplan & M. H. Criqui (eds), *Behavioural Epidemiology and Disease Prevention*, Plenum Press, New York & London.

Landsbergis, P. A. (1988). Occupational stress among health care workers: a test of the job demands–control model, *Journal of Organizational Behavior*, **9**, 217–38.

LaRocco, J. M., House, J. S. & French, J. R. P., Jr (1980). Social support, occupational stress and health, *Journal of Health and Social Behaviour*, **21**, 202–18.

Larson, A. G. & Marcer, D. (1984). The who and why of pain: analysis by social class, *British Medical Journal*, **288**, 883–6.

Lazarus, R. S. & DeLongis, A. (1983). Psychological stress and coping in aging, *American Psychologist*, **38**, 245–54.

Lazarus, R. S., DeLongis, A., Folkman, S. & Gruen, R. (1985). Stress and adaptational outcomes; the problem of confounded measures, *American Psychologist*, July, pp. 770–9.

Leach, C. S. & Rambaut, P. C. (1974). Biochemical responses of the Skylab crewman, *Proceedings of the Skylab Life Sciences Symposium*, **2**, 427–54.

Lebovits, B., Lichter, E. & Moses, V. K. (1975). Personality correlates of coronary heart disease: a re-examination of the MMPI data, *Social Science and Medicine*, **9**, 207–19.

Lebovitis, B. Z., Shekelle, R. B., Ostfeld, A. M. & Paul, O. (1967). Prospective and retrospective psychological studies of coronary heart disease, *Psychosomatic Medicine*, **29**, 265–72.

Lee, R. E. & Schneider, R. F. (1958). Hypertension and arteriosclerosis in executive and non-executive personnel, *Journal of the American Medical Association*, **167**, 1447–50.

Lefcourt, H. M. (1984). Locus of control and stressful life events. In B. S. Dohrenwend & B. P. Dohrenwend (eds), *Stressful Life Events and their Contexts*, Rutgers University Press, New York.

Lehman, E. W. (1967). Social class and coronary heart disease: a sociological assessment of the medical literature, *Journal of Chronic Diseases*, **20**, 381–91.

Lehr, I., Messinger, H. B. & Rosenman, R. H. (1973). A sociobiological approach to the study of coronary heart disease, *Journal of Chronic Diseases*, **26**, 13–30.

Lehrer, S. (1980). Life change and gastric cancer, *Psychosomatic Medicine*, **42**, 499–502.

Lei, H. & Skinner, H. A. (1980). A psychometric study of life events and social adjustment, *Journal of Psychosomatic Research*, **24**, 57–65.

LeShan, L. (1959). Psychological states as factors in the development of malignant disease: a critical review, *Journal of the National Cancer Institute*, **22**, 1–18.

LeShan, L. (1977). *You Can Fight for Your Life: Emotional Factors in the Causation of Cancer,* M Evans, New York.

Levine, S. & Cohen, C. (1959). Differential survival to leukaemia as a function of infantile stimulation in DBA/2 mice, *Proceedings of the Society of Experimental Biology and Medicine*, **102**, 53–4 (summary).

Lewis, C. & Knapp, C. (1989). Family adjustment after relocation: a study of secondary-school age pupils and their parents. Unpublished report to Nationwide Anglia Relocation Ltd.

Lewis, S. & Cooper, C. L. (1983). The stress of combining occupational and parental roles: a review of the literature, *Bulletin of the British Psychological Society*, **36**. 341–5.

Lichtenstein, M. J., Shipley, M. J. & Rose, G. (1985). Systolic and diastolic blood pressures as predictors of coronary heart disease mortality in the Whitehall study, *British Medical Journal*, **291**, 243–5.

Liem, R. & Liem, J. H. (1984). Relations among social class, life events, and mental illness: a comment on findings and methods. In B. S. Dohrenwend & B. P. Dohrenwend (eds), *Stressful Life Events and their Contexts*, Rutgers University Press, New York.

Light, K. C. (1985). Cardiovascular and renal responses to competitive mental challenges. In J. F. Orlebeke, G. Mulder & L. J. P. Van Doornen (eds), *Psychophysiology of Cardiovascular Control*, Plenum Press, New York and London.

Light, K. C. & Obrist, P. A. (1983). Task difficulty, heart rate reactivity and cardiovascular responses to an appetitive reaction time task, *Psychophysiology*, **20**, 301.

Lilienfield, A. M. (1980). *Foundations of Epidemiology*, 2nd edn, Oxford University Press, New York.

Linn, B. S. & Jensen, J. (1983). Age and immune response to a surgical stress, *Archives of Surgery*, **118**, 405–9.

Lipowsky, S. J. (1975). Psychiatry of somatic diseases: epidemiology, pathogenesis, classification, *Comparative Psychiatry*, **16**, 105–24.

Little, J. B. (1977). Radiation transformation in vitro: implications for mechanisms. In H. H. Hiatt, J. D. Watson & J. A. Winston (eds), *Origins of Human Cancer, Book B*, Cold Spring Harbor, New York.

Littler, W. A., Honour, A. J., Carter, R. D. & Sleight, P. (1975). Sleep and blood pressure, *British Medical Journal*, **iii**, 346.

Long, N. R. & Voges, K. E. (1987). Can wives perceive the source of their husbands' occupational stress?, *Journal of Occupational Psychology*, **60**, 235–42.

Lorimer, R. J., Justice, B., McBee, G. W. & Weinman, M. (1979). Weighting events in life-events research (comment on Dohrenwend *et al.*, June 1978), *Journal of Health and Social Behavior*, **20**, 306–7.

Lown, B., Verrier, R. L. & Rabinowitz, S. H. (1977). Neural and psychologic mechanisms and the problem of sudden cardiac death, *American Journal of Cardiology*, **39**, 890–902.

Lundberg, U. (1983). Note on type A behavior and cardiovascular responses to challenge in 3- to 6-year-old children, *Journal of Psychosomatic Research*, **27**, 39–42.

Lundberg, U. & Theorell, T. (1976). Scalings of life changes: differences between three diagnostic groups and between recently experienced and non-experienced events, *Journal of Human Stress*, **1**, 7–17.

Lundberg, V., Theorell, T. & Lind, E. (1979). Life changes and myocardial infarction: individual differences in life change scaling, *Journal of Psychosomatic Research*, **19**, 17–32.

Lynch, H. T. (1981). *Cancer Genetics*, Charles C. Thomas, Springfield, IL.

MaClean, D. & Reichlin, S. (1981). *Psychoneuroimmunology*, **12**, 475.

MacDougall, J. M., Dembroski, T. M. & Krantz, D. S. (1981). Effects of types of challenge on pressor and heart rate responses in Type A & B women, *Psychophysiology*, **18**, 1–9.

MacIver, J. (1969). The epidemiology of mental illness in industry, *Journal of International Psychiatric Clinicians*, **6**, 271–6.

MacKenzie, W. F. & Gardner, F. M. (1973). Comparison of neoplasms in six sources of rats, *Journal of the National Cancer Institute*, **50**, 1243–57.

MacMahon, B. & Pugh, T. F. (1965). Suicide in the widowed, *American Journal of Epidemiology*, **81**, 23–31.

McGrath, J. E. (1970). *Social and Psychological Factors in Stress*, Holt, Rinehart & Winston, New York.

McLaughlin, A. I. G. (1966). Chronic bronchitis and occupation, *British Medical Journal*, **ii**, 101–2.

McLean, A. A. (1979). *Work Stress*, Addison-Wesley, Reading, Massachusetts.

McQueen, D. V. & Siegrist, J. (1982). Social factors in the etiology of chronic disease: an overview, *Social Science and Medicine*, **16**, 353–67.

Maddox, J. (1984). Psychoimmunology before its time, *Nature*, **309**, 400.

Maggini, C., Guazzelli, M., Castrogiovanni, P., Mauri, M., Di Lisio, G. F. Chierchia, S. & Cassano, G. B. (1976/77). Psychological and physiopathological study on coronary patients, *Psychotherapy and Psychosomatics*, **27**, 210–16.

Mai, F. M. M. (1968). Personality and stress in coronary heart disease, *Journal of Psychomatic Research*, **12**, 275.

Mannheim, B. & Schiffrin, M. (1984). Family structure, job characteristics, rewards and strains as related to work-role centrality of employed and self-employed professional women with children, *Journal of Occupational Behavior*, **5**, 83–101.

Manuck, S. B., Corse, C. D. & Winkelman, P. A. (1979). Behavioral correlates of individual differences in blood pressure reactivity, *Journal of Psychosomatic Research*, **23**, 281–8.

Manuck, S. B., Kaplan, J. R. & Clarkson, T. B. (1983). Behaviorally-induced heart rate reactivity and atherosclerosis in cynomologous monkeys, *Psychosomatic Medicine*, **45**, 95–108.

Margolis, B. L., Kroes, W. H. & Quinn, R. P. (1974). Job stress: an unlisted occupational hazard, *Journal of Occupational Medicine*, **16**, 659–61.

Markowe, H. L. J., Marmot, M. G., Shipley, M. J., Bulpitt, C. J., Meade, T. W., Stirling, Y., Vickers, M. V. & Semmence, A. (1985). Fibrinogen: a possible link between social class and coronary heart disease, *British Medical Journal*, **291**, 1312–14.

Marmorston, J. (1966). Urinary hormone metabolite levels in patients with cancer of the breast, prostate and lung, *Annals of the New York Academy of Sciences*, **125**(3), 959–73.

Marmorston, J., Geller, P. J. & Weiner, J. M. (1969). Pre-treatment urinary hormone patterns and survival in patients with breast cancer, prostate cancer, or lung cancer, *Annals of the New York Academy of Sciences*, **164**(2), 483–93.

Marmot, M. G. (1983). Stress, social and cultural variations in heart disease, *Journal of Psychosomatic Research*, **27**, 377–84.

Marmot, M. G. & Khaw, K. T. (1982). Implications for population studies of the age trend in blood pressure, *Contributions to Nephrology*, **30**, 101–7.

Marmot, M. G. & Syme, S. L. (1976). Acculturation and coronary heart disease in Japanese-Americans, *American Journal of Epidemiology*, **104**, 225–47.

Marmot, M. G., Rose, G., Shipley, M. & Hamilton, P. J. S. (1978). Employment grade and coronary heart disease in British civil servants, *Journal of Epidemiology and Community Health*, **32**, 244–9.

Marsh, G. N. & Channing, D. M. (1986). Deprivation and health in general practice, *British Medical Journal of Clinical Research*, **292** (6529), 1173–6.

Marsh, J. T., Lavender, J. F., Chang, S. S. & Rasmussen, A. F. (1963). Poliomyelitis in monkeys: decreased susceptibility after avoidance stress, *Science*, **140**, 1414–15.

Maschewsky, W. (1982). The relation between stress and myocardial infarction: a general analysis, *Social Science and Medicine*, **16**, 455–62.

Mason, J. W. (1968). A review of psychoendocrine research on the pituitary–adrenal cortical system, *Psychosomatic Medicine*, **30**, 576–607.

Mason, J. W. (1975). A historical view of the stress field, *Journal of Human Stress*, June, pp. 22–36.

Masuda, M. & Holmes, T. H. (1978). Life events: perceptions and frequencies, *Psychosomatic Medicine*, **40**, 236–61.

Matthews, K. A. (1983). Psychological perspectives on the type A behaviour pattern, *Psychological Bulletin*, **91**, 293–323.

Matthews, K. A. (1985). Assessment of Type A behavior anger and hostility in epidemiological studies of cardiovascular disease. In A. M. Ostfield & E. D. Eaker (eds), *Measuring Psychosocial Variables in Epidemiologic Studies of Cardiovascular Disease: Proceedings of a Workshop*, US Department of Health and Human Services.

Matthews, K. A. (1988). Coronary heart disease and type A behaviors: update on and alternative to the Booth-Kewley and Friedman (1987) quantitative review. *Psychological Bulletin*, **104**, 373–80.

Matthews, K. A. & Angulo, J. (1980). Measurement of the type A behavior pattern in children: assessment of children's competitiveness, impatience–anger, and aggression, *Child Development*, **51**, 466–75.

Matthews, K. A. & Glass, D. C. (1984). Type A behaviour, stressful life events, and coronary heart disease. In B. S. Dohrenwend & B. P. Dohrenwend (eds), *Stressful Life Events and their Contexts*, Rutgers University Press, New York.

Matthews, K. A. & Siegel, J. M. (1983). Type A behaviors by children, social comparison, and standards for self-evaluation, *Developmental Psychology*, **19**, 135–40.

Matthews, K. A., Glass, D. C., Rosenman, R. H. & Bortner, R. W. (1977). Competitive drive, Pattern A, and coronary heart disease: a further analysis of some data from the Western Collaborative Group Study, *Journal of Chronic Diseases*, **30**, 489–98.

Matthews, K. A., Jamison, J. W. & Cottington, E. M. (1985). Assessment of type A, anger, and hostility: a review of scales through 1982. In A. M. Ostfeld & E. D. Eaker (eds), *Measuring Psychosocial Variables in Epidemiologic Studies of Cardiovascular Disease*, NIH Publication No. 85–2270.

Meade, T. W., Vickers, M. V., Thomson, S. G. & Seghatchian, M. J. (1985). The effect of physiological levels of fibrinogen on platelet aggregation, *Thrombosis Research*, **38**, 527–34.

Mechanic, D. (1974). Discussion of research programs on relations between stressful life events and episodes of physical illness. In B. S. Dohrenwend & B. P. Dohrenwend (eds), *Stressful Life Events; their Nature and Effects*, John Wiley & Sons, New York.

Medalie, J. H. (1985). Personality characteristics: content discussion. In A. M. Ostfeld & E. D. Eaker (eds), *Measuring Psychosocial Variables in Epidemiologic Studies of Cardiovascular Disease*, US Department of Health & Human Services. NIH Publication No. 85–2270.

Medalie, J. H. & Goldbourt, U. (1976). Angina pectoris among 10,000 men. II. Psychosocial and other risk factors as evidenced by a multivariate analysis of a five-year incidence study, *American Journal of Medicine*, **60**, 910–20.

Medalie, J. H., Snyder, M., Groen, J. J., Neufeld, H. N., Goldbourt, U. & Riss, E. (1973a). Angina pectoris among 10,000 men: 5 year incidence and univariate analysis, *American Journal of Medicine*, **55**, 583–94.

Medalie, J. H., Kahn, H. A., Neufeld, H. N., Goldbourt, U., Riss, E., Perlstein, T. & Oron, D. (1973b). Myocardial infarction among 10,000 adult males over a 5 year period. I. Prevalence, incidence and mortality experience, *Journal of Chronic Disability*, **26**, 68.

Medical Research Council Working Party (1985). MRC trial of treatment of mild hypertension: principal results, *British Medical Journal*, **291**, 97–104.

Mellstrom, D., Nilsson, A., Oden, A., Rundgren, A. & Svanborg, A. (1982). Mortality among the widowed in Sweden, *Scandinavian Journal of Social Medicine*, **10**, 33–41.

Meyer, R. J. & Haggerty, R. J. (1962). Streptococcal infections in families, *Paediatrics*, **29**, 539–49.

Miller, P. M., Ingham, J. G. & Davidson, S. (1976). Life events, symptoms and social support, *Journal of Psychosomatic Research*, **20**, 515–22.

Minter, R. E. & Kimball, C. P. (1978). Life events and illness onset: a review, *Psychosomatics*, **19**, 334–9.

Moller, G. & Moller, E. (1978). Immunological surveillance against neoplasia. In J. E. Castro (ed.), *Immunological Aspects of Cancer*, MTP Press, Lancaster.

Monjan, A. A. & Collector, M. I. (1977). Stress-induced modulation of the immune response, *Science*, **196**, 307–8.

Monk, M. (1980). Psychologic status and hypertension, *American Journal of Epidemiology*, **112**, 200–8.

Monroe, S. M. (1982). Assessment of life events. retrospective vs concurrent strategies, *Archives of General Psychiatry*, **39**, 606.

Morgenstern, H. (1985). Socioeconomic factors: concepts measurement, and health effects. In A. M. Ostfeld & E. D. Eaker (eds), *Measuring Psychosocial Variables in Epidemiologic Studies of Cardiovascular Disease*, US Department of Health and Human Services. NIH Publication No. 85–2270.

Moss, A. (1979). Mortality and general susceptibility: a study of heart disease and cancer mortality in Alameda Co., California. Unpublished Ph.D. thesis, University of California, Berkeley.

Mott, P. E., Mann, F. C., McLoughlin, Q. & Warwick, D. P. (1965). *Shift Work : The Social, Psychological and Physical Consequences*, University of Michigan Press, Ann Arbor, MI.

Mueller, E. F., Kasl, S. V., Brooks, G. W. & Cobb, S. (1970). Psychosocial correlates of serum urate levels, *Psychological Bulletin*, **73**(4), 238–57.

Muhlbock, O. (1951). Influence of environment on the incidence of mammary tumors in mice, *Acta International Union Against Cancer*, **7**, 351.

Muslin, H. L., Gyarfas, K. & Pieper, W. J. (1966). Separation experience and cancer of the breast, *Annals of the New York Academy of Sciences*, **125**, 802–6.

Myers, A. & Dewar, H. A. (1975). Circumstances attending 100 sudden deaths from coronary artery disease with coroner's necropsies, *British Heart Journal*, **37**, 1133–43.

Myers, J., Lindenthal, J. & Pepper, M. (1974). Social class, life events and psychiatric symptoms: a longitudinal study. In B. S. Dohrenwend & B. P. Dohrenwend (eds), *Stressful Life Events: their Nature and Effects*, John Wiley & Sons, New York.

Myrtek, M. & Greenlee, M. W. (1984). Psychophysiology of Type A behaviour pattern: a critical analysis, *Journal of Psychosomatic Research*, **28**, 455–66.

Nemeth, G. & Mezei, A. (1963). Personality traits of cancer patients compared with benign tumors on the basis of the Rorschach test. In D. Kissen & L. L. LeShan (eds), *Psychosomatic Aspects of Neoplastic Disease*, Pitman, London.

Neugebauer, R. (1984). The reliability of life-event reports. In B. S. Dohrenwend & B. P. Dohrenwend (eds), *Stressful Life Events and their Contexts*, Rutgers University Press, New York.

Newberry, B. H. (1978). Restraint-induced inhibitions of 7,12-dimethylbenz(a)-anthracene-induced mammary tumours: relation to stages of tumour development, *Journal of the National Cancer Institute*, **61**, 725–9.

Newberry, B. H. (1981). Stress and mammary cancer. In K. Bammer & B. H. Newberry (eds), *Stress and Cancer*, C. J. Hogrefe, Ontario.

Newberry, B. H., Frankle, B., Beatty, P. A., Maloney, B. D. & Gilchrist, J. C. (1972). Shock stress and DMBA-induced mammary tumours, *Psychosomatic Medicine*, **34**, 295–305.

Newberry, B. H., Gildow, J., Wogan, J. & Reese, R. L. (1976). Inhibition of Huggins tumours by force restraint, *Psychosomatic Medicine*, **38**, 155–62.

Newton, G., Bly, C. G. & McCrary, C. (1962). Effects of early experience on the response to transplanted tumour, *Journal of Nervous and Mental Disease*, **134**, 522–7.

Newton, T. J. & Keenan, A. (1985). Coping with work-related stress, *Human Relations*, **38**(2), 107–26.

Nieburgs, H. E., Weiss, J., Navarrete, M., Strax, P., Teirstein, A., Grillione, C. & Siedlecki, B. (1979). The role of stress in human and experimental oncogenesis, *Cancer Detection and Prevention*, **2**, 307–66.

Oatley, K. & Bolton, W. (1985). A social-cognitive theory of depression in reaction to life events, *Psychological Review*, 1985, **92**, 372–88.

Obrist, P. A. (1981). *Cardiovascular Psychophysiology: a Perspective*, Plenum Press, New York and London.

Obrist, P. A. (1985a). Beta-adrenergic hyperresponsivity to behavioural challenges: a possible hypertensive risk factor. In J. F. Orlebeke, G. Mulder & L. J. P. Van Doornen (eds), *Psychophysiology of Cardiovascular Control*, Plenum Press: New York and London.

Obrist, P. A. (1985b). General overview of the area of cardiovascular psychophysiology in relation to stress and disorder. In J. F. Orlebeke, G. Mulder & L. J. P. Van Doornen (eds), *Psychophysiology of Cardiovascular Control*, Plenum Press, New York and London.

Obrist, P. A. (1985c). Cardiovascular reactivity. In A. M. Ostfeld & E. A. Eaker (eds), *Measuring Psychosocial Variables in Epidemiologic Studies of Cardiovascular Disease*, Department of Health and Human Services, NIH Publication No. 88–2270.

Obrist, P. A., Gaebelein, C. J., Shanks-Teller, E., Langer, A. W., Grignold A., Light, K. C. & McCubbin, J. A. (1978). The relationship between heart rate, carotid dP/dt, and blood pressure in humans as a function of the type of stress, *Psychophysiology*, **15**, 102.

Oliver, D. J. (1984). Detecting asymptomatic hypertensive patients, *The Practitioner*, **228**, 599–600.

O'Looney, B. A. (1984). The assessment of type A behavior and the prediction of coronary heart disease: a review, *Current Psychological Research and Review*, Winter.

OPCS (1971). *Registrar General's Decennial Supplement, England and Wales, 1961, Occupational Mortality Tables*, HMSO, London.

OPCS (1978). *Registrar General's Decennial Supplement, England and Wales, 1970–72, Occupational Mortality*, Series DS, No. 1, HMSO, London.

OPCS (1980). *Classification of Occupations and Coding Index*, HMSO, London.

OPCS (1986a). *Occupational Mortality 1979–80, 1982–2: Decennial Supplement*, Part 1, Commentary. Series DS, No. 6, HMSO, London.

OPCS (1986b). *Occupational Mortality 1979–80, 1982–3, Decennial Supplement*, Part II, Microfiche tables, Series DS, No. 6, HMSO, London.

Ortmeyer, C. F. (1974). Variations in mortality, morbidity, and health care by marital status. In L. Erhardt & J. E. Berlin (eds), *Mortality and Morbidity in the United States*, Harvard University Press, Cambridge, MA.

Osler, W. (1910). The Lumleian lectures on angina pectoris, *The Lancet*, **i**, 839–44.

Ostfeld, A. M. & Eaker, E. D. (eds) (1985). *Measuring Psychosocial Variables in Epidemiologic Studies of Cardiovascular Disease*, US Department of Health and Human Services, NIH Publication No. 85–2270.

Ostfeld, A. M., Lebovits, B. Z., Shekelle, R. B. & Paul, O. (1964). A prospective study of the relationship between personality and coronary heart disease, *Journal of Chronic Diseases*, **17**, 265.

Otis, L. S. & Scholler, J. (1967). Effects of stress during infancy on tumour development and tumour growth, *Psychological Reports*, **20**, 167–73.

Paffenbarger, R. S. Jr, Wolfe, P. A., Notkin, J. *et al.* (1966). Chronic disease in former college students. 1. Early precursors of fatal coronary disease, *American Journal of Epidemiology*, **83**, 314–28.

Paffenbarger, R. S., Hale, W. E., Brand, R. J. & Hyde, R. T. (1977). Work-energy level, personal characteristics, and fatal heart attack: a birth cohort effect, *American Journal of Epidemiology*, **105**(3), 200–13.

Paffenbarger, R. S., Hyde, R. T., Wing, A. L. & Steinmetz, C. H. (1984). A natural history of athleticism and cardiovascular health, *Journal of the American Medical Association*, **252**, 491–5.

Page, I. H. (1977). Some regulatory mechanisms of renovascular and essential arterial hypertension. In J. Genest, E. Koiw & O. Kuchel (eds), *Hypertension: Physiopathology and Treatment*, McGraw-Hill, New York.

Page, I. H. & McCubbin, J. W. (1966). The physiology of arterial hypertension. In W. F. Hamilton & P. Dow (eds), *Handbook of Physiology: Circulation*, (section 2, vol. 1). American Physiological Society, Washington, D.C.

Palmblad, J. (1981). Stress and immunologic competence: studies in man. In R. Ader (ed.), *Psychoneuroimmunology*, Academic Press; Harcourt Brace Jovanovich, New York.

Palmblad, J., Cantell, K., Strander, H., Froberg, J., Karlsson, C. G., Levi, L., Granstrom, M. & Unger, P. (1976). Stressor exposure and immunological response in man: interferon-producing capacity and phagocytosis, *Journal of Psychosomatic Research*, **20**, 193–9.

Palmblad, J., Karlsson, C. G., Levi, L. & Lidberg, L. (1979a). The erythrocyte sedimentation rate and stress, *Acta Medica Scandinavica*, **205**, 517–20.

Palmblad, J., Petrini, B., Wasserman, J. & Akerstedt, T. (1979b). Lymphocyte and granulocyte reactions during sleep deprivation, *Psychosomatic Medicine*, **41**, 273–8.

Pancheri, P., Bellaterra, M., Reda, G., Matteoli, S., Santarelli, E., Publiese, M. & Mosticoni, S. (1980). Psycho-neuro-endocrinological correlates of myocardial infarction. Paper presented at the NIAS International Conference on Stress and Anxiety, Wassenaar, Netherlands, June.

Parkes, C. M., Benjamin, B. & Fitzgerald, R. G. (1969). Broken heart: a statistical study of increased mortality among widowers, *British Medical Journal*, **i**, 740–3.

Parkes, K. R. (1982). Occupational stress among student nurses: a natural experiment, *Journal of Applied Psychology*, **67(b)**, 789–96.

Parkin, D. M. (1979). The management of hypertension—study records in general practice, *Journal of the Royal College of General Practitioners*, **29**, 583–7.

Parry, G., Shapiro, D. A. & Davies, L. (1981). Reliability of life event ratings: an independent replication, *British Journal of Clinical Psychology*, **20**, 133–4.

Parsonnet, V. (1982). The proliferation of cardiac pacing: medical, technical and socioeconomic dilemmas, *Circulation*, **65**, 841–5.

Pavlidis, N. & Chirigos, M. (1980). Stress-induced impairment of macrophage tumoricidal function. *Psychosomatic Medicine*, **42**, 47–54.

Paykel, E. S. (1974). Life stress and psychiatric disorder: applications of the clinical approach. In B. S. Dohrenwend & B. P. Dohrenwend (eds), *Stressful Life Events: their Nature and Effects*, John Wiley & Sons, New York.

Paykel, E. S. (1978). Contribution of life events to causation of psychiatric illness, *Psychological Medicine*, **8**, 245–53.

Paykel, E. S. (1983). Methodological aspects of life events research, *Journal of Psychosomatic Research*, **27**, 341–52.

Paykel, E. S. & Rao, B. M. (1984). Methodology in studies of life events and cancer. In C. L. Cooper (ed.), *Psychosocial Stress and Cancer*, John Wiley & Sons, Chichester.

Paykel, E. S., Myers, J. K., Dienelt, M. N., Klerman, G. L., Lindental, J. J. & Pepper, M. P. (1969). Life events and depression: a controlled study, *Archives of General Psychiatry*, **21**, 753–60.

Paykel, E. S., Prusoff, B. A. & Myers, J. K. (1975). Suicide attempts and recent life events, *Archives of General Psychiatry*, **32**, 327–33.

Paykel, E. S., Prusoff, B. A. & Uhlenhuth, E. H. (1971). Scaling of life events, *Archives of General Psychiatry*, **25**, 340–47.

Payne, R. L. (1979). Demands, supports, constraints and psychological health. In C. J. Mackay & T. Cox (eds), *Responses to Stress: Occupational Aspects*, International Publishing Corporation, London.

Payne, R. L. & Fletcher, B. (C) (1983). Job demands, supports and constraints as predictors of psychological strain among schoolteachers, *Journal of Vocational Behaviour*, **22**, 136–47.

Payne, R. L. & Jones, J. G. (1987). Measurement and methodological issues in social support. In S. V. Kasl & C. L. Cooper (eds), *Stress and Health: Issues in Research Methodology*, John Wiley & Sons, Chichester.

Payne, R. L. & Rick, J. T. (1986a). Heart rate as an indicator of stress in surgeons and anaesthetists, *Journal of Psychosomatic Research*, **30**(4), 411–20.

Payne, R. L. & Rick, J. T. (1986b). Psychobiological markers of stress in surgeons and anaesthetists. In T. H. Schmidt, T. M. Dembroski & G. Blumchen (eds), *Biological and Psychological Factors in Cardiovascular Disease*, Springer-Verlag, Berlin.

Payne, R. L., Jick, T. D. & Burke, R. J. (1982). Whither stress research?: an agenda for the 1980s, *Journal of Occupational Behaviour*, **3**, 131–45.

Payne, R. L., Warr, P. & Hartley, J. (1984). Social class and psychological ill-health during unemployment, *Sociology of Health and Illness*, **6**(2), 152–74.

Payne, R. L., Rick, J. T., Smith, G. H. & Cooper, R. (1984). Multiple indicators of stress in an 'active' job: cardiothoracic surgery, *Journal of Occupational Medicine*, **26**, 805–8.

Pearlin, L. I. (1989). The sociological study of stress, *Journal of Health and Social Behavior*, **30**, 241–56.

Pearson, K. & Lee, A. (1903). On the laws of inheritance in man. I: Inheritance of physical characteristics, *Biometrika*, **2**, 357–462.

Pell, S. & D'Alonzo, C. A. (1963). Acute myocardial infarction in a large industrial population, *Journal of the American Medical Association*, **185**, 831–8.

Pennebaker, J. W., Gonder-Frederick, L., Stewart, H., Elfman, L. & Skelton, J. A. (1982). Physical symptoms associated with blood pressure, *Psychophysiology*, **19**, 201–10.

Perper, J. A., Kuller, L. H. & Cooper, M. (1975). Arteriosclerosis of coronary arteries in sudden, unexpected deaths, *Circulation*, **51–52** (Suppl. 3), 27–33.

Perrewe, P. L. & Ganster, D. C. (1989). The impact of job demands and behavioral control on experienced job stress, *Journal of Organizational Behavior*, **10**, 213–29.

Peters, L. J. & Kelley, M. (1977). The influence of stress and stress hormones on the transplantability of a non-immunogenic syngeneic murine tumour, *Cancer*, **39**, 1482–8.

Peters, R. K., Benson, H. & Peters, J. M. (1977). Daily relaxation response breaks in a waking population: II. Effects on blood pressure, *American Journal of Public Health*, **67**, 946–53.

Pittner, M. S. & Houston, B. K. (1980). Response to stress, cognitive coping strategies, and the type A behaviour pattern, *Journal of Personality and Social Psychology*, **39**, 147–57.

Plant, M. A. (1977). Alcoholism and occupation: a review, *British Journal of Addiction*, **72**, 309–16.

Plumb, M. M. & Holland, J. (1977). Comparative studies of psychological functioning in patients with advanced cancer. I. Self-reported depressive symptoms. *Psychosomatic Medicine*, **39**, 264–76.

Pollack, E. S. & Horm, J. W. (1980). Trends in cancer incidence and mortality in the United States, *Journal of the National Cancer Institute*, **64**, 1091–1103.

Pradhan, S. N. & Ray, P. (1974). Effects of stress on growth of transplanted and 7, 12-dimethylbenz(*a*)anthracene-induced tumors and their modification by psychotropic drugs, *Journal of the National Cancer Institute*, **53**, 1241–5.

Pratt, J. (1978). Perceived stress among teachers: the effects of age and background of children taught, *Educational Review*, **30**, 3–14.

Price, V. A. (1982). What is Type A? A cognitive social learning model, *Journal of Occupational Behaviour*, **3**, 109–29.

Public Health Reports (1977). Advance data from NCHS surveys on blood pressure and hypertension, Jan.-Feb, **91**(1), 91.

Purchase, I. F. H. (1980). Inter-species comparisons of carcinogenicity, *British Journal of Cancer*, **41**, 454–68.

Quinn, R. P. & Staines, G. L. (1979). *The Quality of Employment Survey*, Institute for Social Research, Ann Arbor, MI.

Rabkin, J. G. & Struening, E. L. (1976). Life events, stress, and illness. *Science*, **194**, 1013–20.

Raglan, D. R. & Brand, R. J. (1988a). Coronary heart disease mortality in the Western Collaborative Group Study: follow-up experience of 22 years, *American Journal of Epiemiology*, **127**(3), 462–75.

Raglan, D. R. & Brand, R. J. (1988b). Type A behaviour and mortality from coronary heart disease, *New England Journal of Medicine*, **318**(2), 65–9.

Rahe, R. H. (1972). Subjects' recent life changes and their near-future illness reports: a review, *Annals of Clinical Research*, **4**, 250–65.

Rahe, R. H. (1974). The pathway between subjects' recent life changes and their near future illness reports: representative results and methodological issues. In B. S. Dohrenwend & B. P. Dohrenwend (eds), *Stressful Life Events: their Nature and Effects*. John Wiley & Sons, New York.

Rahe, R. H. (1978). Life change measurement clarification (editorial), *Psychosomatic Medicine*, **40**, 95–8.

Rahe, R. H. (1984). Development in lifechange measurement: subjective life change unit scaling. In B. S. Dohrenwend & B. P. Dohrenwend (eds), *Stressful Life Events and their Contexts*, Rutgers University Press, New York.

Rahe, R. H. (1988). Life-change measurement as a predictor of illness, *Proceedings of the Royal Society of Medicine*, **61**, 1124–6.

Rahe, R. H. & Arthur, R. J. (1978). Life change and illness studies: past history and future directions, *Journal of Human Stress*, **4**, 3–15.

Rahe, R. H. & Paasikivi, J. (1971). Psychosocial factors and myocardial infarction. II. An outpatient study in Sweden, *Journal of Psychosomatic Research*, **15**, 33–9.

Rahe, R. H., Romo, M., Bennett, L. & Siltanen, P. (1974). Recent life changes, myocardial infarction and abrupt coronary death, *Archives of Internal Medicine*, **133**, 221–8.

Rao, L. G. S. (1970). Discriminant function based on steroid abnormalities in patients with lung cancer, *The Lancet*, **ii**, 441–5.

Rasmussen, A. F. Jr, Spencer, E. S. & Marsh, J. T. (1959). Decrease in susceptibility of mice to passive anaphylaxis following avoidance-learning stress, *Proceedings of the Society for Experimental Biology and Medicine*, **100**, 878–9.

Rassidakis, N. C., Kelepouris, M., Goulis, K. & Fox, S. (1971). Malignant neoplasm as a cause of deaths among psychiatric patients. I: *International Mental Health Research Newsletter*, **13**, 3–6.

Rassidakis, N. C., Kelepouris, M., Goulis, K. & Karaiossefidis, K. (1972). Malignant neoplasms as a cause of death among psychiatric patients. II: *International Mental Health Research Newsletter*, **14**, 3–6.

Rassidakis, N. C., Erotokristov, A., Volidou, M. & Collarou, T. (1973). Anxiety, schizophrenia and carcinogenesis, *International Mental Health Newsletter*, **15**, 3–6.

Ray, J. J. (1991). If 'A–B' does not predict heart disease, why bother with it? A comment on Ivancevich & Matteson, *British Journal of Medical Psychology*, **64**, 85–90.

Reed, D., McGee, D., Yano, K. & Feinleib, M. (1983). Social networks and coronary heart disease among Japanese men in Hawaii, *American Journal of Epidemiology*, **117**, 384–96.

Reeder, L. G., Schrama, P. G. M. & Dirken, J. M. (1973). Stress and cardiovascular health: an international cooperative study. I: *Social Science and Medicine*, **7**, 573–84.

Renshaw, J. R. (1976). An exploration of the dynamics of the overlapping worlds of work and family, *Family Process*, **15**, 143–65.

Reznikoff, M. (1955). Psychological factors in breast cancer: a preliminary study of some personality trends in patients with cancer of the breast, *Psychosomatic Medicine*, **17**, 96–110.

Reznikoff, M. & Martin, D. E. (1957). The influence of stress on mammary cancer, *Journal of Psychosomatic Research*, **2**, 56.

Richardson, D. W. Jr., Honour, A. J., Fenton, G. W., Stott, F. H. & Pickering, G. W. (1964). Variation in arterial pressure throughout the day and night, *Clinical Science*, **26**, 445.

Riley, V. (1975). Mouse mammary tumors: alteration of incidence as apparent function of stress, *Science*, **189**, 465–7.

Riley, V. (1979). Cancer and stress: overview and critique, *Cancer Detection and Prevention*, **2**, 163–95.

Riley, V. (1981). Psychoneuroendocrine influences on immuno-competence and neoplasia, *Science*, **217**, 1100–9.

Rime, B., Ucros, C. G., Besten, Y. & Jeanjean, M. (1989). Type A behaviour pattern: specific coronary risk factor or general disease-prone condition, *British Journal of Medical Psychology*, **62**, 229–40.

Rissanen, V., Romo, M. & Siltanen, P. (1978). Premonitory symptoms and stress factors preceding sudden death from ischaemic heart disease, *Acta Medica Scandinavica*, **204**, 389–96.

Rissler, A. (1977). Stress reactions at work and after work during a period of quantitative overload, *Ergonomics*, **20**, 13–16.

Robinson, J. O. (1962). A study of neuroticism and casual arterial blood pressure, *British Journal of Social and Clinical Psychology*, **2**, 56–64.

Rogentine, G. N., Van Kammen, D. P., Fox, B. H., Doherty, J. P., Rosenblatt J. E., Boyd, S. C. & Bunney, W. E. (1979). Psychological factors in the prognosis of malignant melanoma: a prospective study, *Psychosomatic Medicine*, **41**, 647–55.

Rosch, P. J. (1984). Stress and cancer. In C. L. Cooper (ed.), *Psychosocial Stress and Cancer*, John Wiley & Sons, Chichester.

Rose, G. & Marmot, M. G. (1981). Social class and coronary heart disease, *British Heart Journal*, **45**, 13–19.

Rose, R. J., Miller, J. Z. & Grim, C. E. (1982). Familial factors in blood pressure response to laboratory stress: a twin study, *Psychophysiology*, **19**, 583.

Rosenman, R. H. (1978). The interview method of assessment of the coronary-prone behavior pattern. In T. M. Dembrowski, S. M. Weiss, J. L. Shields, S. G. Haynes & M. Feinleib, *Coronary-prone Behavior*, Springer, New York.

Rosenman, R. H. & Chesney, M. A. (1980). The relationship of Type A behaviour pattern to coronary heart disease, *Activitas Nervosa Superior*, **22**, 1–45.

Rosenman, R. H., Friedman, M., Straus, R., Wurm, M., Kositchek, R., Hahn, W. & Werthessen, N. T. (1964). A predictive study of coronary heart disease: the Western Collaborative Group Study, *Journal of the American Medical Association*, **189**, 15–22.

Rosenman, R. H., Friedman, M., Straus, R., Wurm, M., Jenkins, C. D. & Messinger, H. B. (1966). Coronary heart disease in the Western Collaborative Group Study: A follow-up experience of two years, *Journal of the American Medical Society*, **195**, 130–6.

Rosenman, R. H., Friedman, M., Straus, R., Jenkins, C. D., Zyzanski, S. J. & Wurm M. (1970). Coronary heart disease in the Western Collaborative Group Study: a follow-up experience of 4½ years, *Journal of Chronic Diseases*, **23**, 173–90.

Rosenman, R. H., Brand, R. J., Jenkins, C. K., Friedman, M., Straus, R. & Wurm, M. (1975).

Coronary heart disease in the Western Collaborative Group Study: final follow-up experience of 8½ years, *Journal of the American Medical Association*, **233**, 872–7.

Rosenman, R. H., Brand, R. J., Sholtz, R. I. & Friedman, M. (1976). Multivariate prediction of coronary heart disease during 8.5-year follow-up in the Western Collaborative Group Study, *American Journal of Cardiology*, **37**, 903–10.

Roszman, T. L., Cross, R. J., Brooks, W. H. & Markesberry, W. R. (1982). Hypothalamic–immune interactions. 2: The effect of hypothalamic lesions on the ability of adherent spleen cells to limit blastogenesis, *Immunology*, **45**, 737–42.

Rozanski, A., Bairey, C. N., Krantz, D. S., Friedman, M. D., Resser, K. J., Morell, M., Hilton-Chalfen, S., Hestrin, L., Bietendorf, J. & Berman, D. S. (1988). Mental stress and the induction of silent myocardial ischemia in patients with coronary artery disease, *New England Journal of Medicine*, **318**(16), 1005–11.

Ruff, M. R., Pert, C. B., Weber, R. J., Wahl, L. M., Wahl, S. M. & Paul, S. M. (1985). Benzodiazepine receptor-mediated chemotaxis of human monocytes, *Science*, **229**, 1281–3.

Russek, H. I. (1962). Emotional stress and coronary heart disease in American physicians, dentists and lawyers, *American Journal of Medical Science*, **243**, 716–25.

Russek, H. I. (1965). Stress, tobacco and coronary disease in North American professional groups, *Journal of the American Medical Association*, **192**, 189–94.

Russek, H. I. & Zohman, B. L. (1958). Relative significance of heredity, diet and occupational stress in coronary heart disease of young adults, *American Journal of Medical Science*, **235**, 266–75.

Rustin, R. M., Dramaiz, M., Kittel, F., Degre, C., Kornitzer, M., Thilly, C. & De Backer, G. (1976). Validation de techniques d'evaluation du profil comportemental 'A' utilisées dans le 'Projet Belge de Prevention des affections cardiovasculairs' (PBP), *Revue Epidémiologie et Santé Publique*, **24**, 497–507.

Saba, T. M. & Antikatzides, T. G. (1976). Decreased resistance to intravenous tumour challenge during reticuloendothelial depression following surgery, *British Journal of Cancer*, **34**, 381–9.

Sabine, J. R., Horton, B. J. & Wicks, M. B. (1973). Spontaneous tumours in C3H-A and C3H-A fB mice: high incidence in the United States and low incidence in Australia, *Journal of the National Cancer Institute*, **50**, 1237–42.

Sarason, I. G. & Sarason, B. R. (1984). Life changes, moderators of stress and health. In A. Baum, S. E. Taylor & J. E. Singer (eds), *Handbook of Psychology and Health*, Vol. IV: *Social Psychological Aspects of Health*, Lawrence Erlbaum, Hillsdale, NJ.

Sarason, I. G. & Sarason, B. R. (eds) (1985). *Social Support: Theory, Research and Applications*, Martinus Nijhoff, The Hague.

Sarason, I. G., Johnson, J. H. & Siegel, J. M. (1978). Assessing the impact of life changes: development of the Life Experiences Survey, *Journal of Consulting and Clinical Psychology*, **46**, 932–46.

Satin, D. G. (1972). Life stresses and psychosocial problems in the hospital emergency unit, *Social Psychiatry*, **7**, 119–26.

Schar, M., Reeder, L. G. & Dirken, J. M. (1973). Stress and cardiovascular health: an international cooperative study. II: The male population of a factory in Zurich. *Social Science and Medicine*, **7**, 585–603.

Scherwitz, L., Berton, K. & Leventhal, H. (1978). Type A behavior, self-involvement, and cardiovascular response, *Psychosomatic Medicine*, **40**, 593–609.

Schleifer, S. J., Keller, S. E., Camerino, M., Thornton, J. C. & Stein, M. (1983). Suppression of lymphocyte stimulation following bereavement, *Journal of the American Medical Association*, **250**, 374–7.

Schmale, A. H. (1972). Giving up as a final common pathway to changes in health, *Advances in Psychosomatic Medicine*, **8**, 20–40.

Schmale, A. H. & Iker, H. P. (1964). The effect of hopelessness in the development of cancer: I. The prediction of uterine cancer in women with a typical cytology, *Psychosomatic Medicine*, **26**, 635–54.

Schmale, A. H. & Iker, H. P. (1966a). The effect of hopelessness and the development of cancer, *Journal of Psychosomatic Medicine*, **28**, 714–21.

Schmale, A. H. & Iker, H. P. (1966b). The psychosocial setting of uterine cervical cancer, *Annals of the New York Acadamy of Sciences*, **125**, 807–13.

Schmale, A. H. & Iker, H. P. (1971). Hopelessness as a predictor of cervical cancer, *Social Science and Medicine*, **5**, 95–100.

Schmid, I., Scharfetter, C. & Binder, J. (1981). Lebensereignisse in Abhangigkeit von soziodemographiscen variablen, *Social Psychiatry*, **16**, 63.

Schonfield, J. (1975). Psychological and life-experience differences between Israeli women with benign and cancerous breast lesions, *Journal of Psychosomatic Research*, **19**, 229–34.

Schonfield, J. (1977). Psychological factors related to recovery from breast cancer *Psychosomatic Medicine*, **39**, 51.

Schuler, R. S. (1982). An integrative transactional process model of stress in organisations, *Journal of Occupational Behaviour*, **3**, 5–19.

Seer, P. (1979). Psychological control of essential hypertension: review of the literature and methodological critiques, *Psychological Bulletin*, **86**, 1015–43.

Seidenberg, R. (1975). *Corporate Wives—Corporate Casualties*, Anchor Press, New York.

Sekaran, U. (1985). The paths to mental health: an exploratory study of husbands and wives in dual-career families, *Journal of Occupational Psychology*, **58**, 129–37.

Seligman, M. E. P. (1975). *Helplessness: On Depression, Development and Death*, W. H. Freeman, San Francisco.

Selye, H. (1936). A syndrome produced by diverse noxious agents, *Nature*, **138**, 32.

Selye, H. (1946). The general adaptation syndrome and disease of adaptation, *Journal of Clinical Endocrinology and Metabolism*, **6**, 117–30.

Selye, H. (1936). *The Stress of Life*, McGraw-Hill, New York.

Selye, H. (1979). Correlating stress and cancer, *American Journal of Proctology, Gastroenterology, Colon and Rectal Surgery*, **30**(4), 18–28.

Selye, H. (1983). The stress concept: past, present and future. In C. L. Cooper (ed.), *Stress Research*, John Wiley & Sons, Chichester.

Sexton, M. M. (1979). Behavioural epidemiology. In O. V. Pomerlean & J. P. Brady (eds), *Behavioural Medicine: Theory and Practice*, Williams & Wilkins, Baltimore, MD.

Shaffer, J., Duszynski, K. R. & Thomas, C. B. (1982). Family attitudes in youth as a possible precursor of cancer among physicians: a search for explanatory mechanisms, *Journal of Behavioural Medicine*, **5**, 143–64.

Shaper, A. G., Pocock, S. J., Walker, M., Phillips, A. N., Whitehead, T. P. & MacFarlane, P. W. (1985). Risk-factors for ischaemic heart disease: the prospective phase of the British Regional Heart Study, *Journal of Epidemiology and Community Health*, **39**, 197–209.

Shapiro, A. P. (1983). The non-pharmacologic treatment of hypertension. In D. S. Krantz, A. Baum & J. E. Singer (eds), *Handbook of Psychology and Health*, Lawrence Erlbaum, London.

Shek, P. N. & Sabiston, B. H. (1983). Neuroendocrine regulation of immune processes: change in circulating cortiscosterone levels induced by the primary antibody response in mice. *International Journal of Immunopharmacology*, **5**, 23–33.

Shekelle, R. B. (1976). Status inconsistency, mobility and CHD: A reply to Horan and Gray. *Journal of Health and Social Behaviour*, **17**, 83–7.

Shekelle, R. B. & Liu, S. C. (1978). Public beliefs about causes and prevention of heart attacks, *Journal of the American Medical Association*, **240**, 756–8.

Shekelle, R. B., Ostfeld, A. M. & Paul, O. (1969). Social status and incidence of coronary heart disease, *Journal of Chronic Diseases*, **22**, 381–94.

Shekelle, R. B., Raybnor, W. J., Ostfeld, A. M., Garron, D. C., Bielauskas, L. A., Lin, S. C., Maliza, C. & Paul, O. (1981). Psychological depression and the 17-year risk of death from cancer, *Psychosomatic Medicine*, **43**, 117–25.

Shrout, P. E. (1984). Scaling of stressful life events. In B. S. Dohrenwend & B. P. Dohrenwend (eds), *Stressful Life Events and their Contexts*, Rutgers University Press, New York.

Siegel, J. M. (1985). Personality and cardiovascular disease: prior research and future directions. In A. M. Ostfeld & E. D. Eaker (eds), *Measuring Psychosocial Variables in Epidemiologic Studies of Cardiovascular Disease: Proceedings of a Workshop*, US Department of Health and Human Services.

Siegel, J. M. & Leitch, C. J. (1981). Assessment of the type A behavior pattern in adolescents, *Psychosomatic Medicine*, **43**, 45–6.

Singer, A. (1982). What causes squamous carcinoma of the cervix. In A. Jordon, F. Sharp & A Singer (eds), *Pre-clinical Neoplasia of the Cervix*, Royal College of Obstetricians and Gynaecologists, London.

Skegg, D. C. G., Corwin, P. A., Paul, C. & Doll, R. (1982). Importance of the male factor in cancer of the cervix, *The Lancet*, **ii**, 581–3.

Skinner, H. A. & Lei, H. (1980). The multidimensional assessment of stressful life events, *Journal of Nervous and Mental Disease*, **168**, 535–41.

Sklar, L. S. & Anisman, H. (1979). Stress and coping factors influence tumour growth, *Science*, **205**, 513–15.

Sklar, L. S. & Anisman, H. (1980). Social stress influences tumor growth, *Psychosomatic Medicine*, **42**, 347–65.

Sklar, L. S. & Anisman, H. (1981). Stress and cancer, *Psychological Bulletin*, **89**, 369–406.

Slaga, T. J., Thomson, S. & Smuckler, E. A. (1975). Prolonged inhibition of mouse epidermal DNA synthesis by dexamethasone, *Journal of the National Cancer Institute*, **54**(4), 931–6.

Sloan, S. & Cooper, C. L. (1986). *Pilots under Stress*, Routledge, New York and London.

Smith, E. B. & Staples, E. M. (1981). Haemostatic factors in human aortic intima, *The Lancet*, **i**, 1171–4.

Smith, G. R. & McDaniel, S. M. (1983). Psychologically mediated effect on the delayed hypersensitivity reaction to tuberculin in humans, *Psychosomatic Medicine*, **45**, 65–70.

Smith, R. E., Johnson, J. H. & Sarason, I. G. (1978). Life change, the sensation-seeking motive, and psychological distress, *Journal of Consulting and Clinical Psychology*, **46**, 348–9.

Smith, R. T. (1979a). Role of social resources in cardiovascular rehabilitation, *Proceedings of the Workshop on Physical Conditioning and Rehabilitation*, National Heart, Lung and Blood Institute, London, May.

Smith, R. T. (1979b). Rehabilitation of the disabled: the role of social networks in the recovery process, *International Rehabilitation Medicine*, **1**, 63–72.

Smith, W. R. & Sebastian, H. (1976). Emotional history and pathogenesis of cancer, *Journal of Clinical Psychology*, **32**(4), 863–6.

Snell, L. & Graham, S. (1971). Social trauma as related to cancer of the breast, *British Journal of Cancer*, **25**, 721–34.

Solomon, G. F. (1969). Stress and antibody response in rats, *International Archives of Allergy and Applied Immunology* **35**, 97–104.

Solomon, G. F. (1981). Emotional and personality factors in the onset and course of autoimmune disease, particularly rheumatoid arthritis. In R. Ader (ed.), *Psycho-neuroimmunology*, Academic Press, New York.

Solomon, G. F. (1985). The emerging field of psychoneuroimmunology, *Behavioral and Brain Sciences*, **8**(3), 4–11.

Solomon, G. F. & Amkraut, A. A. (1979). Neuroendocrine aspects of the immune response and their implications for stress effects on tumor immunity, *Cancer Detection and Prevention*, **2**, 197–223.

Solomon, G. F., Levine, S. & Kraft, J. K. (1968). Early experience and immunity, *Nature*, **220**, 821–2.

Solomon, G. F., Merigan, T. C. & Levine, S. (1967). Variation in adrenal corticoid hormones within physiologic ranges: stress and interferon production in mice, *Proceedings of the Society for Experimental Biology and Medicine*, **126**, 74–9.

Solomon, Z., Mikulincer, M. & Habershaim, N. (1990). Life events, coping strategies, social resources and somatic complaints among combat stress reaction casualties, *British Journal of Medical Psychology*, **63**, 137–48.

Spielberger, C. D., Gorsuch, R. L. & Lusherne, R. E. (1970). *STAI Manual*, Consulting Psychologists Press, Palo Alto, CA.

Staines, G. L. (1980). Spillover versus compensation: a review of the literature on the relationship between work and nonwork. *Human Relations*, **33**, 111–29.

Staines, G. L. & Peck, J. H. (1984). Non-standard work schedules and family life, *Journal of Applied Psychology*, **69**, 515–23.

Stamler, J., Lindberg, H. A., Berkson, D. M., Shaffer, A., Miller, W. & Poindexter, A. (1960). Prevalence and incidence of coronary heart disease in a strata of the labor force of a Chicago industrial corporation. *Journal of Chronic Diseases*, **11**, 405–20.

Steele, G. P., Henderson, S. & Duncan-Jones, P. (1980). The reliability of reporting adverse experiences, *Psychological Medicine*, **10**, 301.

Stein, M., Keller, S. & Schleifer, S. (1979). Role of the hypothalamus in mediating stress effects on the immune system. In B. A. Stoll (ed.), *Mind and Cancer Prognosis*, John Wiley, London.

Stein, M., Schleifer, S. J. & Keller, S. E. (1981). Hypothalamic influences on immune responses. In R. Ader (ed.), *Psychoneuroimmunology*, Academic Press, New York.

Steptoe, A. (1981). *Psychological Factors in Cardiovascular Disorders*, Academic Press, London.

Steptoe, A. & Mathews, A. (1984). *Health Care and Human Behaviour*, Academic Press; Harcourt Brace Jovanovich, New York.

Steptoe, A., Melville, D. & Ross, A. (1982). Essential hypertension and psychological functioning: a study of factory workers, *British Journal of Clinical Psychology*, **21**, 303–11.

Stevens, G. & Featherman, D. L. (1981). A revised socioeconomic index of occupational status, *Social Science Research*, **10**, 369–95.

Stevens, S. S. (1966). A metric for the social consensus, *Science*, **151**, 530–41.

Stone, F. W. (1985). Measures to reduce stress at work. Unpublished Ph.D. thesis, University of Aston in Birmingham.

Stout, C., Morrow, J., Brandt., E. N. Jr & Wolf, S. (1964). Unusually low incidence of death from myocardial infarction: study of an Italian-American community in Pennsylvania. *Journal of the American Medical Association*, **188**, 845–9.

Stroebe, M. S., Stroebe, W., Gergen, K. J. & Gergen, M. (1981/82). The broken heart: reality or myth, *Omega*, **12**(2), 87–105.

Sullivan, P. A., Schoentgen, S., DeQuattro, V., Procci, W., Levine, D., Van Der Meulen, J. & Bornheimer, J. F. (1981a). Anxiety, anger and neurogenic tone at rest and in stress in patients with primary hypertension, *Hypertension*, **3**, 119–23.

Sullivan, P. A., Procci, W., DeQuattro, V., Schoentgen, S., Levine, D., Van Der Meulen, J. & Bornheimer, J. F. (1981b). Anger, anxiety, guilt and increased basal and stress-induced-neurogenic tone: cause or effect in primary hypertension?, *Clinical Science*, **61**, 389–92.

Syme, S. L. (1985). Socioeconomic factors: content discussion. In A. M. Ostfeld & E. D. Eaker (eds), *Measuring Psychosocial Variables in Epidemiologic Studies of Cardiovascular Disease: Proceedings of a Workshop*, US Department of Health and Human Services.

Syme, S. L. & Seeman, T. E. (1983). Sociocultural risk factors in coronary heart disease. In J. A. Herd & S. M. Weiss (eds), *Behavior and Arteriosclerosis*, Plenum, New York.

Syme, S. L., Borhani, N. O. & Buechley, R. W. (1965). Cultural mobility and coronary heart disease in an urban area. *American Journal of Epidemiology*, **82**, 334–46.

Syme, S. L., Hyman, M. M. & Enderline, P. E. (1964). Some social and cultural factors associated with the occurrence of coronary heart disease, *Journal of Chronic Diseases*, **17**, 277–89.

Taffinder, A. P. & Taffinder, G. A. (1984). An audit of hypertension in general practice, *Practitioner*, **228**, 595–8.

Tarlau, M. & Smalheiser, I. (1951). Personality patterns in patients with malignant tumors of the breast and cervix, *Psychosomatic Medicine*, **13**, 117–21.

Temoshok, L. & Heller, B. W. (1984). On comparing apples, oranges and fruit salad: a methodological overview of medical outcome studies in psychosocial oncology. In C. L. Cooper (ed.), *Psychosocial Stress and Cancer*, John Wiley & Sons, Chichester.

Tennant, C. & Andrews, G. (1976). A scale to measure the stress of life events, *Australia and New Zealand Journal of Psychiatry*, **10**, 27–32.

Tennant, C. & Andrews, G. (1977). A scale to measure the cause of life events, *Australia and New Zealand Journal of Psychiatry*, **11**, 163–8.

Tennant, C. & Andrews, G. (1978). The cause of life events in neurosis, *Journal of Psychosomatic Research*, **22**, 41–5.

Tennant, C., Smith, A., Bebbington, P. & Hurry, J. (1979). The contextual threat of life events: the concept and its reliability, *Psychological Medicine*, **9**, 525–8.

Theorell, T. & Floderus-Myrhed, B. (1977). Work load and myocardial infarction—a prospective psychological analysis, *International Journal of Epidemiology*, **6**(i), 17–21.

Theorell, T. & Rahe, R. H. (1971). Psychosocial factors and myocardial infarction. I: An inpatient study in Sweden, *Journal of Psychosomatic Research*, **15**, 25–31.

Theorell, T. & Rahe, R. H. (1972). Behavior and life satisfactions: characteristics of Swedish subjects with myocardial infarction, *Journal of Chronic Diseases*, **25**, 139–47.

Theorell, T. & Rahe, R. H. (1975). Life change events, ballistocardiography and coronary death, *Journal of Human Stress*, **1**, 18–24.

Thomas, C. B. (1976). Precursors of premature disease and death, *Annals of Internal Medicine*, **85**, 653–8.

Thomas, C. B. & Duszynski, K. R. (1974). Closeness to parents and the family constellation in a prospective study of five disease states: suicide, mental illness, malignant tumour, hypertension, and coronary heart disease, *Johns Hopkins Medical Journal*, **134**, 251–70.

Thomas, C. B. & Greenstreet, R. L. (1973). Psychobiological characteristics in youth as predictors of five disease states: suicide, mental illness, malignant tumour, hypertension, and coronary heart disease, *Johns Hopkins Medical Journal*, **132**, 16–43.

Thomas, C. B. & McCabe, O. L. (1980). Precursors of premature disease and death: habits of nervous tension, *Johns Hopkins Medical Journal*, **147**, 137–45.

Thomas, C. B., Duszynski, K. R. & Shaffer. J. W. (1979). Family attitudes reported in youth as potential predictors of cancer, *Psychosomatic Medicine*, **41**, 287–302.

Turner, D. B. & Stone, A. J. (1979). Headache and its treatment: a random sample survey, *Headache*, **19**(2), 74–7.

Uemura, K. & Pisa, Z. (1985). Recent trends in cardiovascular disease mortality in 27 industrialised countries, *World Health Statistics Quarterly*, **38**, 142–62.

Uhlenhuth, E. H., Haberman, S. J., Balter, M. D. & Lipman, R. S. (1977). Remembering life events. In J. S. Strauss, H. M. Batigcan & M. Roff (eds), *The Origins and Course of Psychopathology: Methods of Longitudinal Research*, Plenum Press, New York.

Ulf, D. F. (1975). Life change patterns prior to death in ischemic heart disease: a study on death-discordant twins. *Journal of Psychosomatic Research*, **19**, 273–8.

Van Harrison, R. (1978). Person–environment fit and job stress. In C. L. Cooper & R. L. Payne (eds), *Stress at Work*, John Wiley & Sons, New York.

Van Sell, M., Brief, A. P. & Schuler, R. S. (1981). Role conflict and role ambiguity: Integration of the literature and directions for future research, *Human Relations*, **34**, 43–71.

Verrier, R. L., Calvert, A. & Lown, B. (1975). Effect of posterior hypothalamic stimulation on ventricular fibrillation threshold, *American Journal of Physiology*, **228**, 923–7.

Verrier, R. L., De Silva, R. A. & Lown, B. (1983). Psychological factors in cardiac arrhythmias and sudden death. In D. S. Krantz, A. Baum & J. E. Singer (eds), *Handbook of Psychology and Health* Lawrence Erlbaum, London

Visintainer, M. A., Volpicelli, J. R. & Seligman, M. E. P. (1982). Tumour rejection in rats after inescapable or escapable shock, *Science*, **216**, 437–9.

Wadsworth, M. E. J., Cripps, H. A., Midwinter, R. E. & Colley, J. R. T. (1985). Blood pressure in a national birth cohort at the age of 36 related to social and familial factors, smoking and body mass, *British Medical Journal*, **291**, 1534–8.

Waldron, I. (1977). Sex differences in the coronary-prone behavior pattern, *Proceedings of the Forum on Coronary-prone Behavior*, US Department of Health Education and Welfare. Publication no. (NIH) 78–1451.

Waldron, I., Nowotarski, M., Freimer, M., Henry, J. P., Post, N. & Witten, C. (1982). Cross-cultural variation in blood pressure: a quantitative analysis of the relationships of blood pressure to cultural characteristics, salt consumption and body weight, *Social Science and Medicine*, **16**, 419–30.

Wall, T. (1980). Group work redesign in context: a two-phase model. In K. D. Duncan, M. M. Gruneberg & D. Wallis (eds), *Changes in Working Life*, John Wiley & Sons, Chichester.

Wall, T. D. & Clegg, C. W. (1981). A longitudinal study of group work redesign, *Journal of Occupational Behaviour*, **2**, 31–49.

Wall, T. D., Clegg, C. W. & Jackson, P. R. (1978). An evaluation of the job characteristics model. *Journal of Occupational Psychology*, **51**, 183–96.

Wallace, E. W., Wallace, H. M. & Mills, C. A. (1942). Effect of climatic environment upon the genesis of subcutaneous tumors induced by methylcholanthrene and upon the growth of a transplantable sarcoma in C3H mice, *Journal of the National Cancer Institute*, **3**, 99–110.

Wallace, E. W., Wallace, H. M. & Mills, C. A. (1944). Influence of environmental temperature upon the incidence and course of spontaneous tumors in C3H mice, *Cancer Research*, **4**, 279–81.

Ward, M. M., Mefford, I. N., Parker, S. D., Chesney, M. A., Taylor, C. B., Keegan, D. L. & Barchas, J. D. (1983). Epinephrine and norepinephrine responses in continuously collected human plasma to a series of stressors, *Psychosomatic Medicine*, **45**, 471–87.

Ward, N. G., Bloom, V. L. & Friedel, R. O. (1979). The effectiveness of tricyclic anti-depressants in the treatment of coexisting pain and depression, *Pain*, **7**, 331–41.

Warner, W. L., Meeker, M. & Eells, K. (1949). *Social Class in America*, Social Science Research Associates, Chicago, IL.

Warr, P. B. (1980). An introduction to models in psychological research. In A. J. Chapman & D. M. Jones (eds), *Models of Man*, BPS Publishers, Leicester.

Warr, P. B. (1982). Psychological aspects of employment and unemployment, *Psychological Medicine*, **12**, 7–11.

Warr, P. B. (1987). *Work, Unemployment and Mental Health*, Oxford University Press, Oxford.

Warr, P. B. & Payne, R. L. (1982a). Experiences of strain and pleasure among British adults, *Social Science and Medicine*, **16**, 1691–7.

Warr, P. B. & Payne, R. L. (1982b). Unpleasant emotional strain and feelings of pleasure: point prevalence, attributions of cause and coping responses, *MRC/ESRC SAPU*, Memo no. 497.

Warr, P. & Payne, R. L. (1983). Affective outcomes of paid employment in a random sample of British workers, *Journal of Occupational Behaviour*, **4**, 91–104.

Waters, W. E. (1970). Community studies of the prevalence of headache, *Headache*, **9**, 178–86.

Waters, W. E. & O'Connors, P. J. (1971). Epidemiology of headache and migraine in women, *Journal of Neurology, Neurosurgery and Psychiatry*, **34**, 148–53.

Watson, C. & Schuld, D. (1977). Psychosomatic factors in the etiology of neoplasms, *Journal of Consulting and Clinical Psychology*, **45**(3), 455–61.

Watson, D. & Pennebaker, J. W. (1989). Health complaints, stress and distress: exploring the central role of negative affectivity. *Psychological Review*, **96**, 234–54.

Weiss, J. M. (1970). Somatic effects of predictable and unpredictable shock, *Psychosomatic Medicine*, **32**, 397–408.

Wells, J. A. (1985). Chronic life situations and lifechange events. In A. M. Ostfeld & E. D. Eakes (eds), *Measuring Psychosocial Variables in Epidemiologic Studies of Cardiovascular Disease*, US Department of Health and Human Services, NIH Publication No. 85–2270.

Whitehead, W. E., Blackwell, B., DeSilva, H. & Robinson, A. (1977). Anxiety and anger in hypertension. *Journal of Psychosomatic Research*, **21**, 383–9.

Williams, R. B. Jr, Friedman, M., Glass, D. C., Herd, J. A. & Schneiderman, N. (1978). Section summary; mechanisms linking behavioral and pathophysiological processes. In T. M. Dembrowski, S. M. Weiss, J. L. Shields, S. G. Haynes & M. Feinleib (eds), *Coronary Prone Behavior*, Springer, New York.

Williams, R. B., Haney, T. L., Lee, K. L., Kong, Y., Blumenthal, J. A. & Whalen, R. E. (1980). Type A behavior, hostility and coronary atherosclerosis, *Psychosomatic Medicine*, **42**, 539–49.

Winnett, R. A. & Neale, M. S. (1981). Flexible work schedules and family time allocation: assessment of a system change on individual behaviour using self-report logs, *Journal of Applied Behaviour Analysis*, **14**, 39–46.

Winnubst, J. A. M., Marcelissen, F. H. G. & Kleber, R. J. (1982). Effects of social support in the stressor-strain relationship: a Dutch sample, *Social Science and Medicine*, **16**, 475–82.

Witzel, L. (1970). Anamnese und Zweityerkrankungen bei patienten mit bosartigen neubildungen [anamnesis and second diseases in patients with malignant tumours], *Medizinische Klinik*, **65**, 876–9.

Wolf, S. (1969). Psychosocial forces in myocardial infarction and sudden death, *Circulation*, **39–40**, Suppl. IV, 74–83.

Wolf, T. M., Sklov, M. C., Wenzl, T. A., Hunter, S. M. & Berenson, G. S. (1982). Validation of a measure of type A behaviour pattern in children: Bogalusa heart study, *Child Development*, **53**, 126–35.

World Health Organisation (1982). *Prevention of Coronary Heart Disease: Report of a WHO Expert Committee*, WHO Technical report Series 678, WHO, Geneva.

Wright, E. O. & Perrone, L. (1977). Marxist class categories and income inequality, *American Sociological Review*, **42**, 32–55.

Wrye, H. (1979). The crisis of cancer: intervention perspectives. Journal writing with women with breast cancer. Read before the 87th American Psychiatric Association Convention, New York, September.

Yager, J., Grant, I., Sweetwood, H. L. & Gerst, M. (1981). Life event reports by psychiatric patients, non-patients, and their partners. *Archives of General Psychiatry*, **38**, 343–7.

Young, M. & Willmott, P. (1973). *The Symmetrical Family: A Study of Work and Leisure in the London Region*, Routledge & Kegan Paul, London.

Young, S. (1958). Effect of temperature on the production of induced rat mammary tumors, *Nature*, **219**, 1254–5.

Zaleznik, A., Kets De Vries, M. F. R. & Howard, J. (1977). Stress reactions in organisations: syndromes, causes and consequences, *Behavioural Science*, **22**, 151–62.

Zyzanski, S. J., Jenkins, D. C., Ryan, T. J., Flessas, A. & Everist, M. (1976). Psychological correlates of coronary angiographic findings, *Archives of Internal Medicine*, **136**, 1234–7.

Index